Han(

MW01063419

Jorge R. Petit, M.D.

Chairman
Department of Psychiatry
North General Hospital
Assistant Clinical Professor
Mount Sinai School of Medicine
New York, New York

LIPPINCOTT WILLIAMS & WILKINS
A **Wolters Kluwer** Company
Philadelphia · Baltimore · New York · London
Buenos Aires · Hong Kong · Sydney · Tokyo

Acquisitions Editor: Charles W. Mitchell
Developmental Editor: Sarah G. Mercure
Production Editor: Jeff Somers
Manufacturing Manager: Ben Rivera
Cover Illustrator: Patricia Gast
Compositor: Circle Graphics
Printer: RR Donnelley Crawfordsville

© **2004 by LIPPINCOTT WILLIAMS & WILKINS**
530 Walnut Street
Philadelphia, PA 19106 USA
LWW.com

Printed in the USA

Library of Congress Cataloging-in-Publication Data

ISBN 0-7817-4382-6

Care has been taken to confirm the accuracy of the information
presented and to describe generally accepted practices. However,
the author and publisher are not responsible for errors or omissions
or for any consequences from application of the information in this
book and make no warranty, expressed or implied, with respect to
the currency, completeness, or accuracy of the contents of the
publication. Application of this information in a particular situation
remains the professional responsibility of the practitioner.

The author and publisher have exerted every effort to ensure
that drug selection and dosage set forth in this text are in
accordance with current recommendations and practice at the
time of publication. However, in view of ongoing research, changes
in government regulations, and the constant flow of information
relating to drug therapy and drug reactions, the reader is urged
to check the package insert for each drug for any change in
indications and dosage and for added warnings and precautions.
This is particularly important when the recommended agent is a
new or infrequently employed drug.

Some drugs and medical devices presented in this publication
have Food and Drug Administration (FDA) clearance for limited use
in restricted research settings. It is the responsibility of the health
care provider to ascertain the FDA status of each drug or device
planned for use in their clinical practice.

10 9 8 7 6 5 4 3 2 1

Contents

Preface

The Emergency Department (ED) and other acute care settings are chaotic environments where acute presentations of psychiatric syndromes often pose difficult diagnostic and management questions. It is estimated that there are over 100 million ED visits in the U.S. a year. On average, anywhere from 2% to 12% of the patients are presenting with a psychiatric complaint. These acute presentations are often confusing because key data are either unavailable or difficult to ascertain. Moreover, these presentations are syndromic (group of signs and symptoms occurring together that may potentially characterize a particular abnormality) but have many underlying causes: psychiatric, medical, or substance-related in nature, requiring a concise approach to their assessment and subsequent treatment. The patients or the patient's network, generally identify these acute manifestations as a significant and acute change in baseline functioning that can occur at any time and is unpredictable. The primary focus in these settings is a systematic evaluation that ensures patient and staff safety. It should include:

- rapid assessment of risk factors
- determination of safety concerns
- diagnostic evaluation
- clinical management
- rational pharmacological interventions
- appropriate disposition planning

This handbook addresses common types of acute psychiatric symptoms based on presenting signs and symptoms as seen in acute settings—the inpatient psychiatric or medical-surgical unit or the emergency department. Such presentations are explored based on frequency, severity, prevalence, and potential lethality/danger to self or others, with a step-by-step approach to each presentation. Acute presentations are alphabetized for quick referencing and include a definition, a description of signs and symptoms, and a list of the necessary questions for clinical assessment and diagnosis. A guideline for assessment follows. An evidence-based approach to the assessment, management, and treatment of these presentations was employed wherever possible; in the absence of such, I have used my own experience to dictate recommended practices.

EDs and other acute care settings have variable staffing patterns and available on-site psychiatric services, thus requiring all physicians in these settings to be well versed in the general psychiatric assessment. Additionally, in some settings, reliance on junior staff, residents in training, and medical students makes the understanding and management of these emergencies crucial. Since the majority of psychiatric patients tend to visit EDs at night, and many EDs, even those with limited psychiatric components, are left without even those basic services at night and on weekends, it is imperative that all staff be adept at performing a basic psychiatric assessment. Additionally, acute care psychiatric settings and specialized psychiatric emergency programs must also have staff well trained in providing appropriate psychiatric assessments on patients presenting acutely.

This handbook describes, for each acute presentation, simple and practical management approaches to the clinical evaluation and stabilization of the patient and psychopharmacological interventions. Medications are listed first by generic name with brand names in parenthesis. Recommended doses, frequency of use, and route are provided as example recommendations, but it is the clinician's judgment that should guide the actual psychopharmacological intervention. Medication management must always be based on clinical judgment and a case-by-case assessment.

This handbook focuses on what to do at the outset and how to gather the necessary information and history to adequately evaluate and manage different acute presentations. Mental status exam and laboratory and physical assessment findings are reviewed as part of the initial assessment component. Common treatment strategies, DSM-IV-TR criteria, and differential medical and psychiatric diagnoses are explored for each type of presentation. Finally, an outline of viable disposition outcomes is provided in each instance (admission v. discharge, involuntary v. voluntary, discharge planning, community agency involvement, etc.).

Wherever clinically indicated, I have included some widely used psychiatric rating scales. Although the ED setting may not be the most conducive environment to perform rating scales, the ones I have mentioned in this book are fast and reliable and can be helpful as a guide for symptom assessment, to determine symptom profile and severity, or as a baseline symptom measure for future reference/use.

This handbook also covers key aspects of psychiatric emergency care, including safety considerations, general assessment guidelines, and a review of the mental status exam. Special consideration is given to seclusion and restraint, child and elder abuse recognition and reporting, and special populations such as adolescents, geriatrics, mentally retarded, and patients with HIV. A brief review of the general legal and forensic issues pertinent to these acute presentation and emergency services is included.

Listed below are some recommended readings and textbooks, which I have used and referenced repeatedly throughout, that explain in more detail some of the areas that are covered in this handbook.

BIBLIOGRAPHY

Allen MH (ed). Emergency Psychiatry (Review of Psychiatry Services, Volume 21, Number 3, Oldham MJ and Riba MB, series editors) Washington, DC, American Psychiatric Publishing, 2002.

Allen MH, Currier GW, Hughes DH, et al. The Expert Consensus Guideline Series: Treatment of Behavioral Emergencies. *Postgrad Med Special Report* 2001:1–90.

American Association of Psychiatry: Practice Guideline for the Treatment of Patients with Eating Disorders (revision). *Am J Psychiatry* 2000;157(Suppl)1:1.

American Psychiatric Association Clinical Resources–Practice Guidelines for the Treatment of Patients with Borderline PD, American Psychiatric Association, Washington, 1999.

American Psychiatric Association Practice Guideline for the Treatment of Patients with Bipolar Disorder, 1994.

American Psychiatric Association Practice Guidelines for the Treatment of Patients with Delirium. *Amer J Psych* 1999.

American Psychiatric Association: Diagnostic and Statistical Manual of Mental Disorders, ed. 4-TR. American Psychiatric Association, Washington, 1999.

American Psychiatric Association: Practice Guideline for Psychiatric Evaluation of Adults. *Am J Psychiatry* 1995;152(Nov suppl).

American Psychiatric Association: Practice Guideline for the Treatment of Patients with Panic Disorder.

American Psychiatric Association: Practice Guideline for the Treatment of Major Depressive Disorder (Second Edition).

American Psychiatric Association: Practice Guideline for the Treatment of Patients With Substance Use Disorders; Alcohol, Cocaine, Opioids.

American Psychiatric Association: Practice Guidelines for the Treatment of Patients with Alzheimer's Disease and Other Dementias of Late Life.

American Psychiatric Association: Practice Guidelines for the Treatment of Patients with HIV/AIDS. *Am J Psychiatry* 2000;157:1–62.

American Psychiatric Association's Practice Guidelines for the Treatment of Patients with Schizophrenia. *Amer J Psych* 1997.

Arana GW, Rosenbaum JF. Handbook of Psychiatric Drug Therapy– 4th ed. Arana GW, Rosenbaum JF eds. Lippincott Williams & Wilkins, Philadelphia, 2000.

Braunwald E et al. Harrison's Principle of Internal Medicine, ed 15th. Eugene Braunwald et al eds. McGraw Hill, 2001.

Dorland's Illustrated Medical Dictionary, ed 28. Saunders Co. Philadelphia, 1994.

Harwood-Nuss AL, et al. The Clinical Practice of Emergency Medicine– ed 2nd, eds Harwood-Nuss AL et al. Lippincott-Raven, 1996.

Kaplan HI, Sadock BJ. Comprehensive Textbook of Psychiatry, ed 8, HI Kaplan, BJ Sadock eds. Williams & Wilkins, Baltimore, 1999.

Kaufman DM. Clinical Neurology for Psychiatrists, 4th ed. Kaufman DM ed. W. B. Saunders, Philadelphia, 1995.

Lowinson JH, Pedro R, Milliman RB, Langrod JG (eds): Substance Abuse: A Comprehensive Textbook, 2nd ed. Baltimore, Williams & Wilkins, 1992.

Marx JA, Hockberger RS, Walls RM. Rosen's Emergency Medicine: Concepts and Clinical Practice, 5th ed. Mosby, Inc. St. Louis. 2002.

Rosen P. Emergency Medicine: Concepts and Clinical Practice, 4th Edition, ed Peter Rosen et al. Mosby-Year Book, Inc. 1998.

Rundell JR, Wise MG. Textbook of Consultation-Liaison Psychiatry, eds Rundell JR, Wise MG. American Psychiatric Press, Inc. Washington, DC, 1996.

Schatzberg AF, Nemeroff CB. Textbook of Psychopharmacology, eds Schatzberg AF, Nemeroff CB. 1995, American Psychiatric Press, Inc. Washington, DC.

Stapczynski JS (eds): Emergency Medicine: A Comprehensive Study Guide, 5th ed. American College of Emergency Physicians. McGraw Hill.

Stoudemire A, Fogel BS, Greenberg D (eds). Psychiatric Care of the Medical Patient, ed 2. New York, Oxford University Press, 1999.

Summers WK, Rund DA, Levin ML. Psychiatric illness in general urban emergency room: daytime versus nighttime population. J Clin Psychiatry 1979;41:340.

Tintinalli JE, Peacock FW, Wright MA: Emergency Evaluation of Psychiatric Patients. *Ann Emerg Med* 1994;23:859–862.

Tintinalli JE, Kelen GD, Stapczynski JS. Emergency Medicine: A Comprehensive Study Guide. McGraw Hill. New York. 2000.

Acknowledgments

It is quite an incredible experience to be able to sit down after all the writing is done and finally acknowledge all those friends and colleagues who have been crucial to this project. The process of finally getting to this stage has been a long and arduous one and a lot of people along the way have been very important in helping me get here. I thank the following people who have been key in making this book happen, either through their direct encouragement and support or for their valuable input in reviewing and offering their comments on the manuscript at different times throughout the writing.

Kenneth Davis, thank you for taking the time to help me conceptualize and ultimately give structure to this project, for making some important initial critiques, and for encouraging me to think it was within the realm of possibility.

Sheldon Jacobson, your constant support of me and the role of psychiatric emergency services in an emergency department have been crucial and deeply appreciated. None of this would have been possible without them and your support of me.

Barbara Richardson, your grace and skill under pressure, your integrity, and your overall clinical acumen have always impressed and inspired me. Thank you for taking the time to review parts of the manuscript; your advice has been very important to me and a lot of it was incorporated into this book.

Andy Jagoda, you were and are a role model. Your integration of the psychiatric emergency service and me into the faculty, the residency, and the overall emergency department was fundamental in making my experience and job as fun and meaningful as it was. I am truly thankful for the comments and overall support you have given me over the years to help me push this project and my career forward.

Deborah Marin, Craig Katz, Eleanor Burlingham, Neal Shipley, and Alexander Kolevzon, thank you so much for your review and insightful comments of the initial drafts of some of the material, all of which proved to be truly invaluable.

Daniel Stewart and Jody Lappin, although the paper we wrote for publication on serotonin discontinuation syndrome was never published, I have used parts of that paper in this book and I'd like to acknowledge and thank you both for the work you did in developing that component of this book. Scott Hill, the work we did on violence and agitation in the ER together is the backbone of part of that chapter. It was a great experience working together on that project.

Andrew Chiodo, you are not only an esteemed colleague but also my friend. Without your help at different times throughout the process of writing, especially with editing, this book might not have been written. You have been amazingly supportive and I thank you.

Andrew Kolodny, you too have been quite instrumental in this process. Your commitment in time and energy to help me review, and review again, a lot of this book as well as provide me with your insights and comments have been meaningful and very appreciated.

There are two people to whom I must give special thanks and who have been an integral part of my medical and psychiatric education and formation. Ricardo Mackintosh, you were my mentor in medical school and a true role model. Thank you for that and for the friendship you have provided me all these years. Dova Marder, you were and still are a true inspiration. I have learned so much from you and without all your support, guidance, love, and encouragement I know that this book would not have been possible. This book reflects a lot of what you have taught and shown me about psychiatric emergency services. Thank you.

Gregory Miller, your understanding and support during the last stages of this book, the deadlines and revisions, were fundamentally important to my being able to complete this book on time. You were accepting and very supportive of my needing time and space to complete this project and I cannot thank you enough.

Sarah Mercure and Charley Mitchell, you have both been wonderful to work with and your help has been most appreciated.

I must also thank my family, most especially my father, for always providing me with support and encouragement. You have always been there and, without you, this and many more things in my life would not have been possible. Los quiero mucho.

Lastly and most importantly, to my partner, Fernando Irausquin, this book is truly a testament to your patience, support, encouragement, love, and dedication. Without you in my life it would not have been possible. You are amazing.

General Psychiatric Assessment Guidelines

When confronted with an acute psychiatric presentation, regardless of the setting, remember these four important steps to the approach and assessment of any acute psychiatric presentation. **SAID, Stabilize, Ask, Identify, Disposition**

- **S**tabilize. Agitation, aggression, violence, and other manifestations of behavioral dyscontrol are a major threat to emergency department (ED) functions and must be dealt with quickly and effectively as a first order of priority. Critical medical stabilization is another crucial preliminary step in immediate patient management. This is discussed in more depth in Safety Considerations (Chapter 3).
- **A**sk questions. Gather as much history from as many different sources as possible.
- **I**dentify the symptoms and behaviors that need immediate attention and treat. **I**dentify and address medical acuity with a thorough review of symptoms and a full physical examination. **I**dentify predictive risk factors and safety concerns.
- **D**isposition. Determine safest and least restrictive disposition, ensuring continuity of care at all times.

Stabilization deals with all the supportive medical interventions—the ABCs (airway, breathing, circulation)—as well as all interventions necessary to assist in the management of dyscontrolled behavior that would prevent or hinder a full evaluation. After stabilization, whether psychiatric or medical, the next step is to **A**sk and gather history. In general, an evaluation must include a face-to-face interview for data gathering, a review of any records available, physical examination, certain diagnostic testing, and further information gathering from collateral sources. Many times, with certain psychiatric patients, whether because of a formal thought disorder, suspiciousness or paranoia, intoxication, uncooperativeness, or behavioral dyscontrol, this might be impossible to achieve. Prehospital providers [emergency medical technicians (EMTs), fire fighters, paramedics] or police officers on the scene can be useful in providing relevant details of the patient's condition, presentation, and/or mode of arrival. Family and friends are otherwise an alternative source of information and should be contacted or spoken with as soon as possible, with the patient's expressed verbal or written consent, if available. Patients may be reluctant to disclose certain key elements (i.e., suicide), which is why family, friends, and significant others are important in the history-taking portion of any evaluation. More than 69% of 134 patients reviewed in one study had mentioned suicide within a year of their suicide, and of those, 60% had communicated to their spouse; 50%, to a relative; and only 18%, to a physician. Other key sources of patient information are prior ED or hospital records, the patient's outpatient therapists, caseworkers, psychiatrist, and primary care physicians, if known and reachable by telephone.

The history should include the following elements:

- Presenting illness
- Psychiatric history
- Medical/surgical history
- Family history
- Substance-abuse history.

These elements are crucial in determining important aspects of the patient's life and potential presenting problem(s). In obtaining the patient's understanding of the current situation and/or condition, it is important to obtain a chronologic picture of the events that led up to the presentation. In many instances, these symptoms and conditions may have progressively and slowly been building up or been precipitated by some recent variable or event. Other elements that may be important to gather information about are potential precipitants, stressors, medication adherence, behavioral changes, dangerous behaviors, illicit drug use, and suicidal and violent ideations.

Step two is to Identify the acute presenting symptoms and arrive at a working diagnosis. Acute psychiatric presentations call for the physician to evaluate quickly and to determine whether the presentation is "functional" or "organic" in etiology (in other words, "psychiatric" vs. "medical"). Although these are arbitrary distinctions and are riddled with contradictions—all psychiatric symptoms have an "organic" etiology—it still is useful to consider these categories to make certain that clinicians in the acute care setting will always assess and think about underlying "organic" or "medical" causes when confronted with an acute psychiatric presentation.

Patients with an alteration in behavior, emotion, cognition, and/or with psychotic symptoms should always be assessed for underlying medical condition(s) or medication interactions before ascribing the symptoms or findings to a primary psychiatric or "functional" disorder. In many cases, these acute psychiatric symptoms may be secondary to an underlying medical condition(s) or medication side effects, but manifest as signs and symptoms consistent with a primary psychiatric disorder such as dementia, delirium, psychosis, mania, anxiety, or depression.

All physicians must be able to differentiate and manage these different scenarios: the stable psychiatric patient who appears in the ED with a medical complaint (e.g., productive cough with sputum and fever); the unknown patient with unknown psychiatric history but with acute medical, psychiatric, and/or behavioral symptoms; or the patients with known prior psychiatric and/or medical illness with exacerbation of either or both conditions. Table 1.1 lists predictors that can assist in the differentiation of medical versus psychiatric etiologies.

Assessing medical conditions must be a standard practice for all patients with psychiatric complaints. The reason this is so important is that a significant bias exists against patients with mental illness (who end up not receiving adequate care), which is usually directly or indirectly related to the need of the ED to assign priorities to and triage the more acute and sicker patients, as well as time constraints and other factors. It is estimated that 25% to 50% of patients with psychiatric illness also have a coexisting medical

Table 1.1. Predictors that can assist in the differentiation of medical versus psychiatric etiologies

Age older than 40 or younger than 12 yr
Abrupt or acute onset
Fluctuating course
Perceptual disturbances, such as visual or olfactory hallucinations
Known medical illness or neurologic symptoms
Cognitive alterations (confusion and disorientation)
Headaches
Loss of consciousness
Speech impairments
Abnormal vital signs
Incontinence
Complicated medication regimen
Alcohol or drug use
No psychiatric history

disorder that contributes to the acute syndromic presentation, and 4% to 12% of psychiatric inpatients have a medical condition that was identified as having precipitated or caused the admission. Many studies and reports have shown that the extent and thoroughness of medical and physical evaluations of psychiatric patients are suboptimal. The large majority of psychiatrists do not routinely perform physical examinations on their inpatients, and patients with psychiatric diagnosis meet the same fate when in the ED. Here are more reasons that this is so important:

- In a recent study, the prevalence of physical illness in psychiatric patients was more than 50%, and in another study, in 8% of the cases, a medical condition was thought to be the cause of the psychiatric complaint and an exacerbating factor in 22% of those cases.
- In an ED study, close to 80% of patients with underlying medical disease were labeled as "medically cleared."
- Another study showed that patients often seek treatment for symptoms of disorders that are usually comorbid conditions rather than their primary or principal condition.
- Different studies looking at the incidence of comorbid physical illness in psychiatric patients have shown a wide variation, from 4% to 60%.

Other studies have reported on the co-occurrence of physical illness in the psychiatric population seen in EDs; the most frequent diagnoses were substance abuse, affective disorders, anxiety disorders, psychotic disorders, antisocial personality, and cognitive disorders. The literature shows that many cases of misdiagnosis of medical and psychiatric illnesses are seen. Because so many possible causes of acute psychiatric presentations exist, I provide a categorization scheme in Appendix A, along with a table of possible psychiatric and medical causes for these types of presentations (see Appendix A).

Carefully assessing patients in an acute setting with psychiatric, behavioral, emotional, or cognitive symptoms is a fundamental part of all patient evaluations. The primary assessment should include vital signs and stat blood sugar, general appearance including evidence of trauma, and general level of alertness. Glucose screening should be part of every initial evaluation; hyperglycemia can cause delirium, and hypoglycemia can manifest itself as anxiety, confusion, agitation, or fatigue. Abnormal vital signs, too often neglected in acute psychiatric presentations, can be indicative of an underlying "organic" process. A short but detailed interview of the patient, family, friends, or other collateral sources of information can provide staff with the necessary information to determine how to focus the eventual management and treatment of the patient. This is crucial in the ultimate disposition of and favorable outcome for an acute patient and in differentiating "psychiatric" versus "medical" causes. It is essential to distinguish quickly between these two to institute treatment and management of both the underlying medical condition and the concomitant psychiatric symptoms. In some cases, this will decrease the potential for symptom relapse and the concomitant worsening of the patient's condition, as well as minimize the possibility of increased morbidity and mortality. It also is important in the formulation process of when and under what circumstances psychiatry consultants might need to be called in for further assessment and management, if not available on site. A clear understanding of the potential and predictive risk factors as well as specific safety concerns is fundamental in this process to arrive at a safe and appropriate disposition plan.

In many instances and depending on the level of sophistication of the actual ED setting with respect to on-site psychiatric staff, "medical clearances" of psychiatric patients before admission, transfer, or discharge are becoming a matter of routine. Patients may be medically assessed and determined to be stable; however, we must keep in mind that this does not mean that the patient is "cleared" of all medical disease; this only emphasizes the need for reevaluations in selected cases. A review of vital signs and a thorough history and physical examination, with the addition of laboratory testing when indicated, can help in the differentiation of medical versus psychiatric causes. Many studies have demonstrated that psychiatric patients with no known medical history or current medical complaints had significant laboratory abnormalities and potential underlying medical causes for their psychiatric presentations. Most experts agree that the most important aspect to "medical clearances" of psychiatric patients is to conduct a complete history and physical examination, with laboratory tests driven by the clinical picture. See Table 1.2 for guidelines to assist in the selection of diagnostic tests required for determining medical stability. Once again, the actual diagnostic testing recommended here is provided only as a guideline and should always be driven by the clinician's judgment, hospital protocols, and the clinical picture. In the absence of a clinical indication, routine laboratory tests have the drawback of producing false positives and unnecessary follow-up testing and workup. Table 1.3 provides some indications for neuroimaging.

Obtaining laboratory values and other ancillary tests in an acute setting, at times expensive and time-consuming, can actually heighten the diagnostic accuracy and address undiagnosed or

Table 1.2. Recommended (minimum) laboratory testing guidelines

All patients	SMA-7
	CBC (with differential and platelets)
	Urine toxicology
	Pregnancy tests
Additional labs/tests to be ordered as clinically indicated	ECG
	Neuroimaging
	Serum alcohol levels
	Serum toxicology screen
	Liver-function tests
	Thyroid-function tests
	Pulse oximetry
	Breathalyzer
	INR
	Acetaminophen and ASA serum levels
	Therapeutic drug levels (i.e., digoxin, lithium, theophylline, carbamazepine, valproic acid)
	Uranalysis

CBC, complete blood count; ECG, electrocardiogram; INR, international normalized ratio; ASA, acetylsalicylic acid.

Table 1.3. Indications for consideration of neuroimaging

Abrupt change in personality (especially after age 50 yr)
Acute onset of affective symptoms
Acute onset of psychosis
Brain edema
Chronic psychosis or mood disorder in which a prior MRI was not obtained, refractory illness, marked change in symptom profile while compliant with medications
CNS infections
Concussive/contusive injuries
Delirium
Dementia
Focal neurologic deficits
Hemorrhage
Increased intracranial pressure
Movement disorders of uncertain cause
Prolonged catatonia
Seizure disorders
Toxic encephalopathies

MRI, magnetic resonance imaging; CNS, central nervous system.

untreated underlying medical conditions in psychiatric patients. In many urban settings, chronic mentally ill patients are marginalized and disenfranchised, thus lacking adequate medical coverage and regular follow-up. These patients often use the ED as a source of primary care, and emergency physicians and psychiatrists become the *de facto* primary care physicians. Diagnostic tests should assist the clinician to rule in or rule out the presence of a disorder or condition, which may have treatment consequences; a test's usefulness will be related to its ability to detect the condition correctly, if present, or identify a condition not present. Diagnostic tests in the ED, although controversial, can assist in the short-term as well as the long-term management of these patients. Renal function tests may guide the decision to start lithium, or a baseline electrocardiogram (ECG) will assist with the initiation of an antipsychotic agent. As a rule of thumb, nothing should be "routine," but instead should be guided by clinical judgment. Laboratory results that will not return on a STAT basis should not be attempted in the ED, but should be ordered for the floor if the patient is admitted or left for an aftercare setting. Chest radiographs (CXRs) should not be done routinely for everyone, especially those that are pregnant or are not symptomatic. If a CXR is not clinically indicated on an emergency basis, it should be considered on admission for those patients who are human immunodeficiency virus–positive (HIV+); homeless; living in an adult home, nursing home, or group residence; or at high risk for tuberculosis (TB). A pregnancy test should be done on all women of child-bearing age for whom medication will be administered, CXRs performed, for whom pregnancy would constitute a serious risk to their overall health or in whom ignorance of a pregnancy would constitute a serious risk to a developing fetus, given the patient's chronic use of prescribed or illicit drugs. ECGs should be considered in patients older than 50 years, with known cardiac disease or treated (or to be treated) with a medication known to increase cardiac conduction times (i.e., some typical and atypical neuroleptics). The value and usefulness of toxicology evaluations in the ED also remains a controversial topic. Urine or serum toxicology results can be helpful in patients with recent exposure to poisonous substances, clinical data pointing to recent alcohol or drug use, or clinical suspicion of an elevated serum level of certain medications. In patients in whom substance abuse is suspected, self-reports can be as predictive as or even more so than toxicologic tests, although studies have shown a wide variation in concordance between self-reported history and drug screen in many cases.

It is recommended that medical evaluations be obtained in all psychiatric patients

- With known underlying medical condition
- With abnormal vital signs
- Who are elderly (see Chapter 6.3)
- With new onset of psychiatric symptoms

Figure 1-1 is an Assessment Algorithm to assist in clinical decision making. Considering "organic" causes will heighten one's level of suspicion: cues may include fluctuating levels of consciousness or changes in attention, repetitive grooming or "picking" behaviors,

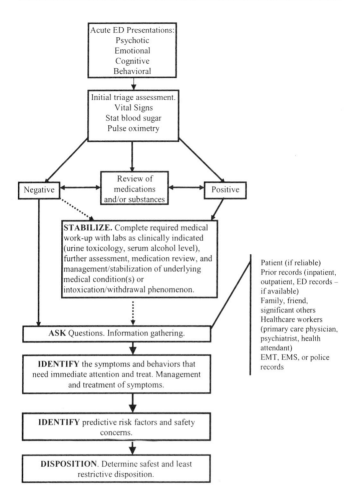

Fig. 1-1. Assessment algorithm.

agitation, vague or undefined perceptual disturbances, disorganized thinking, and confusion. This becomes quite important when confronted with certain patient profiles, in which cursory evaluations tend to occur, such as in the elderly, ED recidivists, the difficult and demanding patient, patients with psychosis or substance use, and HIV/acquired immunodeficiency syndrome (AIDS) patients. As the saying goes, you can't make a diagnosis if you don't think of the diagnosis.

Remember: always maintain a high index of suspicion.

The last step is the determination of a safe **D**isposition plan that will be tailored to the individual's needs and be the least restrictive and safest plan possible. Although no clear guidelines address the variables that must be considered in making a disposition, sound clinical judgment should be the rule. Danger to self (others), impulsivity, depression, ability to care for self, and psychosis are risk factors that must be carefully assessed and addressed thoroughly in making a disposition decision in the ED. In determining a safe and appropriate disposition plan, risk factors mentioned earlier and other safety concerns must be factored in. The provision of adequate continuity of care to these patients is fundamental but usually is driven by the availability of community resources. Social services (if available) should assist in making these plans, and at a minimum, the ED should have lists of community-based programs and, at best, linkages with several programs to ensure a closer and tighter aftercare planning.

Recent data suggest that family caretakers of patients with severe and persistent mental illness have special needs as well; burnout and stress and their impact on the patient's well-being are all very important in many of these cases. Interventions with these caretakers should be attempted, and support resources in their community sought out.

BIBLIOGRAPHY

Allen MH. Definitive treatment in the psychiatric emergency service. *Psychiatr Q* 1996;67:247–262.

American College of Emergency Physicians Clinical Policies Committee. Clinical policy for the initial approach to patients presenting with altered metal status. *Ann Emerg Med* 1999;33:251–281.

Antonowicz JL. Missed diagnosis in consultation liaison psychiatry. *Psychiatr Clin North Am* 1998;21:3.

Broderick KB, Lerner EB, McCourt JD, et al. Emergency physician practices and requirements regarding medical screening examinations of psychiatric patients. *Acad Emerg Med* 2002;9:88–92.

Buckley RA. Differentiating medical and psychiatric illness. *Psych Ann* 1994;24:11.

Claassen CA, Hughes CW, Gilfillan S, et al. The nature of help-seeking during psychiatric emergency service visits by a patient and an accompanying adult. *Psychiatr Serv* 2000;51:924–927.

Dolan JG, Mushlin AI. Routine laboratory testing for medical disorders in psychiatric inpatients. *Arch Intern Med* 1985;145:2085–8.

Hall R, Gardner ER, Popkin MK, et al. Unrecognized physical illness prompting psychiatric admission: a prospective study. *Am J Psychiatry* 1981;138:629–635.

Hammett-Stabler CA, Pesce AJ, Cannon DJ. Urine drug screening in the medical setting. *Clin Chim Acta* 2002;315:125–135.

Henneman PL, Mendoza R, Lewis RJ. Prospective evaluation of emergency department medical clearance. *Ann Emerg Med* 1994;24:672–677.

Hollister LE. Electrocardiographic screening in psychiatric patients. *J Clin Psychiatry* 1995;65:26–29.

Jacobs DG, Jamison KR, Baldessarini RJ. Suicide: clinical/risk management issues for psychiatrists. *CNS Spectrums Int J Neuropsychiatr Med* 2000;5:2, 39.

Knutsen E, DuRand C. Previously unrecognized physical illness in psychiatric patients. *Hosp Community Psychiatry* 1991;42:182–186.

Koranyi EK, et al. Physical illness underlying psychiatric symptoms. *Psychother Psychosom* 1992;38:155.

Korn CS, Currier GW, Henderson SO. "Medical clearance" of psychiatric patients without medical complaints in the emergency department. *J Emerg Med* 2000;18:173–176.

Lagomasino I, Daly R, Stoudemire A. Medical assessment of patients presenting with psychiatric symptoms in the emergency setting. *Psychiatr Clin North Am* 1999;22:819–850.

McIntyre JA, Romano J. Is there a stethoscope in the house (and is it used?). *Arch Gen Psychiatry* 1977;34:1147.

Meyers J, Stein S. The psychiatric interview in the emergency department. *Emerg Clin North Am* 2000;18:173–183.

Olshaker JS, Browne B, Jerrard DA, et al. Medical screening and clearance of psychiatric patients in the emergency department. *Acad Emerg Med* 1997;4:124–128.

Patterson C. Psychiatrists and physical examinations: a survey. *Am J Psych* 1978;135:967.

Perrone J, De Roos F, Jayaraman S, et al. Drug screening versus history in detection of substance use in the ED psychiatric patients. *Am J Emerg Med* 2001;19:49–51.

Reeves RR, Pendarvis EJ, Kimble R. Unrecognized medical emergencies admitted to psychiatric units. *Am J Emerg Med* 2000;18:390–393.

Riba M. Medical clearance: fact or fiction in the hospital emergency room. *Psychosomatics* 1990;31:400–404.

Rund DA. Distinguishing functional from organic brain disorders in the emergency department. *Resid Staff Physician* 1995;41:11–15.

Schiller MJ, Shumway M, Batki SL. Utility of a routine drug screening in a psychiatric emergency setting. *Psychiatr Serv* 2000;51:474–478.

Thienhaus OJ. Rational physical evaluation in the emergency room. *Hosp Community Psychiatry* 1992;43:311–312.

Tintinalli JE, Peacock FW, Wright MA. Emergency evaluation of psychiatric patients. *Ann Emerg Med* 1994;23:859–862.

Way BB, Banks S. Clinical factors related to admission and release decisions in psychiatric emergency services. *Psychiatr Serv* 2001;52:214–218.

Williams ER, Shepherd SM. Medical clearance of psychiatric patients. *Emerg Med Clin North Am* 2000;18:185–198.

Zimmerman M, Mattia JI. Principal and additional DSM-IV disorders for which outpatients seek treatment. *Psychiatr Serv* 2000;51:1299–1304.

Mental Status Exam

The Mental Status Exam (MSE) is the psychiatrist's equivalent of the physical examination. It is an objective measure of several parameters (emotion, behavior, cognition, as well as psychological data), systematically obtained by direct observation and questioning of the patient. It is a cross-sectional view ("snapshot") of the patient at a moment in time and should be able to convey to others a sense ("picture") of the patient. It is a necessary tool for psychiatrists to communicate their findings, and it requires experience as well as a unique lexicon/vocabulary. For nonpsychiatrists, this is, at best, an aspect of their training long forgotten, yet indispensable for any physician dealing with potential psychiatric patients, especially a primary care physician or an emergency department (ED) physician.

Another crucial but neglected aspect of the importance of a psychiatric evaluation of any patient—but especially those with acute psychotic, behavioral, cognitive, and/or emotional symptoms—is the initiation of a future therapeutic relationship. A brief but detailed examination by a physician with time to gather key elements (described later) will give the patient the sense of being listened to, understood, and respected. The physician's style and approach are very influential, but when patients feel they are being listened to and taken into account, adherence to treatment and management will likely improve considerably. Normally, this can be the first and initial step in the creation of a therapeutic alliance; how it is handled will affect the outcome of the patient's ED visit and have a future impact on treatment and aftercare. A smart rule to keep in mind when dealing with patients is to approach them with a calm and soothing voice, demonstrating genuine concern for their problems. If patient feels that the physician is genuine, more information will be forthcoming, and establishing a therapeutic and a more productive working relationship will ensue.

In an ED setting, given the acute nature of the situation, the history and all the information gathered are essential in making a correct working diagnosis and formulating a specific and effective treatment plan. You must strive to gather relevant information from the patient and also, with the patient's explicit verbal or written consent, contact and gather information from other sources. You must take into account and respect the diversity of all the patients you may encounter; being particularly sensitive to ethnicity, place of birth, race, sex, age, gender, social class, sexual orientation, and religious and spiritual beliefs. It is best to adopt an empathic and nonjudgmental attitude about diversity, especially when the patient's characteristics are quite different from your own, and try to remain aware of your biases or prejudices so they do not affect your role as a clinician.

Table 2.1 provides an example of a thorough and comprehensive outline for a psychiatric history. Not all elements listed need be obtained in the acute setting, but the information you have about your patient, whether directly or from collateral sources, will be fundamental to the decision-making process. Information

Table 2.1. Psychiatric evaluation outline

Identifying data
Chief complaint
History of present illness
Psychiatric history
Substance-abuse history
Medical history
Social/Family history
Mental status examination
Assessment
Diagnosis
Miscellaneous or collateral information
Disposition

gathering and appropriate documentation drives the process by which patients are evaluated and treated. It is important to realize that all charting is considered legal documentation, and accuracy and legibility are of utmost importance.

PSYCHIATRIC EVALUATION OUTLINE

Identifying Data

Provide a succinct demographic summary of the patient's age, marital status, race, sex, residence, employment, agency connection, referring source, insurance status or how supported, diagnosis and medications as known, and mode of arrival.

Chief Complaint

In the patient's own words, state why he or she is in the ED and/or the understanding of the current situation.

History of Present Illness

Provide a chronologic picture of the events leading up to the current moment, with an eye on precipitants, stressors, medication adherence, behavioral changes, dangerous behaviors, illicit drug use, and pertinent positives as described by patient, family, or accompanying staff. If the patient is first seen after a suicide attempt, a 24-hour walk-through is important the better to understand the event. If threats are voiced, we must always assess if they are targeted to specific individuals and means of access to a weapon.

Psychiatry History

Summarize all the clinically relevant information that the patient, family, agency, or chart gives on the patient's history, including hospitalizations (including approximate dates, reason for hospitalization, length of hospitalization, medications used while hospitalized, plans on discharge); medication trials; suicide attempts; homicidal ideation; violence; sexual, physical, or domestic abuse; and current follow-up and/or adherence with medications or treatment.

Substance-Abuse History

Carefully assess present alcohol and/or drug history, substance of choice, order of substance preference, and current pattern of use.

Alcohol use details:

Date of first use/quantity
Date of loss of control/quantity
Drinking-pattern details
Tremors
Blackouts
Hallucinations
Seizures
Delirium
Confusional states
Dementia or memory deficits

In cases of patients with alcohol-related problems or suggestions of alcohol-related problems, to assist in making a diagnosis of alcoholism, you may ask four simple questions, commonly known as the CAGE Questionnaire.

- Have you ever . . .
  . . . thought you should **C**ut back on your drinking? (C)
  . . . felt **A**nnoyed by people criticizing your drinking? (A)
  . . . felt **G**uilty or bad about your drinking? (G)
  . . . had a morning **E**ye-opener to relieve hangover or nerves? (E)

If a patient responds with two or three positive responses, a high index of suspicion exists for an alcohol-abuse or alcohol-dependence diagnosis, and four positive responses are almost pathognomonic.

Other drug-use details (note first/last use, quantities, route, effects): amphetamines, cannabis, cocaine, hallucinogens, inhalants, nicotine, opioids, heroin, methadone, phencyclidine, sedatives, hypnotics, anxiolytics, over-the-counter drugs, prescription drugs, or herbal remedies. Also assess past alcohol or drug-treatment history and prior attempts at abstinence, first and last period of abstinence, and longest period of abstinence. Record detoxification (note: inpatient, outpatient, medical vs. nonmedical detoxification, and outcome) and rehabilitations (note inpatient, outpatient, and outcome); disulfiram (Antabuse) treatment and effect; naltrexone (Revia) treatment and effect; methadone maintenance (treatment, dosages, and effect); and 12-step involvement: Alcoholics Anonymous (AA), Narcotics Anonymous (NA), Cocaine Anonymous (CA), or other, as well as home group, sponsor, and their effectiveness.

Medical History

Document all active and past medical problems, medications, allergies, and most current follow-up or physical examination. Include review of systems (ROS) and any positive findings, history of head trauma, human immunodeficiency virus (HIV) and tuberculosis (TB) risk factors and status; recent laboratory values, electrocardiograms (ECGs), and chest radiographs (CXRs) if known or available, and allergies.

Social/Family History

As obtainable, and including assessment of social supports in the community and housing, employment, and interpersonal situations, as well as family history of psychiatric illness including suicides, substance abuse, and alcoholism.

General: born and raised, home life; description of maternal/
paternal or caregiver attention/deprivation; description of childhood/adolescence; quality of significant relationships; siblings and/or children; family functioning; major events or losses

Sexuality: sexual identity, current sexual relationship, current or past sexual problems, safer-sex or high-risk sexual activity

Education: literacy, highest grade achieved, academic performance, emotional/behavioral problems affecting academic performance, special education needs, learning disabilities, General Educational Development (GED), vocational training

Spirituality: organized religion (practices, meaning), alternative spiritual beliefs (practices, meaning)

Vocational/Employment history: current employment, performance, reasons for job terminations, work strengths, deficits, goals, training programs, educational programs, and workfare requirements

Military history: service branch, dates, status, performance, discharge type (honorable/dishonorable), and service connection

Criminal history: arrests (note alcohol/drug associations), misdemeanor convictions, felony convictions, parole or probation status and parole/probation officer name and number, prison history

Sexual/Physical abuse history: Sexual abuse during childhood or adulthood, past perpetrators, circumstances, effects on patient, and actions taken by patient or others. Physical abuse during childhood or adulthood, past perpetrators, circumstances, effects on patient, and actions taken by patient or others. Suspicion or evidence of current sexual or physical abuse by others toward patient, present perpetrators, circumstances, effects on patient, and actions taken by patient or others. Note extent to which alcohol/drug use is a contributing factor in victim or perpetrator status. History of neglect or physical or sexual abuse by patient toward others and/or suspicion or evidence of current neglect, sexual or physical abuse by patient toward others. History of investigation by the local State Children's Protection Services.

Mental Status Exam (see Table 2.2)

Assessment

It is important to assess a patient's level of functioning, especially those patients who have serious and chronic mental disorders, multiple comorbid psychiatric (and medical) conditions, and in the elderly or children/adolescents, in whom their illness may affect their level of functioning. Assessing a patient's functional status (i.e., activities of daily living, ADLs) can be quite helpful in determining the severity of the condition and prognostic and treatment outcomes. These may include inquiring about physical ADLs: eating, toileting, bathing, dressing, or instrumental ADLs (driving, using public transportation, medication taking, shopping, managing money, housekeeping, etc.).

Structured interviews, questionnaires, or rating scales can be helpful in the diagnostic assessment and in the determination of treatment outcomes by allowing quantification of symptom severity and establishment of baseline symptom manifestation, although culture, ethnicity, gender, social, and age variables can bias the interpretation of the results. A few psychiatric rating scales are widely used and helpful in monitoring patient's progress and symptom severity. In the ED, their usefulness is often more limited, but when time permits, these can assist either as a guide in asking and gauging symptom profile and severity or as a tool to establish a baseline for the next level of service and provider(s). The value of these scales, as well as other scales, is their serial/periodic administration to monitor progress and treatment response. Structured interviews, questionnaires, and rating scales should never be a substitute for sound clinical judgment or skills. Recommended scales are discussed in the relevant chapters and listed in Appendix D.

Assessment must include summary and impression of the patient. It should include an assessment of the patient's personality structure or traits. A significant overlap occurs in symptoms between Axis I and II disorders, in addition to the comorbidity that exists among these disorders (more than 50% of patients with borderline personality disorder or schizotypal personality disorder have concurrent depressive disorder). Final assessment and plans must include justification of need for admission; medications received in the ED or recommended for inpatient service; and psychiatry follow-up with date, time, and clinician or agency referred to, including the address, telephone number, and contact person if available at the referring source. Document legal status and discussion of status and rights. Document observational status for admission, and if the patient is discharged, document the patient's safety and discussion of services available with discharge instructions.

Diagnosis

Careful thought must be given to each patient's diagnosis, and a working diagnosis or provisional diagnosis must be provided for each patient. This is the diagnosis to be given to describe the condition chiefly responsible for prompting the current visit or admission and is the main focus of attention or treatment. It is often difficult to determine the provisional diagnosis, and why an expanded differential is expected, with the provisional diagnosis indicated first and the remaining disorders listed in order of focus of attention or treatment. Subtypes and specifiers are provided in *Diagnostic and Statistical Manual of Mental Disorders,* fourth edition, revised (DSM-IV-TR) and must be used for accuracy; subtypes are understood to be "mutually exclusive and jointly exhaustive phenomenological subgroupings within a diagnosis." Specifiers conversely "are not mutually or jointly exclusive and provide a more homogeneous subgrouping of individuals with the disorder who share certain features." Severity and course specifiers also should be applied whenever possible.

Miscellaneous / Collateral Information

Documentation of each contact with patient and family/informant and time spent are required. Phone calls, family meetings, and discussions with other agencies, hospitals, or family members should be made only after the patient has given explicit verbal consent, and should be timed and dated and separated from the rest of the text of the foregoing history. Discussions with other members of the patient's treatment team must be similarly documented. Family meetings should include documentation of who was present, how long it lasted, history obtained, points clarified, goals and objectives met (as previously determined by the team), and concepts communicated/understood by the patient and family. Documentation of request and indication for medical consult, timed and dated, is important. Informal consults also must be documented, and if recommendations of consultant are not followed, the reasons must be stated clearly in the chart.

Mental Status Examination Elements

See Table 2.2 for the basic elements of the psychiatric MSE. They can be used as a guide in directing the questioning and assessment of any patient. The order and the method of questioning are individual skills, gained from repeated evaluations and questioning of patients. Many of the elements of the MSE can be gathered initially and throughout the interview (appearance, attitude, speech, etc.) by direct observation of the patient without requiring a specific line of questioning. Others must be asked more directly, such as suicidality, hallucinations, violence, etc.

Appearance: Dress, grooming, and hygiene are important first indicators. An elderly woman with associated medical findings but with food-stained clothing and smelling of urine can indicate a more severe cognitive disorder like dementia. Other salient characteristics (e.g., tattoos, piercings, odd clothing or make-up) are relevant and should be noted and documented.
Examples: groomed, disheveled, unkempt, or malodorous.

Table 2.2. Mental status examination outline

Appearance
Attitude, eye contact, relatedness
Reliability
Psychomotor activity
Speech
Mood
Affect
Thought process
Thought content
Suicidality
Homicidality
Neurovegetative symptoms
Insight
Judgment
Cognitive functioning

Attitude: A patient's degree of cooperative/uncooperativeness will be easily determined at the outset and will make the evaluation process proceed smoothly or not. Hostile and guarded patients with poor eye contact, who are not forthcoming with any personal information, might be psychotic and/or intoxicated. Also assess a patient's relatedness, impulse control, and reliability as a historian.

Examples: hostile, guarded, apathetic, seductive, evasive, playful, or ingratiating.

Psychomotor activity: A patient's psychomotor behavior is easy to determine by direct observation and refers to the quantitative and qualitative aspects of motor behavior. The patient who is pacing, unable to sit still, coming to the triage or information desk repeatedly, indicates increased psychomotoric activity. This is in direct contrast to a severely depressed patient who is sitting in a chair, slumped over, rigid, and requiring encouragement to engage in conversation.

Examples: psychomotor agitation/retardation, bizarre movements or tics, gestures, or stereotyped movements.

Speech: The physical characteristics of the patient's speech are important to note and must be described in terms of the quantity, rate, rhythm, volume, and quality. Impairments in speech must be included, as well as its spontaneity.

Examples: normal, fluent, loud, soft, fast, pressured, monotone, slow, or incoherent.

Mood is the patient's sustained and predominant internal state of emotion. It should be stated in the patient's own words. A normal mood is described as euthymic with depressed mood and euphoric or elated mood at the opposite extremes. Ask the patient:

How has your mood been?

Have you been feeling sad or blue?

Do you ever feel like crying?

Do you ever feel that you are special?

Have you ever felt as if you were on top of the world?

Do you have any special talents or achievements that no one else has?

If the patient is unable to provide a descriptive adjective to explain the mood state, you can ask her or him to rate the current mood on a scale of 1 to 10 (with 10, the worst mood ever, and 1, the best, or vice versa).

Examples: happy, sad, guilty, scared, upset, empty, or hopeless.

Affect is the externally perceived expression of a patient's mood or emotional state. It is the examiner's objective interpretation of the patient's described mood and has several parameters.

- Stability is the frequency or variation of the emotion (stable or labile, which describes high-frequency emotions, such as switching rapidly from one emotional state to another);
- Intensity is the magnitude of the current emotion (neutral, apathetic, sad, depressed, dysphoric, elevated, manic, irritable, or angry);

- Range is the total magnitude of the emotional state (normal, constricted, blunted, or flat);
- Appropriateness is a measure of the congruence to the stated mood (appropriate/inappropriate).

Thought process: How patients put together ideas and associations.

> *Examples:* logical/illogical, goal-directed, coherent/incoherent, circumstantial, tangential, flight of ideas, loosening of association, thought blocking, derailment, word salad, neologisms, clang association, or verbigeration.

Thought content: This refers to what patients are actually thinking about: ideas, beliefs, preoccupations, obsessions, etc. Question carefully with attention to details about type, frequency, and content, especially of hallucinations. Ask the patient:

> Do you feel safe here?
> Do you ever feel singled out?
> Have you ever felt as if people are trying to hurt you?
> Do you ever hear voices when no one else is around?
> Have you ever heard any strange sounds you can't explain?
> Have you ever seen anything you can't explain?
> Have you ever felt something strange on your skin?
> Have you ever smelled anything when there isn't anything around?
> Do you ever feel that your thoughts are so loud that others can hear them?
> Have you ever heard another person's thoughts?
> Do you ever think that people can place thoughts into your head?
> Can you put thoughts into other people's heads?
> When watching TV, reading a magazine, or listening to the radio, do you ever feel that they are speaking about or to you?
> Are you the kind of person that worries a lot?
> What types of things do you worry about?
> Ever stay up all night worrying?

> *Examples:* paranoid ideation, compulsions, obsessions, phobias, delusions, ideas of reference or influences, or disturbances of perception (hallucinations, sinesthesias, illusions).

Suicidal ideation is a very important aspect of any ED evaluation and an integral part of the psychiatric MSE. This question should be assessed from triage to institute the necessary precautionary procedures as per each institution's policy. Suicidality can be a frequent presenting complaint in the ED and must be elicited by the ED staff if not expressed outright in their questioning. Staff should not feel scared or uncomfortable when inquiring about current or past suicidality. Remember that one of the best prognosticators of future suicidality is past suicide attempts. Patients who might be having suicidal thoughts are potentially relieved if they are asked directly about their thoughts and feel that the staff is interested in their condition. The ED staff must always ask about and assess suicidality (see Chapter 4-21).

Homicidality is another important element of the assessment and one that carries the most medicolegal, emotional, and potentially adverse outcomes if not adequately or thoroughly assessed. All patients should be asked about thoughts of violence or anger toward others, especially with emphasis on access to weapons or possession of weapons. The same procedural issues should be taken into account when initially screening patient's reporting thoughts of wanting to harm others (targeted or nonspecific). Any patient with agitation, angry affect, voicing threats, or with a known history of violence should be thoroughly questioned about

- Plans
- Intent
- Access to weapons
- Current alcohol/drug use
- Target of threat (obtain name, address, and telephone number, if possible)
- History of violence, fights, and incarcerations.

Always remember that patients reporting either suicidality or threats of harm to others require careful documentation of all aspects of the evaluation and the care and assessment process.

Neurovegetative symptoms: All patients require a thorough assessment of the essential neurovegetative parameters: sleep, appetite, energy, and concentration, with special emphasis on any changes from baseline.

Examples: Rate as normal/good/fair/poor or describe changes (e.g., hypersomnia, anorexia).

Insight and judgment: Insight is considered the patient's awareness and understanding of the current condition or situation, as well as diagnoses, need for treatment, or medication adherence. Intellectual insight is different from true emotional insight in which a concordant adaptation of behaviors, thought, and motives is found vis-à-vis the patient's awareness of the illness. Patients can express, on a spectrum, different levels of insight ranging from an absolute denial of illness to true emotional insight. Ask the patient: Do you think that you have a mental/psychiatric illness? If so, do you know what your illness is called? Can you describe some of the symptoms of your illness? Do you think you need treatment? Do you take medications for your illness?

Judgment is a parameter that that can be assessed during the course of the examination with the patient. Does the patient understand the outcomes of behaviors and how that understanding influences behaviors?

Example: How will the patient respond when asked what he or she would do if he or she smelled smoke in a crowded theater?

Cognitive functioning: This portion assesses organic brain functioning and intelligence as well as level of consciousness and memory. A detailed assessment of cognitive functions should be performed on all patients, although the level of detail will be clinically determined.

Many times the family or primary caretakers will provide staff with more information regarding recent or remote memory impairments that a patient might otherwise omit or gloss over if problems exist. The comprehensive evaluation of cognitive functioning and its impairment is a lengthy process that would involve psychological testing as well as more advanced clinical and laboratory workup, but there is a practical and clinically useful screening test: the mini-MSE (MMSE) or Folstein scale (see Table 2.3). The MMSE assesses orientation, attention, memory, verbal fluency, ability to follow complex commands, and visuographic skills. The MMSE is a highly structured, rapid, easy-to-administer test that can be performed at the patient's bedside even by nonclinicians. It is the most widely used scale to monitor cognitive impairment and can determine a cross-sectional "score" of cognitive functioning as well as a useful tracking method of a patient's cognitive state over time. A simple scoring system is provided; of a possible 30 points, 24 to 30 is considered normal, anything less than 24 is considered impairment, and less than 20 is definitive impairment. Normal scores will vary with age and educational level. It is a simple scale and has demonstrated reliability and validity with a high interrater reliability and test–retest reliability for moderate to severe forms of cognitive impairments. Its limitation is its inability to detect milder forms of dementias and cognitive dysfunctions.

- Orientation: Ask the patient the date. Ask specifically for items omitted, and score 1 point for each correct answer.

Table 2.3. Mini-mental status examination

Orientation
  Place: city, state, country, county, floor _____ (5)
  Time: day, date, month, year, season _____ (5)
Registration
  Name three objects and ask patient
    to repeat them _____ (3)
Attention and concentration
  Subtract serial 7s from 100 or spell
    WORLD backward _____ (5)
Recall
  Ask for three objects repeated above _____ (3)
Language
  Name pencil/watch _____ (2)
  Repeat "no ifs, ands, or buts" _____ (1)
  Three-step command (i.e., take paper
    in right hand, fold in half, and place
    on floor) _____ (3)
  Read and obey:
    CLOSE YOUR EYES _____ (1)
  Write a complete sentence _____ (1)
  Copy intersecting pentagons _____ (1)

                              Total: _____ (30)

- Registration: Inform the patient you are going to test his or her memory. Clearly and slowly, about 1 second apart, give the names of three unrelated objects. After all three, ask the patient to repeat them, and score 1 point for each correct item. You may repeat the words until the patient can say all three, up to six trials. If the patient cannot eventually recall all three words, then recall cannot be fully assessed.
- Attention and calculation: Ask the patient to begin with 100 and count backward (subtract) by seven. Stop after five subtractions (93, 86, 79, 72, 65), and score 1 point for each correct answer. If the patient cannot or will not perform this task, ask her or him to spell the word WORLD backward. Score 1 point for each letter in correct order.
- Recall: Ask the patient if he or she can recall the three words you had asked them to remember. Score 1 point for each word remembered correctly.
- Naming: show the patient a wristwatch (or other object) and ask what it is, repeating with a pen or pencil (or other object). Score 1 point for each item named correctly.
- Repetition: Ask the patient to repeat "No ifs, ands, or buts." Score 1 point only if repeated correctly, for one trial only.
- Three-step command: Give the patient a piece of paper and ask her or him to take it in the right (or left) hand, fold it in half, and put it on the floor (or bed or hand it back to you). Score 1 point for each step performed correctly.
- Reading: On a blank paper, write (legibly and large), CLOSE YOUR EYES. Ask the patient to read the sentence and do what it says. Score 1 point only if the patient actually closes the eyes.
- Writing: Give the patient a blank piece of paper and ask him or her to write a sentence. It must be written spontaneously; do not assist or prompt the patient. Score 1 point if sentence has a subject and a verb and makes sense. Grammar and punctuation are not important.
- Copying: On a blank piece of paper, draw two intersecting pentagons and ask the patient to copy them exactly. To score a point, the pentagons must have ten angles, and two must be intersecting.

A patient's *level of consciousness* is determined by the ability to respond to the environmental stimuli. Disturbances of the level of consciousness should make you think of organic causes (e.g., delirium).

Examples: clouding, somnolence, coma, lethargy, or alertness.

Intelligence can be inferred by the patient's interactions with staff, as well as by the patient's ability to learn, integrate, and process new information. Intelligence also is related to vocabulary, general fund of knowledge, patient's socioeconomic status, and schooling.

Remember: Documentation is the key! Write legibly, and thoroughly document every aspect of the history gathered.

BIBLIOGRAPHY

Dziedzic JK, Brady WJ, Lindsay R, et al. The use of the Mini-Mental Status Examination in the ED evaluation of the elderly. *Am J Emerg Med* 1998;16:686–689.

Ewing JA. Detecting alcoholism: the CAGE Questionnaire. *JAMA* 1984;252:1905–1907.

Mini-Mental Status Exam, adapted from Folstein MF, Folstein SE, McHugh PR. "Mini-mental State:" a practical method for grading the cognitive state of patients for the clinician. *J Psychiatr Res* 1975;12:189.

Kirrane RM, Siever LJ. New perspectives on schizotypal personality disorder. *Curr Psychiatr Rep* 2000;2:62–66.

Koenisgberg HW, Anwunah I, New A, et al. Relationship between depression and borderline personality disorder. *Depress Anxiety* 1999;10:158–167.

Rosenberg RC. The therapeutic alliance and the psychiatric emergency room crisis as opportunity. *Psych Ann* 1994;24:610–614.

Wind AW, Schellevis FG, Van Staveren G, et al. Limitations of the Mini-Mental Status Examination in diagnosing dementia in general practice. *Int J Geriatr Psychiatry* 1997;12:101–108.

Safety Considerations

Safety in the emergency department (ED), or any acute care setting, is a very important issue, and staff efforts must always be focused on ensuring patient and staff safety. This is a priority for all staff! Because EDs or acute care settings are all different in size, staff composition, patient-to-staff ratio, room and patient allocation, and security presence, safety considerations are crucial. Additionally, because of the high patient volume and acuity, and especially in training institutions (with the presence of new and untrained staff), safety becomes a top priority. Borrowing from the substance-abuse field:

Always Remember: People, Places, and Things!

- Always make sure you are safe.
- Always make sure patients and staff members are safe.
- Always monitor patients for possible violence.
- Always make certain your environment is safe.
- Always trust your instincts when you feel unsafe.

It is well known that mental health workers are at an increased risk of experiencing work-related violence. The prevalence and incidence of workplace violence in the ED and the mental health sector are quite high and becoming a serious occupational hazard. Even in the prehospital sector, emergency medical service providers are at increased risk for encountering violence; male sex, age, and hour of the day are highly associated with episodes of violence. Nurses, being the front-line staff in patient care—especially ED nurses—also are at increased risk of experiencing emotional, verbal, and at times even physical abuse not only by the patients but by family members and visitors as well. In 1999, the International Council of Nurses recognized workplace violence as a serious occupational hazard for nursing, demonstrating the widespread problem this has become.

Because all EDs or acute care settings are quite different, the following are recommendations for established practices when dealing with acute psychiatric presentations. Once a patient has been triaged, the patient should be changed into hospital pajamas and/or searched for weapons and contraband. This is the first step in assuring safety for the patients and staff. When a patient becomes behaviorally dyscontrolled in an inpatient unit, similar actions should be taken:

- Place the patient on an enhanced observational status
- Conduct a search whenever possible.

Many institutions, at the point of triage or on an initial quick assessment, "eye-balling," will determine which patients need to be searched and placed on some form of enhanced monitoring. Enhanced monitoring should be provided, at a minimum—when clinically determined—when a patient endorses either suicidal or homicidal ideation, command auditory hallucinations, or any aggressive behavior. A staff nurse and/or the physician should conduct the search with the assistance, when possible, of a hospital security officer. The search should involve the removal of all potentially dangerous objects including jewelry, hair appliances, shoestrings, belts, necklaces, and any contraband found. The patient can then be placed into hospital pajamas, or if clothing has been adequately searched, can remain in street clothes less the items confiscated in the search. These items should be placed in a sealed bag marked with the patient's name and stored in a secured cabinet or in some other safe place. Other security measures to consider are a mouth check (for concealed razor blades) and a metal-detector screening, whether with a hand-held metal detector or a full-body metal-detecting apparatus, conducted by hospital security officers. See Fig. 3-1 safety algorithm.

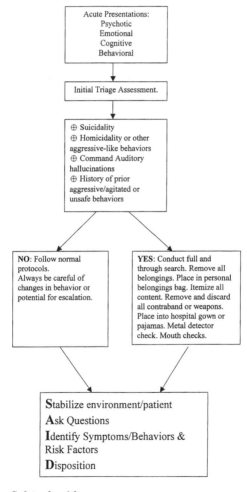

Fig. 3-1. Safety algorithm.

These are some basic tenets of safety that must be adhered to at ALL times in an acute care setting.

- No patients are to be interviewed in an "unsafe" room. Rooms are considered "unsafe" when they contain objects that can potentially be dangerous, such as too many chairs (more than required for the interview), bottles, pens, medical equipment, etc. Any room where a psychiatric interview will be conducted must be uncluttered.
- Staff must make sure that they are personally "safe"—avoid any personal loose jewelry, ties, or clothing that can be used or grabbed by patients.
- No patient deemed in need of some form of enhanced monitoring should be interviewed before conducting a search for contraband.
- Interviews should be conducted in an open room, keeping an easy means of egress, should a patient become acutely agitated. During the interview, keep your chair positioned near the door for a rapid exit.
- When possible, you and the patient should be comfortably seated during the interview.
- In treatment or interview rooms, keep doors open at all times. Other than for purposes of locked seclusion, NO CLOSED DOORS should be allowed at any time.
- Hospital security, if available, should be present during the interview if you do not feel safe with the patient alone. If security personnel are unavailable, ensure that additional staff are present.
- Do not permit or allow an agitated patient hot beverages, glass bottles, cans, cutting utensils, etc.
- Do not allow patients in need of enhanced observation to remain unsupervised while alone.
- Do not allow patients to be unattended in a closed or locked bathroom.
- Do not allow patients to have access to anything that can be potentially dangerous, such as shoelaces, drawstrings, sheets, headphones, pens, pencils, and/or other pointed objects.
- At all times you must trust your instincts, and NEVER do anything that you feel is unsafe or makes you uncomfortable.
- Ask for help or assistance if you feel it is necessary.
- Become familiar with the locations of panic buttons or alarms, if available, as well as the numbers for security assistance or backup.

Because we have a volatile workplace, potentially fraught with danger and at times with violence, it is imperative that safety be a top priority, and education and continuous in-service training of all staff be an ongoing part of an acute care setting (Table 3.1). Studies have shown that educational programs can help to reduce the number of violent events, especially with those staff that are less experienced or have less formal training. Violence-prevention management, in-service training on restraints, careful screening of violence-prone individuals, and security personnel training and response are recognized to be effective methods to improve safety and increase awareness among staff. Many studies have shown that some form of critical incident stress management, an integrated and comprehensive crisis-intervention approach to dealing with staff's psychological aftermath of violence (which usually

Table 3.1.   Ten safety do's and don'ts

Do's	Don'ts
Search all patients for contraband, and remove dangerous objects	Allow patients to keep objects that are potentially dangerous
Keep the door open when interviewing patients	Allow patients to have hot beverages, glass, or sharp objects
Make sure your environment is uncluttered and "safe"	Allow yourself to become trapped or cornered in a room by a patient
Make sure personal belongings are tucked away or in	Feel embarrassed or intimidated to ask for help
Position yourself with a rapid means of egress	Feel you cannot have assistance or help when conducting a patient interview
Know how to get help	
Know where your panic buttons or alarms are located	Allow splitting or inconsistencies
Trust your "gut" feeling about patients and potentially dangerous situations	Conduct an interview if feeling menaced or frightened
	Lay hands on or attempt to restrain the patient if alone or patient is too agitated
Ask patients about suicidal plans and or homicidal thoughts	Use the most restrictive measures before trying less-invasive techniques
Ask patients about access to a weapon	Allow a patient to be alone or unattended

includes preincident training, acute crisis intervention, and postincident response), can significantly reduce staff assaults.

Although physicians in an ED will invariably encounter violent patients, the frequency of these encounters is somewhat dependent on the size and location of the ED. The agitated and belligerent patient should be considered a behavioral emergency with a quick and definitive response. These patients make up a small number of ED visits, but these types of situations require an inordinate amount of time and attention from staff. It is imperative that any physician be ready for and capable of effectively handling the patient that becomes violent as well as able to act definitively to prevent escalation and injury before moving on to further evaluation.

Poor training or inadequate understanding of the management of violence can place both the patients and those around them at significant risk. Prompt assessment of the situation and the immediate deployment of de-escalation techniques (or other management approaches) will ensure an optimal outcome. Because the accurate differential diagnosis of an agitated patient is often not possible in an emergency situation, it is imperative to have a clear understanding of the management approach to uncontrollable patients.

The management of violent patients can be divided into several progressive unified approaches, which are neither mutually exclusive nor absolute in their order of implementation.

These are

- Environmental manipulation
- De-escalation techniques
- Physical restraint/seclusion
- Pharmacologic interventions.

For a stepwise approach in managing the violent patient; the least restrictive yet most effective means of control should always be selected. This is known as the *least-restrictive alternative doctrine.*

Perceived Threat	Action
Low	Search Environmental Manipulations
Moderate	Search Verbal de-escalation Psychoparmacological intervention
High	Search Psychoparmacological intervention Restraints/Seclusion

ENVIRONMENTAL

When agitation is present, it is essential that precautions be taken to ensure the immediate safety of other patients and staff. Several environmental variables can be controlled or modified to decrease the potential for escalation of violence. These include

- Patient comfort
- Relative isolation
- Decreased time of wait
- Staff attitude
- Decreased stimuli.

The patient should be made as comfortable and safe as possible. A quiet room or individual examination room, with a decrease in external stimuli, can assist in the de-escalation of a patient. Offering the patient a chair to sit on or stretcher to lie down, and/or something to drink like a cup of water or juice, conveys caring and respect and can improve a potentially volatile situation.

The ED physicians should never place themselves or any other staff member in an unsafe situation (i.e., in a closed room, access to doors blocked). All items or objects that can be potentially dangerous should be removed or at least taken into account by the staff to prepare for and to minimize the danger of injury. Certain staff approaches should be carefully monitored, especially when dealing with a violent patient. It is important to both maintain a safe distance from an agitated patient and to respect his or her personal space. Prolonged or intense direct eye contact can be perceived as menacing by the patient. Body language and positions such as crossed arms or hands behind the back or hidden also can be considered confrontational and threatening. The most important approach is always maintaining a calm and in-control stance. Staff should closely monitor the patient's behavior for any changes in mood, speech, and psychomotoric activity—any of these can signal an impending loss of control.

DE-ESCALATION

Verbal de-escalation should be one of the first approaches to any agitated patient unless the patient's degree of agitation is such that it indicates an imminent risk of self-harm or harm to others. The concept of de-escalation or "defusing" or "talk down" of an agitated patient might appear to be an intuitive process and a role certain staff might feel comfortable taking on, but it is complex and requires certain skill sets. De-escalation techniques are all the verbal and nonverbal responses from and by staff, which if done or carried out correctly can completely defuse or reduce a potentially violent situation.

The staff member, most often the ED physician, senior nurse, or consultant psychiatrist, should appear calm and in control, speaking to the patient in a nonprovocative, nonconfrontational manner with a soft, soothing tone. Staff provocations may result in further violence. The staff member should be able to convey a sense of control over the situation and appear empathic and concerned.

Empathic statements, such as these, can be very useful.

- I understand you're not feeling well and that you're having a hard time.
- It sounds as if you're in pain and confused.
- Sometimes people get very stressed and need some help.

Statements, such as the ones following, made in the context of genuine desire to assist the patient and attempt to provide and offer safety, can place a potentially violent patient more at ease:

- You're here to get help, and we're going to try to figure out what's going on.
- Allow us to us help you; don't be afraid.
- You're safe now here with us.

Staff members should reinforce that the patient is in a safe environment and that everyone is there to assist in the evaluation and treatment. Verbal limits also can be used, and the patients should be told that they will not be allowed to harm themselves or others, and that safety measures will be taken to ensure the safety and adequate evaluation of their needs. The patient at risk for violence must be told decisively and emphatically that staff will ensure and maintain control. The clinician must set limits with the patient while explaining the consequences of present and future actions. The clinician should be able to provide reasonable, positive reinforcements and propose alternatives to aggressive behavior such as talking with staff, making a phone call, or allowing staff to continue their evaluation. Staff should be consistent in their approach and should be very clear of the management of a potentially violent patient. No room for second-guessing or contradictory approaches can be allowed when a patient is out of control. Overt anger or hostility should never be expressed toward an agitated patient.

When attempting to de-escalate an agitated patient remember to

- Use a calm and soothing tone of voice
- Remain a safe distance from the patient
- Prepare staff or security personnel for the potential for violence
- Be familiar with "emergency or panic" alarms/buttons in the ED.

Security personnel, when available, can be of use for several different reasons: the presence of uniformed hospital security personnel or local police can be a show of force that may calm a patient down considerably. If not, they can be instrumental in the implementation of physical restraints/containment. A well-trained hospital security force can be instrumental in assisting the ED staff with the management of agitated patients.

PHYSICAL RESTRAINTS AND SECLUSION

About 4% of patients are placed in restraints in urban EDs because of combative and dangerous behaviors. Restraints and seclusion should be used as a final response to any and all emergency and imminent dangerous behavior and should be based on the individualized assessment of the patient needs by professional staff that is competent and educated in the use of restraints and/or seclusion (see Chapter 5.2).

Seclusion and restraints should never be used as a means of punishment or retribution for an agitated, demanding, or disruptive patient, or for the convenience of staff, or as a substitute for a treatment program. Implementation of restraints or seclusion can place staff and patients at a higher risk for injury. It is imperative that the staff be prepared and well rehearsed in techniques that can minimize risk. It is crucial to preserve the patient's rights and dignity at all times. This can be achieved by ensuring the patient's privacy as much as possible; by allowing participation and choices in care decisions by the patient and/or significant others; and by providing ongoing assessment and monitoring and the provision of physical care and comfort during the time in restraints and seclusion.

Once the decision has been made to proceed with restraints or seclusion of an agitated patient, choose a predetermined "leader" from among staff. The physician, a senior nurse, or the consultant psychiatrist, with experience in the management and implementation of restraints and/or seclusion, should assume this task. Sufficient competent personnel and hospital security must be present to assure the needed manpower so that the procedure will be carried out effectively. This also becomes important should physical force be warranted if the patient refuses or cannot comply with staff instructions. At all times, the staff should convey confidence and calmness. Staff should proceed with the implementation of restraints or seclusion as if it were a standard and familiar procedure.

PSYCHOPHARMACOLOGIC INTERVENTION

Pharmacologic management of the violent or agitated patient may serve as primary therapy or as an adjunct to the other efforts at de-escalation (Table 3.2). Inquire first or review old records/charts for any history of drug allergies. Consider whether the patient has a history of adverse drug reactions or a medical contraindication exists to using medication. Most patients will prefer (and we hope, agree) to take oral (PO) medication. Oral administration can address the behavioral dyscontrol issues and best retain dignity for all, but if parenteral routes are agreeable, the effects will be more rapid. This approach should be reserved for those patients who are not overtly threatening, in whom relief from anxiety or psychomotor agitation may prevent escalation and obviate the need for physical options. Precautions have to be maintained until the physician is convinced that the threat is defused. Medications should not be a substitute for physical restraint or other imme-

**Table 3.2.   Pharmacologic management
of the violent or agitated patient**

Mild to Moderate Agitation/Cooperative Patient/No Psychosis:
lorazepam (Ativan) 0.5mg to 2mg PO - repeat lorazepam 1mg to
2mg PO every 30 to 60 minutes as needed until sedation.(max
dose 10–15mg in 24h period)

Mild to Moderate Agitation/Cooperative Patient/Psychosis:
lorazepam (Ativan) 0.5mg to 2mg PO
or
haloperidol (Haldol) 1mg to 5mg PO
fluphenazine (Prolixin) 1mg to 5mg PO
Repeat as needed 30 to 60 minutes as needed until sedation. (max dose 25–50mg in 24 h period)
If neuroleptic naïve add: anticholinergic agent (benztropine 0.5 to
2mg PO) to each dosing.
or
risperidone (Risperdal) 0.5 to 2mg PO
Repeat in 60 minutes as needed until sedation (max dose 6–10mg
in 24h period)
or
olanzapine (Zyprexa) 2.5 to 10mg PO
Repeat in 60minutes as needed until sedation (max dose 20–30mg
in 24h period)
or
quetiapine (Seroquel) 25 to 100mg PO
Repeat in 60minutes as needed until sedation (max dose
300–575mg in 24h period)
or
ziprasidone (Geodon) 10 to 20mg PO
Repeat as needed 2 to 4 hours until sedation (max dose 40mg in
24h period)
or
aripiprazole (Abilify) 10 to 15mg PO (max dose 30mg in 24 hour
period)

Moderate to Severe Agitation/Cooperative/With or without psychosis:
lorazepam (Ativan) 1mg to 2mg PO or IM
[either alone or in combination]
haloperidol (Haldol) 5mg to 10mg PO or IM
or
fluphenazine (Prolixin) 5mg to 10mg PO or IM
Repeat above as needed 30 to 60minutes as needed until sedation.
If neuroleptic naïve add: anticholinergic agent (benztropine 0.5 to
2mg PO) to each dosing.
or
ziprasidone (Geodon) 10mg to 20mg PO or IM
Repeat as needed 2 to 4 hours until sedation

Moderate to Severe Agitation/Uncooperative/With or without psychosis:
lorazepam (Ativan) 1mg to 2mg IM
+
haloperidol (Haldol) 5mg to 10mg IM
or
fluphenazine (Prolixin) 5mg to 10mg IM

continued

Table 3.2.   (Continued)

Repeat above as needed 30 to 60minutes as needed until sedation.
If neuroleptic naïve add: anticholinergic agent (benztropine 0.5 to
    2mg PO) to each dosing.
or
ziprasidone (Geodon) 10mg to 20mg IM
Repeat as needed 2 to 4 hours until sedation

diate measures to ensure the safety of the patient or staff. Alternatively, physical restraint may be definitive. As mentioned previously, some individuals may perceive security from restraint and become tranquil enough to cooperate with medical or psychiatric care. However, at times, pharmacologic therapies are necessary in addition to physical restraint. This would include continued threatening or violent behavior, such as spitting, biting, disruptive verbal threats, and struggling against the restraints and medical care (i.e., blood drawing and other testing). This concept is paramount in cases in which a primary medical condition can be complicated by continued struggle or agitation.

The concept of rapid tranquilization evolved as a method of chemically controlling violent, agitated behavior in the acute setting with large doses of antipsychotic medications. The goal of rapid tranquilization is to control behavior, without oversedation, loss of airway, or cardiovascular stability, and enough to permit the evaluation and care to proceed. It is not diagnosis specific; it is effective for behavioral dyscontrol due to psychiatric, emotional, or medical causes.

If the behaviors continue to escalate and violence becomes more imminent, then the offering of medication to assist in regaining control must be attempted. Throughout the encounter and whenever possible, the patient should be given choices, which can assist in their ability to regain some measure of control. The patient can be provided a choice regarding the route of medication application [i.e., PO vs. intramuscular (IM)]. These options should be predetermined by staff, and no bargaining must be allowed on the patient's terms or demands if the outcomes cannot be safely met. Most patient will prefer oral and then parenteral forms of medications when given a choice.

The staff should explain to the patient at all times that choices and consequences result from their behavior. Providing the patient with the option of PO medication can calm an agitated patient by instilling a sense of control over a very chaotic inner state. The option of refusing PO medication can be explained as necessitating the use of more restrictive measures of containment. If the behavior continues to escalate, and these approaches fail, the area must be made secure. The patient must be made aware of the management plan, and staff forces must be gathered and the more restrictive approaches considered.

These medications and their use are NOT considered chemical restraints. The regulations regarding the use of chemical restraints clearly differentiate the pharmacologic intervention as mentioned here from "chemical restraints" as those medications used in "standard treatment" for a patient's medical or psychiatric needs. Medications used on a PRN or STAT basis, including medications to treat aggressive or violent behavior or to induce sleep or sedation, are not considered part of the chemical restraints regulations. Although many of these agents are not Food and Drug Administration (FDA) approved for the management of aggression and/or violence, they are considered part of the "standard treatment" and thus not a chemical restraint. It is important to clarify these issues with the internal hospital policies and established practices at your ED.

Haloperidol has become the standard for rapid tranquilization because of its strength and desirable side-effect profile; it is a powerful antipsychotic with minimal sedating and cardiovascular effects. It may be given PO or IM, and although not FDA approved for intravenous (IV) use, it is commonly given by that route without complications. It has repeatedly been shown to be safe and effective for immediate control of behavior. As mentioned, the predominant side effects are extrapyramidal. The most common, obvious, and at times disconcerting side effect is acute dystonia, usually manifested as torticollis, opisthotonos, or oculogyric crisis (see Chapter 4.1). These side effects are most commonly seen in the first 24 hours, predominantly in young, healthy individuals, and are not dose related.

Droperidol has been used for years in Europe as an antipsychotic, and in the United States for its sedating and antiemetic properties, as an adjunct for general anesthesia. In 2001 the FDA issued a "black box" warning about cases of sudden death at high doses (more than 25 mg) in patients at risk for cardiac arrhythmias. The use of droperidol at present should be approached with care especially in patients with unknown or unclear cardiac history.

A variety of different benzodiazepines (BZDs) have been investigated and found useful for behavior control, and currently the most commonly studied BZD is lorazepam, which has the advantage of safety, rapid IM absorption, and reliability. Although effective and safe in small doses, the BZDs lack the therapeutic index of the psychotropics, and thus the range of titratability. Their real benefit for behavior control is in the combination with psychotropics. In particular, they seem to show a benefit by minimizing the extrapyramidal symptom (EPS) side effects either by allowing a lower dose of antipsychotic or through their own muscle-relaxant properties. This offers the advantage of minimizing the amount of any single drug given and combining the sedation of the BZD with the behavioral-modification properties of the antipsychotic.

Rapid tranquilization has become a standard of care that is safe and effective. Side effects, although not frequent, can occur; EPS side effects, dystonic reactions, akathisia, and hypotension are the most commonly seen, but if anticipated and treated, will rarely cause major problems to the patient. Rapid tranquilization refers to the use of high-potency antipsychotics, alone or in combination with a BZD, given PO, IM, or IV in frequent intervals to achieve sedation.

Oral liquid concentrate and rapidly dissolving tablets of certain atypical antipsychotics are currently available, and most recently, the FDA approved (June 2002) ziprasidone (Geodon), IM form. Olanzapine (Zyprexa) IM is under FDA review. These new options will increase the armamentarium of choices for the use in acute agitation and behaviorally dyscontrolled patients. The advantage with the newer atypical IM agents is their relative lower incidence of EPS side effects (akathisia, dystonia, tremors) and easier transition from IM to PO for long-term aftercare. The data look promising, and the integration of these drugs into the clinical practice is sure to grow.

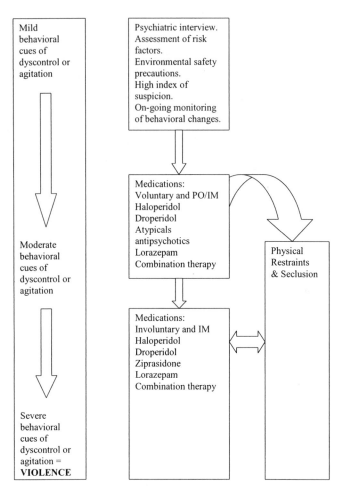

Fig. 3-2. Behavioral dyscontrol management algorithm.

For rapid tranquilization of different types of patients, use "cocktails" as described below; remember always to use sound clinical judgment when making these decisions (Fig. 3-2, Behavioral dyscontrol management algorithm).

BIBLIOGRAPHY

Ayd FJ. Haloperidol: twenty years clinical experience. *J Clin Psychol* 1978;39:807.

Bodkin JA. Emerging uses for high potency benzodiazepines in psychotic disorders. *J Clin Psych* 1990;51(suppl):41.

Brasic JR, Fogelman D. Clinician safety. *Psychiatr Clin North Am* 1999;22:923–941.

Citrome L, Volvaka J. Violent patients in the emergency setting. *Psychiatr Clin North Am* 1999;23:789–801.

Cressman WA, Plostnieks J, Johnson PC. Absorption, metabolism, and excretion of droperidol in human subjects following IM and intravenous administration. *Anesthesiology* 1973;38:363.

Currier GW. Atypical antipsychotic medications in the psychiatric emergency service. *J Clin Psychiatry* 2000;61(suppl 14):21–26.

Currier GW, Allen MH. Physical and chemical restraints in the psychiatric emergency service. *Psychiatr Serv* 2000;51:717–719.

Daniel DG, Potkin SG, Reeves KR, et al. Intramuscular (IM) ziprasidone 20 mg is effective in reducing acute agitation associated with psychosis: a double-blind, randomized trial. *Psychopharmacology* 2001;155:128–134.

Donlon PT, Hopkin J, Tupin JP. Overview: safety and efficacy of rapid neuroleptization method with injectable haloperidol. *Am J Psych* 1979;136:273.

Dubin WR, Feld JA. Rapid tranquilization of the violent patient. *Am J Emerg Med* 1989;7:313.

Educate your staff to prevent assaults. *ED Manag* 2001;13:101–103.

Erdos BZ, Hughews DH. A review of assaults by patients against staff at psychiatric emergency centers. *Psychiatr Serv* 2001;52:1175–1177.

Fernandes CM, et al. The effect of an educational program on violence in the emergency department. *Ann Emerg Med* 2002;39:47–55.

Flannery RB. The Assaulted Staff Action Program (ASAP): ten year empirical support for critical incident stress management (CISM). *Int J Emerg Ment Health* 2001;3:5–10.

Flannery RB et al. Characteristics of staff victims of patient assault: ten year analysis of the Assaulted Staff Action Program (ASAP). *Psychiatr Q* 2001;72(3):237–248.

Grange JT, Corbett SW. Violence against emergency medical services personnel. *Prehosp Emerg Care* 2002;6:186–190.

Here's how to prevent assaults on staff. *ED Manag* 2001;13 (suppl 1–2):66–69.

Hill S, Petit J. The violent patient. *Emerg Med Clin North Am* 2000;18:301–315.

Hillard JR. Choosing antipsychotics for rapid tranquilization in the ER. *Curr Psychiatry* 2002;1:22–29.

JCAHO. *Comprehensive accreditation manual for hospitals.* Oakbrook Terrace: JCAHO, 1996.

Lavoi FW. Consent, involuntary treatment, and the use of force in an urban emergency department. *Ann Emerg Med* 1992;21:25–32.

Lesem MD, Zajecka JM, Swift RH, et al. Intramuscular ziprasidone, 2mg versus 10mg, in the short-term management of agitated psychotic patients. *J Clin Psychiatry* 2001;62:12–18.

Lyneham J. Violence in New South Wales emergency department. *Aust J Adv Nurs* 2001;18:8–17.

May DD, Grubbs LM. The extent, nature and precipitating factors of nurse assault among three groups of registered nurses in a regional medical center. *J Emerg Nurs* 2002;28:11–17.

Mendoza R, Djenderedjian AH, Adams J, et al. Midazolam in acute psychotic patients with hyperarousal. *J Clin Psych* 1987;48:291.

Modell JG, Lenox RH, Weiner S. Inpatient clinical trial of lorazepam for the management of manic agitation. *J Clin Psychopharm* 1985;5:109.

Presley D, Robinson G. Violence in the emergency department: nurses contend with prevention in the healthcare arena. *Nurs Clin North Am* 2002;37:161–169, viii–ix.

Reischel UA, Shih RD. Evaluation and management of psychotic patients in the emergency department. *Hosp Physician* 1999:26–38.

4

Acute Psychiatric Presentations

Chapter 4-1 Abnormal Movements

Akathisia
Catatonia
Dystonic Reactions
Parkinsonism
Postural tremor
Tardive Dyskinesia

A group of movement disorders—some medication induced—can become the focus of clinical attention and can lead a patient to the emergency department (ED). Catatonia is a type of presentation characterized by abnormal movements, although it is not medication related. It is important to assess and differentiate these movement disorders adequately from other psychiatric disorders as well as possible underlying or causative medical and/or neurologic disorders.

The neuroleptic-induced movement disorders, commonly called extrapyramidal side effects (EPSs), were frequently encountered with the use of conventional or typical antipsychotic agents more so than with the newer agents—called atypical because of their reduced risk of EPS. An atypical neuroleptic is defined as an antipsychotic drug that is therapeutically more effective in both positive and negative symptoms of schizophrenia than are the conventional agents and that cause fewer acute and chronic EPS symptoms. Atypical antipsychotic drugs also have been shown to reduce the frequency of EPS-related patient medication non-adherence, as well as the need for concomitant antiparkinsonian drug use. EPS symptoms are caused by the D_2 blockade of the medication in the nigrostriatal pathways, which are involved in refined movements and motor control. This blockade leads to emergence of acute extrapyramidal symptoms that appear as akathisia, dystonia, and parkinsonism, or chronic extrapyramidal symptoms such as tardive dyskinesia. In an estimated 50% to 90% of patients, EPS develop in the course of neuroleptic therapy and can result in high levels of nonadherence. Chronic forms of EPS can develop in as high as 15% to 20% of patients receiving conventional antipsychotics.

The new atypical antipsychotics generally show a decrease in EPS-related side effects, thought to be due to the decreased degree of D_2 antagonism in the nigrostriatal pathways. See Table 4-1.1 for common subjective (mental) and objective (motor) symptoms of EPS, which can have serious consequences for the patient and the treatment. *Diagnostic and Statistical Manual of Mental Disorders,* fourth edition, revised (DSM-IV-TR) includes these disorders under the category of Medication-Induced Movement Disorders, which are classified under "other conditions."

Commonly in practice or clinic setting, these side effects are monitored and tracked, whenever someone is taking a neuroleptic, by the Abnormal Involuntary Movement Scale (AIMS). This

Table 4-1.1. Extrapyramidal symptoms: a comparison

	Motor	Mental	Consequences	Differential
Akathisia	Pacing, rocking back and forth, shifting foot to foot lifting the feet as if marching in place, or other repetitive purposeless actions	Restlessness, inability to relax, poor concentration, agitation, irritability, aggressivity	Lower rates of improvement and poorer outcomes; higher rates of TD	Psychotic agitation, restless-legs syndrome
Dystonia	Briefly sustained or fixed abnormal postures of the eyes, tongue (protrusion or dysfunction), jaw (trismus), face, neck (torticolli or retrocolli), limbs, trunk	Fear, anxiety	Noncompliance and potential for relapse	Manipulation, hysteria, seizures, catatonia, focal or segmental dystonia
Parkinsonism	Tremor, rigidity, bradykinesia (akinesia), masked facies, decreased arm swing	Bradyphrenia, cognitive impairment	Secondary dysphoria, mental clouding (bradyphrenia), cognitive impairment	Negative symptoms, depression, Parkinson disease

TD, tardive dyskinesia.

scale is helpful in determining a baseline measure of abnormal movements, and through serial repetitions of the scale, to determine any worsening or improvement in symptom severity. In the ED, time permitting, the AIMS can be used either as a guide for assessing abnormal movements or as a baseline measure to assist inpatient (or outpatient) staff in determining the patient's current status. The scale is easy to administer (see Appendix D); you must discretely observe the patient at rest (e.g., in the waiting room) before conducting the rest of the examination. Try to use a chair that is hard and firm but without arms. Then follow these instructions:

- Ask the patients to remove anything in their mouths (i.e., gum, candy).
- Ask the patients about the current condition of their teeth and if they wear dentures. Ask if the teeth or dentures bother them currently.
- Ask the patients whether they notice any movement in the mouth, face, hands, or feet, and if so, to describe and indicate how it may bother them or interfere with their activities.

After observing the patient and conducting the rest of the examination, rate on a scale of 0 (none), 1 (minimal), 2 (mild), 3 (moderate), and 4 (severe), according to the severity of symptoms. The higher the score, the more severe the neuroleptic-induced movement disorder.

Antipsychotic-induced movement disorders are a particular problem in the elderly. Studies have shown that the incidence and prevalence of parkinsonism and tardive dyskinesia (TD) are greater in the elderly, although dystonia seems to be fairly uncommon among the elderly. Elderly patients with preexisting EPSs and those with dementia are at higher risk of developing significant drug-induced movement disorders. These rates are lower when atypical antipsychotic agents are used; in recent studies, some evidence supports the use of these atypical agents in the treatment of existing drug-induced movement disorders. Predictors of favorable outcomes in EPSs are younger age, use of atypical antipsychotic agents, and the concomitant use of anticholinergic medications.

AKATHISIA

Definition

Akathisia is a condition of motor restlessness in which there is a feeling of muscular quivering, an urge to move about constantly, and an inability to sit still. It is a common extrapyramidal side effect of neuroleptic drugs. It is considered a subjective feeling of restlessness with an objective motor component, most commonly caused by neuroleptic medication—especially high-potency agents.

Presentation

Akathisia can go undetected because it is a subjective complaint of restlessness, exacerbated by anxiety or stress, or is misdiagnosed as breakthrough agitation or increased irritability. Patients will complain of needing to move around, inability to find a comfortable position, feeling anxious, or feeling as if they are crawling out of their skin. Patients will frequently need to pace or rock from foot to foot, and cross and uncross their legs while seated.

These feelings can affect their sleep and add another layer of complexity to their clinical presentation. Because the most common underlying diagnosis (based on its treatment with antipsychotics) is schizophrenia, agency workers or family members, because of the increase in restlessness or even agitation, often bring these patients to the ED. Some patients, in mild cases of akathisia, may exhibit only the objective signs of akathisia and either may be unable to express or simply do not have the subjective symptoms. Patients will usually appear anxious, uncomfortable, and even dysphoric, making the differential quite challenging.

Management

A careful evaluation and high clinical suspicion of akathisia is very important. In almost 20% to 50% of patients taking antipsychotic medication, akathisia develops, and 50% of patients with akathisia will have other parkinsonian side effects as well. Akathisia can occur in the first weeks of therapy, most commonly seen in elderly women. It is important to determine if the symptoms are of recent onset after the initiation of neuroleptic medication or if the patient is taking maintenance antipsychotic medication. Because of the intense anxiety and distressing nature of akathisia, it is a major cause of medication nonadherence. The need to diagnose akathisia adequately is fundamental; many times akathisia will be mistakenly treated with increased neuroleptic medication. This tends to worsen the clinical picture and can precipitate further restlessness and agitation. The symptoms of akathisia can easily mimic a worsening of the underlying disorder being treated. In patients with schizophrenia, these symptoms can develop because of the medication, or substance abuse, or an undiagnosed medical illness, or a psychosocial stressor, or nonadherence with the medications, or plainly because of a worsening of the illness despite medication adherence. Akathisia also can be easily mistaken for a manic state of excitement, in which the patient is unable to sit still and needs to move around constantly. The difference with mania is that patients with akathisia feel very uncomfortable and find this state of restlessness quite unpleasant. The dysphoria and anxiety can be mistaken for a depressive disorder, and some patients even express suicidal ideation because of this intense discomfort.

The obvious treatment of choice is to reduce the dose of the neuroleptic agent. Because patients in the ED with akathisia need immediate relief, consider sedation with benzodiazepines. Relief usually occurs in minutes and is complete, although the symptoms can recur after initial relief, requiring repeated doses.

lorazepam (Ativan), 1 to 2 mg, PO or IM; repeat if necessary after reevaluation of patient.

Akathisia tends not to respond as well to anticholinergic agents typically used to treat other parkinsonian side effects, although if they are present, the use of benztropine (Cogentin) can prove to be effective. Alternative treatment strategies, although not for immediate management, include β-adrenergic blockers (propranolol), benzodiazepines, diphenhydramine, clonidine, or even amantadine.

Disposition

Recurrence must be anticipated when patients are discharged from the ED and psychoeducation provided for this possibility.

The patient should be cautioned and provided with a few doses of benzodiazepines, such as lorazepam (Ativan) or diphenhydramine (Benadryl). Additionally, the use of an anticholinergic agent, such as benztropine (Cogentin), can be useful if other EPS symptoms are present. Immediate follow-up with the outpatient psychiatrist for medication management, reduction in the neuroleptic dose, or change in medication class is crucial.

CATATONIA

Definition

Catatonia is a condition in which an alteration in the muscular tone occurs, and it covers a broad group of psychomotor abnormalities characteristically found in, but not limited to, psychotic disorders.

Presentation

Catatonia, although not medication induced, has motor manifestations that appear as abnormal movements and can be the focus of an ED visit. It is commonly thought to be a psychiatric manifestation, and a subtype of schizophrenia, but in reality, it can be seen in both psychiatric and medical conditions, such as frontal lobe, extrapyramidal, and toxic–metabolic disorders. Because of this conceptualization of catatonia as a psychiatric illness, it is unrecognized and underdiagnosed. Catatonia can occur in association with a wide range of psychiatric disorders—10% of patients with severe acute psychiatric illness can have catatonia. It can be seen in schizophrenia, mania, depression, or anxiety disorders, as well as neurologic disorders (disorders of the basal ganglia, limbic system, diencephalon, and frontal lobes), systemic metabolic disorders, toxic drug states, and as a consequence of certain medications. These alterations in psychomotor behavior can be considered the motoric component—characteristically affecting the muscle tone—of the underlying disease state. Often a concerned family member, agency worker, or other caretaker will bring patients with catatonic symptoms to the ED. About 10% of patients with severe acute psychiatric illness can have extremes of motor behavior—from extreme psychomotoric retardation to catatonic excitement. Other common symptoms include

- *Catalepsy* occurs when a patient remains immobile and maintains an awkward body posture or position for a prolonged period.
- *Waxy flexibility* (*cerea flexibilitas*) describes when a patient can be moved and molded into any position that will be maintained, despite its awkward or uncomfortable position. Patient's limbs are reported as feeling as if they were made of wax.
- *Catatonic stupor* describes a patient's lack of reaction to or awareness of the surroundings. A patient will have severely decreased or slowed psychomotoric behavior, almost to the point of immobility.
- *Catatonic excitement* occurs when the patient exhibits excessive motor activity and restlessness that is apparently purposeless and not influenced by external stimuli.
- *Negativism* describes the patient's resistance to any attempts to be moved or follow commands. *Mutism* can be considered part of the negativism observed in catatonic patients. Patients

will not respond to verbal cues without any underlying organic cause for such.

- *Catatonic posturing* is similar to the other abnormal movements that catatonics assume; here the patient adopts a bizarre posture and maintains it for long periods.
- *Stereotypies* are repetitive patterns of speech or behavior.
- *Mannerisms* are characteristic habitual movements that the patient makes, such as grimaces, staring, or other facial and body habits.
- *Echopraxia* occurs when the patient imitates or repeats what the interviewer is doing, such as imitating the interviewer writing notes in the chart, scratching his head, or other behaviors and postures.

Although not a motor symptom *per se,* another symptom often seen in catatonic patients is *echolalia,* when the patient imitates or repeats what the interviewer is saying or asking.

Management

A thorough physical examination and medical workup is warranted to rule out any underlying medical or neurologic condition that causes the catatonia. Patients with catatonia, despite their otherwise detached or even stuporous presentation, maintain full awareness, so the physician should always assume that the patient is cognizant of what is transpiring. A study comparing psychiatric catatonic with medical catatonic symptoms and presentations demonstrated little difference between the two, thus making the medical assessment an even more important role in the ED.

Catatonia normally responds to anticholinergic agents, barbiturates, benzodiazepines, and electroconvulsive therapy. If the patient has a known psychiatric condition and is taking psychiatric medication, consider using anticholinergic medications to treat any EPS.

benztropine (Cogentin), 0.5 to 2 mg, PO or IM

If the patient has catatonic schizophrenia, the treatment will be geared to minimizing the agitation and/or anxiety in the ED. Atypical antipsychotic medications are thought to be more beneficial in treating ongoing schizophrenic patients with a predisposition to catatonia than are the other agents.

haloperidol (Haldol), 0.5 to 5 mg, PO or IM; can repeat within 30 minutes
fluphenazine (Prolixin), 1 to 5 mg, PO or IM; can repeat within 30 minutes
olanzapine (Zyprexa), 5 to 10 mg, PO
risperidone (Risperdal), 0.5 to 2 mg, PO
quetiapine (Seroquel), 25 to 50 mg, PO
lorazepam (Ativan), 0.5 to 2 mg PO/IM/IV; repeat every 4 to 6 hours if needed

If an underlying organic etiology is present, then consider using a sedative agent such as a benzodiazepine.

lorazepam (Ativan), 1 to 2 mg, PO/IM, or even IV, can be given every 4 to 6 hours

Differential diagnosis of catatonia should include

- Lethal catatonia
- Neuroleptic malignant syndrome
- Serotonin syndrome
- Delirium
- Mania
- Benign stupor.

Disposition

If the underlying etiologic factor is organic, a medical admission for further evaluation and monitoring is warranted. Treatment of the underlying medical cause is the recommended strategy. If the cause is psychiatric, depending on the severity of the symptoms and the impairment they cause, an admission might be required as well. For cases of less severity or intensity with minimal impairments and favorable response to treatments provided in the ED, a discharge to the patient's established outpatient aftercare setting might be considered.

DYSTONIC REACTIONS

Definition

Dystonic reactions are movement disorders, resulting as a side effect of neuroleptic medication, characterized by dyskinetic movements or muscular contractions due to disordered tonicity of the muscles.

Presentation

This is a common presenting complaint; in about 10% of psychiatric patients taking neuroleptics, this side effect develops. Dystonias can occur within the first couple of days of treatment, have a rapid onset, and are generally painful and very frightening to the patient.

The dystonia can involve different muscle groups:

- Neck (torticollis or retrocollis)
- Eyes (oculogyric crisis)
- Jaw (trismus or feeling as if one's jaw is locked)
- Tongue (protrusion, stiffness, or twisting)
- Entire body (opisthotonus or pleurothotonus, slight rotation of the trunk and tonic lateral flexion).

Patients can have the outward manifestations of dystonia as described or have dysarthria, from involvement of the tongue and jaw musculature. Patients can have writhing movements of the extremities or trunk, grimacing, or respiratory distress, depending on the muscle groups involved. If the laryngeal muscles are affected, it can become life threatening. This is a frightening and very uncomfortable experience for the patient and can lead to medication nonadherence. Patients will often report that they are allergic to certain neuroleptics, and it is usually because of a dystonic reaction they had in the past and not because of a true allergic reaction to the medication.

Dystonic reactions occur most frequently with high-potency neuroleptics, such as haloperidol or fluphenazine, although they can be caused by any medication that has dopamine-blockade action. They occur most commonly within the first week or so of treatment—estimated 50% within the first 2 days—or after an IM injection of a neuroleptic agent. Men younger than 40 years and patients with traumatic brain injuries or children are most vulnerable.

Management

Patients with any of these dystonic reactions must be treated immediately. Assess whether the patient has a psychiatric history and is currently receiving any neuroleptic treatments. Recent initiation of neuroleptic treatment, changes in regimen, or recent IM neuroleptic use should make you think of an acute dystonic reaction. Carefully assess which muscle groups are affected, and remember that the musculature involved is unique to the patient and is important to document carefully for future occurrences. Psychoeducation about the symptoms as a medication side effect with fast-acting treatments can help allay some of the fear and concern at the moment.

Treatments must be rapid and preferably IM or IV with anticholinergic agents, antihistaminergic agents, or benzodiazepines.

benztropine (Cogentin), 1 to 2 mg, IM or IV; repeat within 15 minutes if no effect.

diphenhydramine (Benadryl), 25 to 50 mg, IM or IV; repeat within 15 minutes if no effect.

lorazepam (Ativan), 1 to 2 mg, IM or IV (especially in laryngeal dystonias with benztropine)

The most important aspect of neuroleptic use is, first and foremost, psychoeducation of the patient about the medication's possible side effects. Second is the prophylactic use of anticholinergic agents with a high-potency medication or with a patient with high-risk factors for dystonia. You can use anticholinergic agents as an effective adjunct to high-potency neuroleptic treatments:

benztropine (Cogentin), 0.5 to 2 mg, PO, BID

Differential diagnosis of acute dystonic reactions should include

- Other dystonias: torsion dystonia or focal dystonia
- Spastic torticollis
- Occupational spasms
- Seizures
- Tetany
- Tetanus
- TD
- Encephalitis
- Metabolic disorders
- Catatonic or psychotic posturing.

Disposition

Hardly ever are these symptoms severe enough to require more intensive interventions, and rarely must a patient with laryngeal dystonia be intubated. The symptoms are frightening and very disconcerting for the patient and a major reason for medication non-adherence. After the dystonia has been treated, psychoeducation must take place with the patient about medication adherence and the importance of continued medication adherence. Adding an anticholinergic agent to the medication regimen is something to consider. Speak to or leave message with the patient's treating psychiatrist or other treating physician if you decide to add a medication. Help the patient regain confidence and trust in the medication, and explain that with the appropriate anticholinergic agent, little chance is found of recurrence of the dystonia.

PARKINSONISM

Definition

Characterized by signs and symptoms traditionally observed in Parkinson disease, which are caused by neuroleptic medication.

Presentation

Parkinsonism can be difficult to differentiate from actual Parkinson disease. Commonly, these patients will have cogwheel rigidity, shuffling gait, masked facies, tremor, drooling, and decreased arm swing. Parkinsonian symptoms can be a manifestation of Parkinson disease, a neuroleptic medication side effect, sequelae of a traumatic brain injury or other neurologic disorder, or result from exposure to toxins, such as N-methyl-4-phenyl-1,2,3,6,-tetrahydropyridine (MTPT, an illicit IV opioid).

In medication-induced parkinsonism, the patient has an underlying psychiatric history and is either taking neuroleptic medication or was recently started on neuroleptic medication, usually a high-potency agent.

Management

A thorough assessment with a neurologic examination is indicated. Determine the patient's history and medication regimen. If rigidity is severe, look for dystonias, or think about neuroleptic malignant syndrome.

Treatment recommendations range from decreasing the dose of the antipsychotic drug, changing the medication to a lower potency or atypical agent, to adding an anticholinergic medication.

For rapid relief, consider

benztropine (Cogentin), 1 to 2 mg, PO or IM/IV

Disposition

Once the initial distress over the symptoms has been managed, most patients will be safe for discharge to their homes. Recommendations for medication changes or additions of an anticholinergic agent should be made to the patient's treating physician. It is important to try to speak to or leave message with the treating physicians to inform them of the patient's complaint and proposed treatment options, as discussed with the patient. A note or copy of the evaluation can help if the physician is within the hospital's network. A prescription for an anticholinergic or antiparkinsonian agent can help alleviate the symptoms until the treating physician can see the patient. See Table 4-1.2 for a list of commonly used anticholinergic medications.

Table 4-1.2.   List of medications commonly considered to have anticholinergic properties

The term antiparkinsonian describes a category of drugs whose original or most common use and intended therapeutic effect is to control or prevent symptoms of or Parkinson disease or syndrome.

Akineton (biperiden)
Artane (trihexyphenidyl)
Benadryl (diphenhydramine)
Cogentin (benztropine)
Comtan (entacapone)
Kemadrin (procyclidine)
Mirapax (pramipexole)
Parlodel (bromocriptine)
Permax (pergolide)
Sinemet (carbidopa + levodopa)
Symmetrel (amantadine)
Tasmar (tolcapone)

POSTURAL TREMOR

Definition

Tremor is considered an involuntary rhythmic oscillation of certain parts of the body (fingers, hand, wrist, or head).

Presentation

Many causes of tremors are known, including anxiety, fatigue, drug related (alcohol, benzodiazepines, caffeine, cocaine, hallucinogens, opioid, or stimulants), hyperthyroidism, Parkinson disease, Wilson disease, cerebellar disorders, other metabolic and toxic causes, and even a form of benign or senile tremor. Many medications [antipsychotics, steroids, β-adrenergic stimulants (isoproterenol), lithium, antidepressants, valproate] also can produce tremors as a side effect.

If the tremors are the main focus of the patient's concern and visit, you must reassure them that treatments are available and are often very effective. The tremors are usually faster than one beat per minute and are most noticeable in the upper extremities.

Management

Ask the patient to hold out the hands in front, palms down, and observe. Tremors can subside when the patient is relaxed or asleep and worsen under stress. If a patient is exhibiting tremors, medical and neurologic workups are indicated to assist in the differential diagnosis.

Treatment will be dependent on the cause. Reassurance and supportive interventions are always helpful. In drug-related causes, intoxication, or withdrawal, observation is the norm, unless the tremors are associated with other physiological signs that warrant drug-specific intervention (see subchapters 4.14 and 4.24). Tremors due to antipsychotic medication can be easily treated with:

benztropine (Cogentin), 0.5 to 2 mg, PO or IM
diphenhydramine (Benadryl), 25 to 50 mg, PO or IM

Outpatient management of anxiety (performance)-related tremors can use β-blockers, such as:

atenolol (Tenormin), 50 mg, PRN or BID

The outpatient management of medication-induced tremors should include

- Reassessing the actual medication (switching may be called for)
- Reducing the dose of the medication to the lowest effective dose
- Managing external stressors (to minimize exacerbations)
- Taking medication at bedtime.

Disposition

Patients with tremors hardly ever require hospitalization; unless the tremor is part of a more serious intoxication or withdrawal phenomenon or is an associated finding of a more serious medical/neurologic condition.

The use of standing medications for the management can be considered, such as benztropine (Cogentin) or atenolol (Tenormin), but must be discussed with the patient, and preferably the patient's outpatient provider or primary physician will make that determination along with the earlier recommendation.

TARDIVE DYSKINESIA

Definition

Dyskinesia is a distortion or impairment of voluntary movements, as in tic, spasm, or myoclonus. TD, which can become irreversible, is an iatrogenic extrapyramidal disorder produced by long-term administration of antipsychotic medication.

Presentation

It is the most serious of the medication-induced side effects. Patient will have a variety of symptoms and severity of symptoms. These can be

- Repetitive, involuntary, hyperkinetic movements such as chewing or protrusion or vermicular motion of the tongue
- Side-to-side or rotatory jaw movements
- Oral/buccal dyskinesias that usually resemble continual chewing movements, lip smacking, puckering, and pursing
- Paroxysms of rapid eye blinking
- Choreathetoid hyperkinetic movements in the limbs and trunk
- Respiratory involvement, although uncommon, can produce aerophagia, irregular rates of respiration, or belching/grunting noises.

The oral/buccal movements are the earliest signs and the most common. The more severe symptoms can be quite painful, disfiguring, and can cause significant disability.

TD can appear within several months of treatment with the antipsychotic drugs and will disappear after the medication is discontinued, although in others, the symptoms may persist indefinitely. Additionally, it can appear as tardive dystonia (sustained abnormal posture or positions) or tardive akathisia. The symptoms of TD tend to improve when the patient is asleep and to worsen under stress. TD can persist for weeks and months after antipsychotic medications have been discontinued and ultimately can be irreversible. The consequences of not diagnosing or anticipating TD can include disfiguring and painful effects, medication nonadherence, increased morbidity and mortality, and worst of all, they may be potentially irreversible.

Management

The best method of prevention is to monitor carefully the patient by using the AIMS and by using the smallest effective optimal dose of the antipsychotic. Patients should be thoroughly apprised of the risks of TD before treatment is initiated. The first signs of TD should prompt the treating physician either to reduce the dose of the antipsychotic or to change the medication to an alternative agent, such as clozapine or an atypical agent. Mild cases and those detected in the earliest stages have the best chance of improving once the antipsychotic is discontinued. Atypicals have reduced likelihood of inducing TD and show antidyskinetic properties in patients with preexisting TD. In these patients, the atypicals have been shown to help resolve the symptoms of TD.

In patients with signs and symptoms of TD, consider a full medical and neurologic workup, laboratory evaluations, and computed tomography (CT) or magnetic resonance imaging (MRI) of the head. Establish the psychiatric history and the use of antipsychotic medication. Conduct an AIMS rating. Contact the patient's family or treating physician to determine the history and length of time receiving antipsychotic treatment and recent changes, stressors, or precipitants.

Anticholinergic agents do not help and may even aggravate the symptoms of TD. Reductions in medications or changes should not take place in the ED setting. Speak to or leave a message with the patient's treating physician to discuss treatment options. Speak with the patient and provide information about TD and treatment options. Make sure the information is conveyed in a positive and nonjudgmental fashion so that the patient's relationship with the primary physician is not disrupted or jeopardized.

Differential diagnosis of TD should include the following:

- Bruxism
- Idiopathic dystonias (blepharospasm, mandibular dystonia, facial tics)
- Dystonia musculorum deformans
- Torsion dystonia
- Postanoxic or postencephalitic extrapyramidal symptoms
- Edentulous dyskinesia
- Huntington chorea
- Brain neoplasms
- Meige disease (spontaneous oral dyskinesias)
- Parkinson disease

- Perioral (rabbit) syndrome
- Senile chorea
- Sydenham chorea
- Tourette disorder
- Wilson disease
- Fahr syndrome.

Certain medications and toxic agents must also be ruled out in the differential diagnosis of TD, including antidepressants, lithium, anticholinergics, phenytoin, L-Dopa and dopamine agonists, amphetamines and related stimulants, and magnesium and other heavy metals.

Disposition

Patients with TD seldom require an inpatient hospitalization unless they have other comorbid conditions that would require a hospitalization. Psychoeducation is fundamental for the patient and family. Remind the patient that this is a common, if unfortunate, side effect of the medication and can be dealt with as an outpatient. If the patient is very anxious, the use of a benzodiazepine may be appropriate, with a prescription for a few days provided on discharge.

Management of patients requiring long-term antipsychotic medication requires that you think about what medication and what dosages you are going to use before initiating treatment. Several known risk factors exist for the development of TD, which you must be familiar with and think about before starting someone on a medication that can cause an irreversible side effect. These risk factors are listed in Table 4-1.3. The use of atypical antipsychotic agents has been shown to reduce the probability of causing TD and may even assist in reducing TD in these patients. Predictors of favorable outcomes once TD has developed are lower doses of neuroleptic and concomitant use of anticholinergic medication. Research into calcium-channel blockers and γ-aminobutyric acid (GABA) agonists, such as baclofen, progabide, muscimol, valproic acid, or tetrahydroisoxazolopyridine (THIP) for the treatment of TD has been inconclusive.

Table 4-1.3. Risk factors for developing tardive dyskinesia

Gender: women are at greater risk than men
Age: elderly more at risk than younger patients
Race: African Americans more at risk
Cognitive impairment
Affective disorders
Comorbid medical conditions such as diabetes
Alcohol and nicotine abuse
History of neuroleptic use
    Cumulative amount and duration of use of neuroleptics
    Early incidence of EPS during treatment
    Concomitant use of anticholinergic agents

EPS, extrapyramidal side effect.

BIBLIOGRAPHY

Caligiuri MR, Jeste DV, Lacro JP. Antipsychotic-induced movement disorders in the elderly: epidemiology and treatment recommendations. *Drugs Aging* 2000;17:363–384.

Caroff SN, Mann SC, Campbell EC, et al. Movement disorders associated with atypical antipsychotic drugs. *J Clin Psychiatry* 2002;63 (suppl 4):12–19.

Carroll BT, Kennedy JC, Goforth HW. Catatonic signs in medical and psychiatric catatonias. *CNS Spectrum* 2000;5:66–69.

Casey DE. Tardive dyskinesia and atypical antipsychotic drugs. *Schizophr Res* 1999;35(suppl):S61–S66.

Casey DE. Will the new antipsychotics bring hope of reducing the risk of developing extrapyramidal syndromes and tardive dyskinesia? *Int Clin Psychopharmacol* 1997;12(suppl 1):S19–S27.

Casey DE, Keeper GA. Neuroleptic side effects: acute extrapyramidal syndromes and tardive dyskinesia. *Psychopharmacol Bull* 1988;24: 471–475.

Fink M, Taylor MA. The many varieties of catatonia. *Eur Arch Psychiatry Clin Neurosci* 2001;251(suppl 1):I8–13.

Guy W. *ECDEU assessment manual for psychopharmacology.* Washington, DC: Department of Health, Education, and Welfare, 1976.

Jeste DV, et al. Risk of tardive dyskinesia in older patients. *Arch Gen Psychiatry* 1995;52:756–765.

Jibson MD, Tandon R. New atypical antipsychotic medications. *J Psychiatr Res* 1998;32:215–228.

Kamin J, Manwani S, Hughes D. Extrapyramidal side effects in the psychiatric emergency service. *Psychiatr Serv* 2000;51:287–289.

Kruger S, Braunig P. Catatonia in affective disorders: new findings and a review of the literature. *CNS Spectrum* 2000;5:48–53.

Lohr JB, Caligiuri MP, Edson R, et al. Treatment predictors of extrapyramidal side effects in patients with tardive dyskinesia: results from Veterans Affairs Cooperative Study 394. *J Clin Psychopharmacol* 2002;22:196–200.

Soares KV, McGrath JJ. Calcium channel blockers for neuroleptic-induced tardive dyskinesia. *Cochrane Database Syst Rev* 2001;1: CD000206.

Soares KV, McGrath JJ, Deeks JJ. Gamma-aminobutyric acid agonists for neuroleptic-induced tardive dyskinesia. *Cochrane Database Syst Rev* 2001;2:CD000203.

Chapter 4-2 Agitation/ Aggressive Behavior

DEFINITION

Agitation is considered the state of heightened mental and motor excitation and activity. Aggression is a form of behavior that leads to self-assertion, which may arise from innate drives and/or as a response to frustration. Aggression can be manifested by destructive and attacking behaviors or covert attitudes of hostility and obstructionism. It is a forceful or assaultive verbal or physical action toward another person that can result in harm or hurt to others.

It is the motor component of the affects of anger, hostility, or rage, and most often implies an intention to harm or injure others.

PRESENTATION

Aggression is most often internally directed, usually focused on oneself or on inanimate objects. However, at times, agitation and aggressive acts can be triggered by a trivial event or may be unprovoked and find an external expression. In these instances, aggression and ultimately violence can be directed toward others, hospital staff, or other patients in the ED setting. Agitation and aggression are behaviors that cut across many clinical, both medical and psychiatric, conditions. They can fluctuate and overlap with many other conditions. These behaviors are a manifestation of psychic and motor discomfort with a more reactive response to stimuli, increased levels of irritability, and intense psychomotor activity.

Many psychiatric disorders have agitation as an associated component, including depression with concurrent anxiety, dementia, intermittent explosive disorder, psychosis (related to positive symptoms), and akathisia. See Table 4-2.1 for a list of common disorders with associated aggression. See Table 4-2.2 for a list of aggression/agitation symptoms and behaviors. Patients with antisocial behavior and those that meet criteria for antisocial personality disorder, grouped in the Cluster B Personality Disorders, are more prone to act out their aggressive impulses and become violent. Antisocial individuals, from childhood onward, regularly disregard and violate the rights of others and can get into serious trouble by breaking laws or rules, or by deceit or theft. The prevalence rates vary from 5% to 15%, although they are much higher— as to be expected—in prison populations. A significant comorbidity is found with other primary Axis I disorders, including substance-related disorders and posttraumatic stress disorder (PTSD).

Significant life events, whether positive or negative, can cause severe emotional and psychological stress. The consequent development of symptoms, especially aggressivity, and impairment in functioning can be seen in an adjustment disorder with disturbance of conduct or with mixed disturbance of emotions and conduct.

Certain general medical conditions can produce persistent changes in personality characteristics, with, for example, aggression, lability, or disinhibition. These personality changes, commonly seen after a traumatic brain injury or in temporal lobe epilepsy, for example, can appear in the ED as a primary complaint or be part of a larger and more complex picture.

MANAGEMENT

Patients that exhibit agitation and aggressive behavior are at risk of hurting themselves as well as others and require quick assessment and treatment. Safety is the number one priority, and all efforts should be made to assess the immediate situation and try to prevent further escalation. Generally speaking, the focus of an agitated or aggressive patient in the ED should be first to rule out all medical causes before ascribing the behavior to a psychiatric condition. Determine, if possible, underlying causes of agitation (psychiatric, medical, drug-related, situational, etc.); this

Table 4-2.1. Disorders associated with aggressive behaviors

AIDS
Akathisia
Alcohol intoxication or withdrawal
Alzheimer disease
Amphetamine intoxication or amphetamine-induced psychotic disorder
Analgesics
Anticholinergic delirium
Antisocial personality disorder
Anxiolytic disinhibition
Attention deficit/hyperactivity disorder
Bipolar disorder
Borderline personality disorder
Brain tumors
Brief psychotic disorder
Cerebrovascular disease/stroke
Cocaine intoxication or cocaine-induced psychotic disorder
Conduct disorder
Delirium
Delirium, dementia, and other cognitive disorders
Delusional disorder
Encephalitis
Huntington disease
Hyper- or hypothyroidism
Hypoglycemia
Intermittent explosive disorder
Meningitis
Mental retardation
Multiple sclerosis
Oppositional defiant disorder
Parkinson disease
Porphyria
Posttraumatic stress disorder
Schizoaffective disorder
Sexual sadism
SLE
Steroid-induced mood disorder (mania) or delirium
Substance-related disorders
TBI
Vitamin deficiencies
Wilson disease

AIDS, acquired immunodeficiency syndrome; SLE, systemic lupus erythematosus; TBI, traumatic brain injury.

**Table 4-2.2. Common aggression/
agitation symptoms and behaviors**

Disorder	Symptom	Behavior
Schizophrenia	Avolition Blunted affect Delusions Disorganized thinking Hallucinations Social withdrawal	Abnormal motor behaviors Anxiety Disinhibition Irritability Verbal and physical aggression Wandering
Bipolar	Delusions Elated/irritable mood Hallucination Racing thoughts Sleep disturbances	Grandiosity Impulsivity Pressured speech Psychomotor agitation
Dementia/ Delirium	Apathy Confusion Delusions Hallucinations Misperceptions Social withdrawal	Abnormal motor behaviors Anxiety Disinhibition Verbal and physical aggression Wandering
Substance- related	Confusion Delusions Euphoria or elated mood Hallucinations Sensorial hypersensitivity	Anxiety Bizarre behaviors Disinhibition Impulsivity Irritability Panic Verbal and physical aggression

will help with the intervention and possible psychopharmacologic choice. Mild traumatic brain injury must be assessed carefully—moderate to severe brain injury is a medical emergency. In patients with sudden changes in personality and aggressivity, inquire about head injuries, loss of consciousness, and posttraumatic amnesia. Look for neurologic symptoms, headaches, dizziness, and nausea as associated findings in mild traumatic brain injury. Follow up with skull radiographs to rule out fractures and neuroimaging to verify any intracranial injuries. Risk factors for traumatic brain injury complications include patients with coagulopathy, alcohol and drug use, prior neurosurgical interventions, seizure disorders, and the elderly.

A recent study found that depressive symptoms in men are strongly associated with aggressivity, more so than current alcohol-abuse symptoms. Obtain a complete medical and psychiatric history, especially about substance-related issues. Evaluate medication toxicity or drug–drug interactions. Complete medical and neurologic examinations with the clinically indicated laboratory examinations also are important.

Medication management, traditionally with typical antipsychotics, such as haloperidol in combination (most often) with lorazepam, is still a treatment mainstay. Newer atypical antipsychotics are somewhat better in their side-effect profile, although rapid-onset and parenteral forms are still unavailable for most agents. Oral solutions, rapidly dissolving tablets, and the introduction of IM (olanzapine and ziprasidone) preparations may help in the treatment of agitation and aggression in an ED setting by increasing the armamentarium of possible medication choices. Oral risperidone and lorazepam were found to be comparable in effect to IM haloperidol and lorazepam in the management of agitated psychotic patients.

The Overt Aggression Scale (OAS) can help to document and measure specific aspects of aggression. It is divided into four categories:

- Verbal aggression
- Physical aggression against objects
- Physical aggression against self
- Physical aggression against others.

The OAS, listed in Appendix D, can help in determining a baseline score for aggression before initiating psychopharmacologic interventions and thereafter to document the efficacy, or lack thereof, of any therapeutic intervention. It also can be a guideline in the ED for the types of behaviors that cause concern and require closer attention, especially as the behaviors escalate. Although this scale is more useful in an inpatient setting where the serial monitoring of the behaviors is clinically advantageous, in the ED, it can serve as an indication of aggressivity as well as a baseline score for the inpatient team to follow.

Disposition

Patient's disposition will vary according to the underlying condition causing the agitation. Agitation and aggressivity in the context of akathisia, anxiety, depression, and often antisocial behavior may require immediate management and observation with a likely discharge back to the community for aftercare treatment. Conversely, aggression due to paranoia, delusions, mania, abuse of a substance, or a medical condition may require an inpatient hospitalization. The process for admission remains the same, and the plans for continued management on the floor must be decided and/or discussed with the admitting team. Many medications are currently in use for the management of agitation/aggressivity, including mood stabilizer (carbamazepine, valproate, topirimate, lithium, etc.), β-adrenergic–receptor antagonists, and dopamine-receptor antagonists, among others.

BIBLIOGRAPHY

Allen MH. Managing the agitated psychotic patient: a reappraisal of the evidence. *J Clin Psychiatry* 2000;61(suppl 14):11–20.
Bacaner N, Kinney TA, Biros M, et al. The relationship among depressive and alcoholic symptoms and aggressive behavior in adult male emergency department patients. *Acad Emerg Med* 2002;9:120–129.
Breier A, Meehan K, Birkett M, et al. A double-blind, placebo-controlled dose-response comparison of intramuscular olanzapine and haloperi-

dol in the treatment of acute agitation in schizophrenia. *Arch Gen Psychiatry* 2002;59:441–448.

Brieden T, Ujeyl M, Naber D. Psychopharmacological treatment of aggression in schizophrenic patients. *Pharmacopsychiatry* 2002;35: 83–89.

Centers for Medicare and Medicaid Services (CMS). *Medicare conditions of participation for hospitals on patients' rights* (42 CFR Section 482.13).

Currier GW, Simpson GM. Risperidone liquid concentrate and oral lorazepam versus intramuscular haloperidol and intramuscular lorazepam for treatment of psychotic agitation. *J Clin Psychiatry* 2001;62:153–157.

Currier GW, Trenton A. Pharmacological treatment of psychotic agitation. *CNS Drugs* 2002;16:219–228.

De Kruijk JR, Twijnstra A, Leffers P. Diagnostic criteria and differential diagnosis of mild traumatic brain injury. *Brain Inj* 2001;15: 99–106.

Labbate LA, Warden DL. Common psychiatric syndromes and pharmacologic treatments of traumatic brain injury. *Curr Psychiatry Rep* 2000;2:268–273.

Lesem MD, Zajecka JM, Swift RH, et al. Intramuscular ziprasidone, 2 mg versus 10 mg, in the short-term management of agitated psychotic patients. *J Clin Psychiatry* 2001;62:12–18.

Lindenmayer JP. The pathophysiology of agitation. *J Clin Psych* 2000;61:5–10.

Overt Aggression Scale (OAS) Source: Reprinted from Yudovsky SC, Silver JM, Jackson M, et al. The Overt Aggression Scale: an operationalized rating scale for verbal and physical aggression. *Am J Psychiatry* 1986;143:35–39.

Servadei F, Teasdale G, Merry G, and Neurotraumatology Committee of the World Federation of Neurosurgical Societies. Defining acute mild head injury in adults: a proposal based on prognostic factors, diagnosis, and management. *J Neurotrauma* 2001;18:657–664.

Chapter 4-3 Agoraphobia

DEFINITION

Agoraphobia is an abnormal fear or anxiety about feeling helpless in an embarrassing situation in which help may not be available, in the event of having an unexpected or situationally predisposed panic attack or panic-like attack. Agoraphobia is characterized especially by the avoidance of open or public places, crowds, standing in line, being on a bridge, or traveling on a bus, train, or automobile.

PRESENTATION

Rarely does someone with agoraphobia appear in a setting like the ED unless he or she is brought in by someone for an evaluation, or agoraphobia is uncovered as part of the interview and evaluation of another condition. In two thirds of patients with agoraphobia, it is associated with panic attacks or panic disorder, as well as other anxiety disorders such as phobias, obsessive–compulsive disorders (OCDs), and depressive disorders.

Agoraphobia places a huge strain on the person's social and occupational functioning and on interpersonal relationships and the social network. It is important to assess the impact that agoraphobia has on a person's life, such as financial or employment hardships and the possibility of an increase in the use of alcohol or drugs. Patients with agoraphobia will seldom leave the home without a friend or family member. Patients will go to great lengths to avoid all situations that might leave them without help or where they might have another panic attack or panic-like symptoms.

MANAGEMENT

If agoraphobia is associated with panic-like symptoms, it is imperative to conduct a full medical workup (see Chapter 4.4). Anxiety disorders, like panic disorder, have been shown to increase one's risk of suicide. Assess carefully and inquire about coping mechanisms, family support system, and future-oriented plans. Reassure the patient that with adequate treatment, the agoraphobia will resolve; explain that it may take some time for the medication and/or therapy to resolve the symptoms fully. If agoraphobia is associated with other psychiatric conditions, these must be assessed, diagnosed, and treated as well.

In making the differential diagnosis, you must assess whether agoraphobia is associated with panic disorder and rule out other commonly associated disorders such as depressive disorders and other anxiety disorders, especially social phobia. Social phobia, although similar in certain aspects, is related to anxiety around social or performance situations in which the patient fears scrutiny by others and possible embarrassment. Agoraphobia conversely is related to the fear of being out in the open and having panic symptoms.

Consider paranoia and delusional thinking in assessing whether fear of leaving the home is psychotic. Substance abuse, as with personality disorders, also can be associated and must be adequately assessed and managed. People with avoidant, paranoid, schizoid, or schizotypal personality disorder also may exhibit fears of leaving their homes.

As with panic disorder treatment, the use of anxiolytics and selective serotonin reuptake inhibitors (SSRIs) are the current mainstays. The Food and Drug Administration (FDA) has approved several medications for the use in panic disorder, and consequently they are effective for agoraphobia as well. Cognitive/behavioral therapy (CBT), such as applied relaxation, respiratory training, and even *in vivo* exposure, is indicated for panic disorders and has been shown to be effective.

In the ED, immediate resolution of anxiety symptoms in a patient with agoraphobia can be achieved with short-acting benzodiazepines, such as

alprazolam (Xanax), 0.25 to 1 mg, PO
lorazepam (Ativan), 0.5 to 2 mg, PO

DISPOSITION

Once a diagnosis of agoraphobia has been reached, seldom do these patients need hospitalization. Rarely does a person with agoraphobia with associated anxiety and depressive disorder require hospitalization. Referral to an experienced outpatient mental health professional is indicated. Psychoeducation is important for the patient and the family. A prescription for a 3- or 4-day course of benzodiazepines may be warranted if the anxiety symptoms are severe, and a dose of the medication in an ED setting has been successful in mitigating the anxiety:

alprazolam (Xanax), 0.25 to 1 mg, PO, TID, or lorazepam (Ativan), 0.5 to 2 mg, PO, TID

The prescription must be accompanied by a referral to an outpatient setting. Assess carefully substance-abuse history and determine the risk and benefits of providing benzodiazepines from an ED setting. Make certain that this decision is made with clinical foresight and taking into account the possibility of satisfying a patient's drug-seeking behavior or becoming a setting that prescribes benzodiazepines in the face of aftercare nonadherence. If outpatient care can be guaranteed and an appointment made, at times it may be possible, with thorough psychoeducation provided about the illness and the medication, to start a low-dose SSRI, helping to jump-start the treatment. Unless you can be assured that the person has an appointment and is likely to keep it, initiation of SSRI treatment should be left for the outpatient setting. Combination therapy can be very effective, and couples and family therapy may be indicated as well.

Of note and in general, benzodiazepine use in the ED is a controversial topic and one that is fraught with many misconceptions and potential problems. Recently the use of benzodiazepines from an ED setting has increased because of overall improved psychiatric diagnostic accuracy, greater availability of different benzodiazepines (short- and long-acting with more specific clinical indications), research that showed that disinhibition is relatively rare, heightened awareness of benzodiazepine abuse potential, and the introduction of flumazenil, which has decreased the mortality in benzodiazepine overdose. The judicious use of benzodiazepines in the ED to manage acute anxiety, agitation, substance-related (cocaine, amphetamine, hallucinogen) intoxication symptoms, substance-related (alcohol, benzodiazepines, cocaine, amphetamine, hallucinogen, opioid) withdrawal symptoms, medication-induced movement disorders, catatonia, acute stress, and PTSD must be weighed against the consideration of abuse potential, oversedation, cognitive and motor impairment (especially in the elderly), teratogenicity, and the abrupt withdrawal phenomenon. The prescription of benzodiazepines from the ED also must be thought through carefully; the continuation of ongoing benzodiazepines treatment on discharge should not be interrupted because of the possibility of benzodiazepine withdrawal.

BIBLIOGRAPHY

Ashton H. Guidelines for the rational use of benzodiazepines: when and what to use. *Drugs* 1994;48:25–40.

Dietch JT, Jennings RK. Aggressive dyscontrol in patients treated with benzodiazepines. *J Clin Psychiatry* 1988;49:184–188.

Meador KJ. Cognitive side effects of medication. *Neurol Clin* 1998;16: 141–155.

Parran T Jr. Prescription drug abuse: a question of balance. *Med Clin North Am* 1997;81:967–978.

Shaner R. Benzodiazepines in the psychiatric emergency setting. *Psych Ann* 2000;30:268–275.

Uhlenhuth EH, Balter MB, Ban TA, et al. International study of expert judgment on therapeutic use of benzodiazepines and other psychotherapeutic medications: pharmacotherapy of anxiety disorders. *J Affect Disord* 1995;35:153–162.

Chapter 4-4 Anxiety

DEFINITION

Anxiety is considered an unpleasant emotional state consisting of psychophysiologic responses to anticipation of real or imagined danger. Anxiety is a normal part of growth, change (experiential and existential), and is very different from pathologic anxiety, which is considered an inappropriate and maladaptive response (in either its intensity or duration) to an external, perceived or real, stimulus.

PRESENTATION

Anxiety can be a response to a situational or external event/stimuli; it can be a manifestation of an underlying medical or psychiatric condition; or it can be a sign of a medication- or substance-related effect. Anxiety is characterized by its combined physiological symptoms, indicative of a hyperactive autonomic nervous system response, and psychological manifestations.

Physiological signs:

Autonomic hyperactivity: flushing, pallor, tachycardia, palpitations, sweating, cold hands, diarrhea, dry mouth, urinary frequency
Dizziness or light-headedness
Back- or headaches
Difficulty swallowing
Fatigability
Increased startle response
Restlessness
Hyperreflexia
Muscle tension
Paresthesias
Shortness of breath and/or hyperventilation
Trembling, twitching or feeling shaky.

Psychological symptoms:

Butterflies in stomach
Decreased libido
Difficulty concentrating
Distractibility
Feelings of dread or doom
Hopelessness
Hypervigilance
Insomnia
Irrational fears
Lump in throat
Worries

Most patients with anxiety, whatever the underlying cause, will most likely seek help for the physiological manifestations from their internist or medical specialist before seeing a psychiatrist. Many ED visits with vague somatic complaints and unclear physical findings can be, in part, due to an undiagnosed or unrecognized anxiety disorder. Panic disorder and social phobia are among the most disabling of the anxiety disorders, with concomitant loss of productivity, increased healthcare costs, and increased work absenteeism. The following are a list of some DSM-IV-TR anxiety disorders and their presenting signs and symptoms.

Acute stress disorder: After a traumatic event, patients may complain of feeling anxious, unable to sleep, feeling detached or numb, with episodes of derealization or depersonalization. Patients may report dissociative feelings with decreased emotional responsiveness, as if being "in a daze." Patients may experience symptoms and marked avoidance of any emotionally painful stimuli, as well as hyperarousal symptoms (see Chapter 4-11).

Agoraphobia without history of panic disorder: Patients will seldom arrive in the ED on their own, most often brought in by a family member or because of an unrelated medical or psychiatric condition. Intense anxiety will be about being out of the home, for fear of having a panic attack. The fear is usually about being in a situation or place where escape is hard or may lead to embarrassment or where no help would be available if another panic attack were to occur (see Chapter 4-3).

Anxiety disorder due to a general medical condition: Patients will appear in the ED with intense anxiety, panic attacks, obsessional thinking, or compulsive behaviors with associated physical complaints and findings.

Generalized anxiety disorder (GAD): Patients will have intense and overwhelming anxiety that interferes with many aspects of their life. The anxiety is characterized by shakiness, restlessness, feeling "on edge or keyed-up," shortness of breath, palpitations, muscle tension, irritability, difficulty concentrating, difficulty sleeping, and easy fatigability. GAD is highly comorbid with depression, with subsequent higher rates of disability and dysfunction and lower treatment-success rates than with either disorder alone.

Obsessive compulsive disorder (OCD): Patients will rarely come to ED unless brought in by others or for another reason. The patient will complain of insistent and persistent thoughts or ideas that invade their consciousness. This will cause the person to have intense anxiety and ultimately lead to the need to counteract the thought or idea by performing an act or behavior (see Chapter 4-17).

Panic disorder: When patients have four or more of the psychological and physiological symptoms listed earlier, developing abruptly and crescendoing within 10 minutes or so, and occurring without an associated stressor and resolving shortly thereafter, this is considered a panic attack. A panic disorder occurs when the patient has one or more panic attacks and at least 1 month of persistent concern or worries about having another attack or a change in behavior because of the panic attacks. Agoraphobia can be a common associated feature (see Chapter 4-3). A series of panic attacks can often progress to the development of phobic avoidance. It is estimated that current and lifetime comorbidity of depression and panic disorder is approximately 10%, with poorer clinical outcomes. Usually greater impairment, more severe panic symptoms and course, and greater rates of suicidal ideation are found.

Posttraumatic stress disorder (PTSD): As in the case of acute stress disorder, patients after a traumatic event may go on to experience anxiety symptoms, as listed earlier, in addition to reexperiencing avoidant and hyperarousal symptoms. If the symptoms persist for more than 1 month and cause significant functional impairment, the patient may have PTSD (see Chapter 4-11).

Phobias: Patients with phobias have intense and irrational fears of specific objects, activities, or situations. This anxiety often leads them to avoid these things, at great personal cost, which further exacerbates the anxiety.

Substance-induced anxiety disorder: Patient may have a wide variety of anxiety symptoms after recent substance use. The actual type of anxiety symptoms will be related to the substance used, the amount, the time of use, and whether the patient is intoxicated or withdrawing from the causative substance.

Stressful life events, whether positive or negative, can cause emotional and psychological distress and ultimately anxiety. The presence of anxiety symptoms and functional impairment after a stressor may be part of an adjustment disorder with anxiety.

MANAGEMENT

Anxiety can be a component of many medical disorders, medication side effects, or effects, and is associated with many other psychiatric disorders, especially anxiety and depressive disorders. See Table 4-4.1 for a list. It is important to determine where comorbid depression exists; studies have demonstrated that if so, anxiety disorders tend to be more chronic and severe, include greater social and occupational dysfunction, higher rates of alcohol and drug use, greater risks of suicide, and poorer response to short- and long-term treatment. Additionally, anxiety and panic with comorbid depression are all serious risk factors for suicide and are often accompanied with impulsivity.

Obtain a thorough history; evaluate normal versus pathologic anxiety. Consider administering the Hamilton Anxiety Scale (see Appendix D). Try to gather information from the patient, family or friends, and coworkers, especially about aspects related to the patient's internal state, behaviors, and ability to function. Is the anxiety a manifestation of a life stressor? Try to determine if precipitants or other identifiable stressors exist, as well as information about the type of anxiety, course, onset, severity, duration, frequency, and other associated characteristics:

- Compulsions?
- Obsessions?
- Depressive symptoms?
- Insomnia?
- Substance use or abuse symptoms?
- Avoidance behavior?
- Personality disorder?
- Medical problems?
- Medications?
- Caffeine intake?

Table 4-4.1. Medical and psychiatric disorders associated with anxiety

Cardiovascular	Arrhythmias, cardiomyopathies, congestive heart failure, coronary insufficiency, mitral valve prolapse, post MI, angina
Deficiency states	Pellagra, vitamin B_{12} deficiency
Endocrine	Adrenal dysfunction/Cushing disease, pheocromocytoma, diabetes, pseudohyperparathyroidism, hypoglycemia/hyperinsulinemia, carcinoid syndrome, hyperparathyroidism, hypoglycemia, hypokalemia, hypothyroidism, pituitary dysfunction
Inflammatory	SLE, rheumatoid arthritis, polyarteritis nodosa, temporal arteritis
Gastrointestinal	Colitis, Crohn disease, irritable bowel syndrome, peptic ulcer disease
Miscellaneous	Hypoxia, anemia, premenstrual syndrome, febrile illness and chronic infections, porphyria, infectious mononucleosis, uremia, posthepatitis syndrome, pancreatic tumor, collagen-vascular disease, brucellosis
Neurologic	AIDS, dementia and delirium, neoplasms, trauma and postconcussive syndromes, seizure disorders, essential tremor, Huntington chorea, subarachnoid hemorrhage, migraine, cerebrovascular disease, lupus cerebritis, multiple sclerosis, Parkinson disease, encephalitis, cerebral syphilis, vestibular dysfunction, Wilson disease, cerebral arteriosclerosis, complex partial seizures
Psychiatric	Acute stress disorder, adjustment disorder with anxious or mixed features, anxiety disorder due to a general medical condition, GAD, OCD, panic disorder, PTSD, depression, mania, schizophrenia; alcohol, amphetamine, caffeine, cannabis use intoxication, withdrawal, and/or induced-anxiety disorder
Respiratory	Asthma, COPD, hyperventilation syndrome, pneumothorax, pulmonary edema, pulmonary embolism, pulmonary insufficiency
Toxic/ Medications	Anesthetics/analgesics, antidepressants, antihistamines, antihypertensives, antimicrobials, bronchodilators, caffeine preparations, calcium-channel blockers, digitalis, estrogen, ethosuximide, heavy metals and toxins, hydralazine, insulin, levodopa, muscle relaxants, antipsychotics, NSAIDs, procaine, procarbazine, sedatives, steroids, sympathomimetics, theophylline, thyroid preparations, vasopressor agents, penicillin, sulfonamides, mercury, arsenic, phosphorus, organophosphates, carbon disulfide, benzene, aspirin intolerance

MI, myocardial infarction; SLE, systemic lupus erythematosus; AIDS, acquired immunodeficiency syndrome; OCD, obsessive-compulsive disorder; PTSD, posttraumatic stress disorder; COPD, chronic obstructive pulmonary disorder; NSAIDs, nonsteroidal antiinflammatory drugs; GAD, generalized anxiety disorder.

Conduct a full physical and medical/neurologic workup. You must rule out any underlying or causative medical disorder. Inquire about psychiatric history and other psychiatric diagnoses. Determine the degree of impairment caused by the anxiety. Once all organic causes have been ruled out, and an anxiety disorder is your working diagnosis, you must try to rule out other comorbid psychiatric conditions. Many possible anxiety disorders are listed in DSM-IV-TR. Based on a patient's history, presentation, and other relevant information, it is important that you narrow the diagnosis and come up with a working diagnosis that best fits the patient's constellation of signs and symptoms.

Treatment consists of supportive and empathic measures, which are usually the most effective in a short-term setting. Offer the patient reassurances and psychoeducation regarding the disorder and the possible treatment options. The use of short-acting benzodiazepines in the short term can help relieve much of the intense anxiety and facilitate a more thorough interview or examination. Short-acting benzodiazepines are the treatment of choice. Occasionally antihistamines can be used as an alternative to benzodiazepines. Nonbenzodiazepines, such as buspirone (BuSpar) or hydroxyzine (Vistaril, Atarax) can be effective in certain anxiety disorder patients. A rational decision about the use of medication in patients with anxiety is best informed by the ultimate findings and the working diagnosis. For patients with anxiety and depression or psychosis, consider an antidepressant or antipsychotic agent. Consider akathisia (see Chapter 4.1) in patients with anxiety and restlessness with a diagnosed psychotic disorder and receiving antipsychotic medication treatment. In patients with PTSD or panic disorder, the use of an antidepressant might be more favorable. Benzodiazepines, preferably short acting, should be given in the short term and in small quantities. Test the patient's response to the anxiolytic agent while in the ED to determine whether symptomatic relief and/or any side effects ensue. Determine which anxiolytic agent you will prescribe, based on the presenting symptom profile and the medication effects. Inquire about insomnia, and consider the use of a longer-acting agent that can serve as a hypnotic as well. Consider carefully the use of benzodiazepines in patients with co-occurring substance abuse or possible malingering. Never prescribe benzodiazepines too liberally from the ED (always a few days' supply, to minimize any potential future drug-seeking behavior from an ED).

Table 4-4.2 lists commonly used benzodiazepines with their dosage forms, onset, and dosage equivalents.

Lorazepam and alprazolam can be given sublingually for more rapid onset of action. Valium comes combined with clidinium bromide (Librax, Clipoxide) and amitriptyline (Limbitrol), so it is imperative that you inquire about these medications to be sure of the patient's benzodiazepine regimen and potential for withdrawal if the medication is discontinued.

DISPOSITION

Most patients with anxiety, once stabilized, can usually be discharged from the ED. In many cases of new-onset anxiety disorders, psychoeducation is important, and referral to an outpatient provider is a must. Those patients with established aftercare

Table 4-4.2. Commonly used benzodiazepines, dosage forms, onset, and dosage equivalents

Generic	Brand	Dosage	Onset (After Oral Dose)	Dose Equivalents
Alprazolam	Xanax	0.25-, 0.05-, 1-, 2-mg tablets	Intermediate	0.5
Chlordiazepoxide	Librium	5-, 10-, 25-mg tablets/capsules	Intermediate	10
Clonazepam	Klonopin	0.5-, 1-, 2-mg tablets	Intermediate	0.25
Clorazepate	Tranxene	3.75-, 7.5-mg tablets/capsules 15-mg tablets	Rapid	7.5
Diazepam	Valium	2-, 5-, 10-mg tablets	Rapid	5
Estazolam	ProSom	1-, 2-mg tablets	Intermediate	0.33
Flurazepam	Dalmane	15-, 30-mg capsules	Rapid–intermediate	30
Lorazepam	Ativan	0.5-, 1-, 2-mg tablets 2 mg/ml and 4 mg/ml parenteral	Intermediate	1
Midazolam	Versed	1 mg/ml, 5 mg/ml parenteral	Intermediate	1.25–1.7
Oxazepam	Serax	15-mg tablets	Intermediate–slow	15
Quazepam	Doral	10-, 15-, 30-mg capsules	Rapid–intermediate	15
Temazepam	Restoril	7.5-, 15-mg tablets	Intermediate	5
Triazolam	Halcion	7.5-, 15-, 30-mg capsules 0.125-, 0.25-mg tablets	Intermediate	0.1

plans must be referred to their primary provider. A note or a call to the providers with any recommendation or suggested changes and the interventions carried out in the ED is quite helpful. Prescriptions for benzodiazepines or other medications should customarily be a few days' worth pending a follow-up appointment with an outpatient provider. Benzodiazepines traditionally were considered the first-line treatments but are now being replaced with the SSRIs as the leading treatment option. The FDA has approved the following antidepressants for their use in the following anxiety disorders: generalized anxiety disorder (venlafaxine), social phobia (paroxetine), and panic disorder (sertraline and paroxetine). Benzodiazepines carry the risk of affecting a patient's cognition, causing physiological abuse, dependence, or withdrawal phenomenon, and are not effective at treating depression as a comorbid condition. Recent evidence backs up the use of SSRIs as a primary treatment option for patients with anxiety disorders, especially those with comorbid depression. Outpatient treatment strategies may include supportive, cognitive–behavioral, or other psychotherapeutic approaches that should be addressed with the patient as part of the psychoeducational component of their ED experience.

BIBLIOGRAPHY

Bruce SE, Machan JT, Dyck I, et al. Infrequency of "pure" GAD: impact of psychiatric comorbidity on clinical course. *Depress Anxiety* 2001;14:219–225.

Davidson JR. Pharmacotherapy of generalized anxiety disorder. *J Clin Psychiatry* 2001;62(suppl 11):46–50.

Davidson JR, Connor KM, Sutherland SM. Panic disorder and social phobia: current treatments and new strategies. *Cleve Clin J Med* 1998;65(suppl 1):SI39–SI44.

Fava M, Rosenbaum JF, Hoog SL, et al. Fluoxetine versus sertraline versus paroxetine in major depression: tolerability and efficacy in anxious depression. *J Affect Disord* 2000;59:119–126.

Fawcett J. Treating impulsivity and anxiety in the suicidal patient. *Ann N Y Acad Sci* 2001;932:94–102; discussion, 102–105.

Gorman JM, Coplan JD. Comorbidity of depression and panic disorder. *J Clin Psychiatry* 1996;57(suppl 10):34–41.

Judd LL, Kessler RC, Paulus MP, et al. Comorbidity as a fundamental feature of generalized anxiety disorders: results from the National Comorbidity Study (NCS). *Acta Psychiatr Scand* 1998; 98(suppl 393):6–11.

Katerndahl DA. Predictors of the development of phobic avoidance. *J Clin Psychiatry* 2000;61:618–624.

Kessler RC, DuPont RL, Berglund P, et al. Impairment in pure and comorbid generalized anxiety disorder and major depression at 12 months in two national surveys. *Am J Psychiatry* 1999;156: 1915–1923.

Kessler RC, McGonale KA, Zhao S, et al. Lifetime and 12-month prevalence of DSM-III-R psychiatric disorders in the United States: results from the national comorbidity survey. *Arch Gen Psychiatry* 1994;51:8–19.

Lecrubier Y. The impact of comorbidity on the treatment of panic disorder. *J Clin Psychiatry* 1998;59(suppl 8):11–14.

Lydiard RB, Brawman-Mintzer O. Anxious depression. *J Clin Psych* 1998;59(suppl 18):10–17.

Merritt TC. Recognition and acute management of patients with panic attacks in the emergency department. *Emerg Med Clin North Am* 2000;18:289–300.

Pollack MH. Exploring the relationship between anxiety disorders and depression: anxiety disorders and major depression: the added challenge of comorbidity. Program and abstracts of Anxiety Disorders Association of America. Austin, TX: 22nd National Conference, 2002.

Pollack MH, Smoller JW. Pharmacologic approaches to treatment-resistant panic disorder. In: Pollack MH, Otto MW, Rosenbaum JF, et al., eds. *Challenges in clinical practice: pharmacologic and psychosocial strategies.* New York: Guilford Press, 1996:89–112.

Schatzberg AF. New indication for antidepressants. *J Clin Psychiatry* 2000;61(suppl 11):9–17.

Vasile RG, Goldenberg I, Reich J, et al. Panic disorder versus panic disorder with major depression: defining and understanding differences in psychiatric morbidity. *Depress Anxiety* 1997;5:12–20.

Wittchen H-U, Carter RM, Pfister H, et al. Disabilities and quality of life in pure and comorbid generalized anxiety disorder and major depression in a national survey. *Int Clin Psychopharmacol* 2000;15:319–328.

Chapter 4-5 Appetite Disturbance

DEFINITION

Obesity and anorexia can be considered the two ends of the spectrum of a disturbance in appetite or weight regulation. Anorexia is the lack or loss of the appetite for food, whereas overeating can be seen as the opposite in behavior toward food. In anorexia nervosa, a psychiatric disorder, a refusal to maintain a normal minimal body weight, intense fear of becoming obese, disturbance in body image, and amenorrhea are found. This disorder is grouped with bulimia and eating disorder not otherwise specified in the DSM-IV-TR. Obesity is considered the excessive accumulation of adipose tissue mass, in excess of 20% of the patient's expected weight by height/weight tables or an elevated body mass index (BMI).

PRESENTATION

Appetite disturbances, excluding anorexia and bulimia, are a common finding in many medical and psychiatric disorders. A patient's loss of appetite or overeating can accompany many disorders and, at times, is an associated finding of a more complex underlying disease state or a medication side effect. A careful review of a patient's eating habits, customs, and actual intake and weight maintenance are an important part of any evaluation. Many patients will lose their appetite and subsequently lose weight or gain weight because of overeating for multiple reasons, including medication side effects. Patients with anorexia or bulimia seldom seek help for themselves or come to the ED unless brought by concerned family members or friends. The patient's symptoms are usually ego-syntonic (in other words, it is acceptable, consonant, and compatible with the person's standards of their "self"), and they feel that they do not have a problem or need any help. Occasionally a patient with anorexia will be so undernourished and medically compromised that she or he might end up in a general adult or pediatric emergency service with significant medical complications. In these instances, a consultation with these services might be required of the psychiatric team, and the need for a full assessment is in order.

At times, a patient with anorexia or bulimia appears in the ED, and this is the opportunity to intervene and assess carefully. In such cases, a patient may seek help for better dieting techniques, complaining of constipation and wanting laxatives, needing diuretics for bloating or edema or for the manifestations of malnourishment (weakness, leg cramps, amenorrhea, depression, or anxiety). See Table 4-5.1 for common medical complications of eating disorders.

Anorexia: The hallmark of a patient with anorexia is the overwhelming need to be thin, with an almost irrational sense that she is too fat or is terrified she will become fat. The patient will completely minimize the weight loss, even when perilously dangerous, and she or he cannot maintain the expected weight for their age and height—85% or less. The patient may report a series of complicated diets, increased physical activity, frequent weighing, limited social interactions due to the dieting, and focus on weight loss. Patients, although they are normal or below normal in weight and appearance, will continue to feel that they look fat and need to continue losing weight. They might have an elaborate set of rules or rituals they follow for their daily weight control and food intake. These patients tend to see dieting and weight control in very concrete fashion—black-or-white thinking about weight—at times even with magical thinking about certain food groups: "good or safe" and "bad or dangerous" foods. In more advanced stages, for women, menstrual periods stop, or in young girls, their menses do not start, whereas with men, their levels of sex hormones will diminish.

Bulimia: Patients with bulimia have an overwhelming fear of and preoccupation with fatness, although their self-loathing and disgust for their body image is greater than that in anorexia. In bulimia, patients might have formerly been obese. Bingeing is frequently seen as a loss of control—unstoppable once started—and usually in response to a low or sad mood. The patient will eat in a short time an enormously larger-than-normal quantity of food in one sitting. This will initially help relieve the depressed mood but will then lead to feelings of guilt, shame, depression, and the overwhelming concern about having gained weight. Patients with bulimia will report feeling out of control while eating and then need to vomit, misuse laxatives, exercise excessively, or fast to get rid of the calories consumed during the binge. These patients will also report dieting when not bingeing. Weight may be normal or near normal unless anorexia also is present, although because of the extreme caloric fluctuations, a patient's weight may fluctuate dramatically from day to day.

Table 4-5.1.   Medical complications of eating disorders

Related to weight loss	Cachexia: loss of fat, muscle mass, low-normal thyroxine (normal TSH), cold intolerance, difficulty in maintaining core body temperature, hypoglycemia, increased cortisol Cardiac: loss of cardiac muscle, small heart, arrhythmias, atrial and ventricular premature contractions, prolonged QT interval, bradycardia, hypotension, ventricular tachycardia, sudden death GI: delayed gastric emptying, bloating, constipation, abdominal pain Reproductive: amenorrhea, low LH and FSH levels, low estrogen or testosterone Dermatologic: lanugo, alopecia, peripheral edema, hypercarotenemia (yellow tint to skin secondary to large consumption of vegetables with vitamin A), acrocyanosis Hematologic: mild normochromic, normocytic anemia, leukopenia (with decreased polymorphonuclear leukocytes) Electrolyte: increased BUN and creatinine, hyponatremia Neuropsychiatric: abnormal taste sensation, depression, anxiety, mild cognitive disorder Skeletal: osteoporosis
Related to purging (vomiting and laxative abuse)	Metabolic: hypokalemia, hypochloremic alkalosis, hypomagnesemia GI: enlargement and inflammation of the salivary glands and pancreas, increased serum amylase, esophageal and gastric erosion, dysfunctional bowel with haustral dilation Dental: erosion of dental enamel and tooth decay Neuropsychiatric: seizures, mild neuropathies, fatigue and weakness, mild cognitive disorder

TSH, thyroid-stimulating hormone; GI, gastrointestinal; LH, luteinizing hormone; FSH, follicle-stimulating hormone; BUN, blood urea nitrogen.

Depression and anxiety are common associated findings, and patients feel unworthy and have significant self-doubt and deeply buried anger. Impulse control may be a problem (e.g., shoplifting, sexual adventurousness, alcohol and drug abuse, and other kinds of risk-taking behavior can be commonly seen as well).

Although not an official DSM-IV-TR diagnosis, binge-eating disorder may be seen in the ED. These patients binge-eat frequently and repeatedly, feeling out of control and unable to stop eating during the binges. They may eat rapidly and secretly, or may snack and nibble all day long and feel guilty and ashamed of binge eating. They may report a history of diet failures and tend to be obese and many times depressed as well. These patients do not regularly vomit, overexercise, or abuse laxatives as do bulimics.

Obesity: Although not specifically a category of eating disorders, nor necessarily related to appetite disturbances, obesity is a very common problem; more than half of the U.S. population is overweight, and 25% meet criteria for obesity. Caloric intake, when it exceeds the body's energy expenditure, translates into increased body weight. This carefully balanced homeostasis, once slightly thrown off, can have significant impact on a person's body weight. How much one eats is regulated by many complex factors, most importantly by the hypothalamus, but also by culture and psychological factors. Obesity carries with it major adverse health effects, with serious increases in morbidity and mortality. Obesity is an associated feature of many medical disorders, such as

- Cushing disease
- Hypothyroidism
- Insulinoma
- Craniopharyngioma and other disorders involving the hypothalamus
- Neuroendocrine disorders (adiposogenital dystrophy or Fröhlich syndrome).

Because appetite and how much one eats often can be related to one's mood state, fluctuations in appetite and weight gain can be commonly seen in psychiatric disorders. Obesity and its myriad accompanying health risks and complications are seldom seen primarily in an ED setting, unless concomitant medical problems are present. See Table 4-5.2 for a list of pathological consequences of obesity. Although as many as half of obese people will have depression, anxiety, or other emotional disturbances, it is uncommon for them to seek help in an ED setting.

In patients with chronic psychiatric problems, especially those taking maintenance antipsychotic medication, weight gain can become a serious problem that may become a focus of clinical attention in an ED setting. The typical and atypical antipsychotic agents can cause weight gain. Of the atypicals, clozapine (Clozaril) and olanzapine (Zyprexa) are associated with the greatest degree of weight gain. Medication-related weight gain and treatment-emergent diabetes are fast becoming serious health concerns facing patients with serious and chronic mental illness. Several high-risk groups are known to be more affected by weight gain and obesity: the poor, African-American women, children, adolescents, and people with serious mental illness. The emergence of diabetes and

Table 4-5.2.   Pathologic consequences of obesity

Hormonal/Metabolic	Hyperinsulinemia and insulin resistance → type 2 diabetes mellitus Hyperuricemia → gout Hypertriglyceridemia and hypercholesterolemia → hyperlipidemias
Reproductive	Males: hypogonadism; plasma testosterone and sex-hormone-binding globulin (SHBG) are decreased; estrogen levels are increased; gynecomastia Females: Menstrual abnormalities → oligomenorrhea; increased androgen production, decreased SHBG, increased estrogen, polycystic ovarian syndrome, increased incidence of uterine cancer
Cardiovascular	Coronary disease, stroke, congestive heart failure, hypertension, left ventricular hypertrophy, angina pectoris, ventricular arrhythmias, venous stasis, varicose veins, cerebrovascular disorders
Pulmonary	Decreased chest-wall compliance, increased work of breathing, increased minute ventilation, decreased total lung capacity and functional residual capacity, obstructive sleep apnea, obesity hypoventilation syndrome, secondary polycythemia, right ventricular hypertrophy
Hepatobiliary	Increased biliary secretions of cholesterol, supersaturation of bile → gallstones, cholecystitis, hepatic steatosis
Bones, joints, skin	Osteoarthritis, acanthosis nigricans, increased skin friability with enhanced risk of fungal and yeast infections, bone spurs of the heel, worsening of postural faults
Renal	Proteinuria, renal vein thrombosis, nephrosis
Cancer	Males: higher incidence of cancer of colon, rectum, prostate Females: higher incidence in gallbladder, bile ducts, breasts, endometrium, cervix, and ovaries

SHBG, sex hormone–binding globulin.

weight gain/obesity have serious medical health risks and increased morbidity and mortality, with such negative consequences as hypertension, dyslipidemias, coronary artery disease, congestive heart failure, and stroke.

Studies done on weight gain in patients taking antipsychotic medication show a wide variety in average weight gained, from minimal weight gain (less than 0.5 kg) with haloperidol (Haldol) and ziprasidone (Geodon) to significant weight gain (more than 3.5 kg) with clozapine (Clozaril) and olanzapine (Zyprexa). Although it does not appear to be dose related and more an issue of increased appetite, the risk to the patients remains high. Although patients will hardly ever appear in the ED with weight gain as a primary complaint, it may be a clinical issue that must be addressed.

Other less familiar diseases, disorders, and problem conditions involve food, eating, and weight, although they are not extensively studied or researched and occasionally quite rare. They are the following.

Muscle dysmorphia (bigorexia): Sometimes called bigorexia, muscle dysmorphia can be thought of as being on the other end of the spectrum from anorexia nervosa. Patients obsess about being small and undeveloped and worry that they are little and too frail. Even if they have good muscle mass, they believe their muscles are inadequate. Compulsive exercising is quite common.

Night-eating syndrome: The person has little or no appetite for breakfast and may delay the first meal for several hours after waking. These patients often get upset over how much they ate the night before, when most of the day's calories were ingested.

Nocturnal sleep-related eating disorder: Thought to be a sleep disorder, not an eating disorder. The patient reports eating while asleep and may sleepwalk as well.

Rumination syndrome: Patient reports eating, swallowing, and then regurgitating the food back into the mouth, where it is chewed and swallowed again. The process may be repeated several times or for several hours per episode and can be voluntary or involuntary. These individuals report that the regurgitated material does not taste bitter, and that it is returned to the mouth with a gentle burp; no violent gagging, retching, or even nausea occurs.

Prader-Willi syndrome: A congenital problem usually associated with mental retardation and behavior problems, including a drive to eat constantly that cannot be denied.

Pica: A craving for nonfood items such as dirt, clay, plaster, chalk, or paint chips.

Cyclic vomiting syndrome: Cycles of frequent vomiting, usually (but not always) found in children. These may be related to, or share neurologic mechanisms with, migraine headaches.

Chewing and spitting: The individual may put food in his or her mouth, taste it, chew it, and then spit it out. Although many think this may be a separate eating disorder, others consider it a calorie-control behavior commonly seen in anorexia nervosa, and sometimes in bulimia and eating disorders not otherwise specified. It is thought to be a creative mechanism that allows some enjoyment of food while avoiding calories.

MANAGEMENT

Gather history from family and friends. Patients with anorexia especially tend to minimize or deny the degree of impairment they may have. Try to ally yourself with the patient and avoid any form of power struggle; anorexic patients have significant control issues—do not challenge them. Regardless of the level of medical severity, it is important to conduct a thorough physical examination and a comprehensive medical workup. Laboratory tests should include

Serum electrolytes
Renal-, liver-, and thyroid-function tests
Glucose
Amylase
Complete blood count (CBC), platelets, and differential
Cholesterol level
Electrocardiogram (ECG)
Uranalysis (with electrolytes)
Serum osmolality
Urine toxicology.

Urine toxicology is important to check for the presence of stimulants, which may be used for weight loss by some patients. It is important to rule out all possible medical causes of weight loss, including tumors and cancer. The assessment also is important to try to determine whether the weight loss is an associated symptom of another psychiatric disorder, such as a depressive disorder, somatization disorder, schizophrenia or delusional disorder, and bulimia (30% to 50% of patients with anorexia have symptoms of bulimia). Amenorrhea or altered menses are a common finding. Keep a high level of suspicion when confronted with unexplained growth retardation, unexplained primary amenorrhea, weight loss of unknown origin, unexplained hypercholesterolemia, and excessive exercising routines when evaluating an adolescent for clues to anorexia.

Patients with bulimia can have normal weight and may or may not exhibit electrolyte abnormalities or other physical findings. In patients that purge frequently or abuse laxatives, hypokalemia, hypomagnesemia, hypochloremic alkalosis, and hyperamylasemia may be found. Menstrual disturbance may occur in patients with bulimia, although it is not a consistent finding. Differential diagnosis of bulimia should include anorexia. It is important to perform a thorough neurologic examination and consider certain neurologic disorders, such as seizure disorders, central nervous system (CNS) tumors, Klüver-Bucy syndrome, or Kleine-Levine syndrome. Although not very common, seldom seen in the ED, and related to these eating disorders only from the perspective of alteration in body image, body dysmorphic disorder is found in some patients. Patients with this somatoform disorder have intense preoccupation with a real or an imagined defect in their bodily appearance.

In the ED, the management is geared toward the medical and psychiatric assessment and provision of support and psycho-education for the patients and family. If anxiety or agitation is present and severe, consider the use of anxiolytic agents, such as lorazepam (Ativan). Use low doses and monitor carefully; many patients with anorexia have compromised medical conditions and may be sensitive to these agents. As with the elderly or medically ill, remember: use small doses and go slowly.

Treatment-emergent weight gain/obesity and diabetes must be addressed. Case series report an incidence of treatment-emergent diabetes at approximately 1%; screening in the ED in these high-risk groups is becoming a must. Ask these patients about their risk factors for diabetes (such as family history, being in a high-risk ethnic group, BMI greater than 27, history of gestational diabetes, hypertension, and dyslipidemias), which if present, warrant a more thorough workup and assessment.

DISPOSITION

Anorexia: The accepted and widely held medical consensus has restoration to 90% of predicted weight as the primary goal in patients with anorexia. This is often rejected by the patient, fearing that the weight gain will lead to obesity and that the patient will be "out of control." Psychoeducation about the treatment options and the medical complications with the patient and family, as well as reassurances of optimal weight maintenance through a program, can be helpful. The family's frustration and concern must be addressed and allayed as well as possible. Hospitalization should be strongly considered in patients with less than 75% of their expected body weight or more than 30% loss in a 3-month period. Other indications for hospitalization include severe metabolic disturbances, serious depression, suicidal ideation, psychosis, or prior outpatient treatment failures. During hospitalization, it is important to correct electrolyte imbalances, dehydration, and nutritional restoration, in addition to assessing and correcting any related complications of starvation.

In less severely affected patients, an outpatient setting or partial hospitalization program, if available, can be appropriate. Family and individual therapy, especially CBT, is a mainstay of such programs, along with psychopharmacologic interventions. These can range from using ciproheptadine (Periactin) to other agents such as amitriptyline (Elavil), clomipramine (Anafranil), fluoxetine (Prozac), pimozide (Orap), or chlorpromazine (Thorazine).

Bulimia: A patient with bulimia can usually be treated as an outpatient; cognitive/behavioral approaches—among the most useful—are indicated, but also to be considered are group, family, or interpersonal therapy. Only one of the SSRIs has been FDA approved for the use in bulimia: fluoxetine (Prozac), at higher doses than usually used to treat depression. It is thought that the SSRI can help decrease the binge eating and the purging. Other antidepressants and even mood stabilizers have been used in treating patients with bulimia, with mixed results. Remember that it is important to consider any existing comorbid conditions and treat those as well.

Obesity: Obesity is to be considered a chronic medical condition; the goal is to attain a normal weight without causing iatrogenic treatment-related morbidity. This goal is a difficult one to achieve and involves many approaches including CBTs, reduced caloric intake through dieting, exercise, surgery, and certain psychopharmacologic agents. The treatment and management of obesity is an outpatient, multidisciplinary approach. Because more than half of the patients with obesity have either anxiety or depression, treatment of these disorders is crucial in assisting the rest of the outpatient plans to be more effective.

Treatment-emergent weight gain/obesity and diabetes must be referred for specialized aftercare; psychoeducation and nutritional education, exercise routines, and other behavioral approaches are essential in these patient.

BIBLIOGRAPHY

Allison DB, Mentore JL, Heo M, et al. Antipsychotic-induced weight gain: a comprehensive research synthesis. *Am J Psychiatry* 1999;156: 1686–1696.

Aquila R. Management of weight gain in patients with schizophrenia. *J Clin Psychiatry* 2002;63(suppl 4):33–36.

Basson BR, Kinon BJ, Taylor CC, et al. Factors influencing acute weight changes in patients with schizophrenia treated with olanzapine, haloperidol, or risperidone. *J Clin Psychiatry* 2001;62:231–238.

Dixon L, Weiden P, Delahanty DC. Prevalence and correlates of diabetes in national schizophrenia samples. *Schizophr Bull* 2000;26: 903–912.

Goldstein LE, Henderson DC. Atypical antipsychotics and diabetes mellitus. *Prim Psychiatry* 2000;7:65–68.

Gray MCG, Witter J, Mehler PS. Detection and management of eating disorders in the emergency setting. *J Am Assoc Emerg Psychiatry* 1997;3:73–77.

Hetherington MM, Rolls BJ. Dysfunctional eating in the eating disorders. *Psychiatr Clin North Am* 2001;24:235–248.

Johnson JG, Cohen P, Ksaen S, et al. Eating disorders during adolescence and the risk for physical and mental disorders during early adulthood. *Arch Gen Psychiatry* 2002;59:545–552.

Kiess W, Reich A, Muller G, et al. Clinical aspects of obesity in childhood and adolescence: diagnosis, treatment and prevention. *Int J Obes Relat Metab Disord* 2001;25(suppl 1):75–79.

Kinon BJ, Basson BR, Gilmore JA, et al. Long-term olanzapine treatment: weight changes and weight-related health factors in schizophrenia. *J Clin Psychiatry* 2001;62:92–100.

Kotler LA, Walsh BT. Eating disorders in children and adolescents: pharmacological therapies. *Eur Child Adolesc Psychiatry* 2000;9 (suppl 1):108–116.

Kruger S, Kennedy SH. Psychopharmacotherapy of anorexia nervosa, bulimia nervosa, and binge-eating disorder. *J Psychiatry Neurosci* 2000;25:497–508.

Malhotra S, McElroy SL. Medical management of obesity associated with mental disorders. *J Clin Psychiatry* 2002;63(suppl 4):24–32.

McIntyre RS, McCann SM, Kennedy SH. Antipsychotic metabolic effects: weight gain, diabetes mellitus, and lipid abnormalities. *Can J Psychiatry* 2001;46:273–281.

Mitchell JE, Peterson CB, Myers T, et al. Combining pharmacotherapy and psychotherapy in the treatment of patients with eating disorders. *Psychiatr Clin North Am* 2001;24:315–323.

Nielsen S. Epidemiology and mortality of eating disorders. *Psychiatr Clin North Am* 2001;24:201–214.

Robb AS. Eating disorders in children: diagnosis and age-specific treatment. *Psychiatr Clin North Am* 2001;24:259–270.

Russel JM, Mackell JA. Bodyweight gain associated with atypical antipsychotics: epidemiology and therapeutic implications. *CNS Drugs* 2001;15:537–551.

Russell GF. Involuntary treatment in anorexia nervosa. *Psychiatr Clin North Am* 2001;24:337–349.

Schatzberg AF. New indications for antidepressants. *J Clin Psychiatry* 2000;61(suppl 11):9–17.

Sussman N. Review of atypical antipsychotics and weight gain. *J Clin Psychiatry* 2001;62(suppl 23):5–12.

Wetterling T. Bodyweight gain with atypical antipsychotics: a comparative review. *Drug Saf* 2001;24:59–73.

Wirshing DA, Wirshing WC, Kysar L, et al. Novel antipsychotics: comparison of weight gain liabilities. *J Clin Psychiatry* 1999;60:358–363.

Wonderlich S, Mitchell JE. The role of personality in the onset of eating disorders and treatment implications. *Psychiatr Clin North Am* 2001;24:249–258.

Chapter 4-6 Confusion/ Disorientation

DEFINITION

Confusion or disorientation is a state of disturbed orientation in regard to time, place, or person, affecting the clarity and coherence of one's thinking. Both of these conditions affect cognitive functioning and are a disturbance in consciousness most often associated with organic brain causes.

Cognitive disorders, characterized by a significant deficit in cognition, orientation, or memory, can be medical in origin as well as psychiatric. DSM-IV-TR lists several cognitive disorders: delirium, dementia, and amnestic disorders. We here discuss delirium and other acute confusional states. Many confusing, vague, and ill-defined terms have been used in the past to describe delirium, including organic brain syndrome, acute confusion, clouded states, pseudosenility, acute brain syndrome, encephalopathy, and toxic psychosis.

PRESENTATION

Although confusion is considered a hallmark of organic disorders, it can be seen in certain psychiatric conditions, such as schizophrenia, delirium, dementia (Alzheimer's disease), amnestic disorders, and other disorders. Delirium is often underdiagnosed by physicians, and when diagnosed, it is usually late in the course of the disease state, increasing the morbidity and mortality. Patients with confusion and disorientation are most often brought to the ED by a concerned family member or caretaker. Occasionally agency workers bring them in from adult or nursing homes because of worsening of the confusion and possible dangerous wandering or agitated behavior.

One of the most common reasons for an acute confusional state in the ED is usually delirium. See Table 4-6.1 for a list of some of the common cause of delirium/acute confusional states. Delirium is an acute, reversible organic mental syndrome characterized by reduced ability to maintain attention to external stimuli and reduced levels of consciousness; sensory misperceptions; disturbances in sleep and level of psychomotor activity; disorientation to time, place, and person; and memory impairment. Delirium is classified as a mental disorder because it involves a fluctuating level of consciousness and is associated with significant impairments in mental, behavioral, and emotional functioning. Delirium is usually of short-term onset and temporary duration, and is always because of a medical/organic cause. Several prodromal

Table 4-6.1.   Common causes of acute confusional states

Infectious and inflammatory	Abscess, encephalitis, meningitis, vasculitis, SLE, febrile illnesses, and infections in general
Metabolic	Hypo- or hypernatremia, hypercalcemia, hypercarbia, hepatic encephalopathy, hypo- or hyperglycemia, hypoxia, thiamine deficiency (Wernicke encephalopathy), hypo- or hyperthyroidism, uremia
Neoplastic	Deep midline tumors, CNS primary or metastatic tumors, increased intracranial pressure
Neurologic	Absence status epilepticus, complex partial status epilepticus, postictal state, subdural or epidural hematomas, normal-pressure hydrocephalus
Postsurgical	Analgesics, electrolyte imbalance, fever, hypoxia, preoperative atropine
Cardiac	Congestive heart failure, arrhythmia, pulmonary embolus, myocardial infarction, hypertension
Systemic	Pneumonia, urinary tract infection, anemia, acute bowel infarction, appendicitis, volvulus
Toxic	Drug intoxication or withdrawal, nonprescription drugs, prescription drugs such as steroids, anticholinergic medications, cardiac medications, antihypertensives, anticonvulsants, cimetidine, nonnarcotic and narcotic analgesics
Traumatic	Concussion, severe traumatic brain injury
Vascular	Stroke, subarachnoid hemorrhage

SLE, systemic lupus erythematosus; CNS, central nervous system.

signs and symptoms can precede a delirious state; these include anxiety, restlessness, drowsiness or insomnia, disturbing dreams, and transient hallucinations. Delirium is a common cause of agitation and confusion in hospitalized patients and a primary reason for psychiatric consultation. Delirium occurs in more than 15% of all general hospital admissions, with higher rates (20% to 30%) in the elderly, especially those with preexisting cognitive impairments. Although these rates are quite high, this condition goes undetected more than half the time. See Table 4-6.2 for a list of possible medical causes of delirium. The morbidity and mortality from delirium cannot be overstated; this is a serious and potentially life-threatening condition that must be assessed and managed quickly. Your level of suspicion for delirium must always be high in patients with fluctuating courses of orientation and confusion.

The history of a patient with confusion and disorientation is usually obtained from collateral sources, such as family, friends, caretakers, guardians, and even hospital nursing staff, because the patient is often a poor historian. Patients will have impairment in their level of awareness of their environment, and difficulty in focusing and/or sustaining or shifting attention. These fluctuations will vary over the course of the day, with lucid peri-

Table 4-6.2.   Causes of delirium

Central nervous system disorder	Degenerative diseases
	Head trauma (especially concussion)
	Meningitis or encephalitis
	Neoplasms
	Seizures and postictal states
	Temporal lobe seizures
	Vascular disease (e.g., hypertensive encephalopathy)
Metabolic disorder	Acid–base imbalance
	Anemia
	Endocrinopathies (thyroid, parathyroid, pituitary, pancreas, adrenal)
	Fluid or electrolyte imbalance
	Hepatic failure
	Hypoglycemia
	Hypoxia
	Renal failure (e.g., uremia)
	Thiamine deficiency
Cardiopulmonary disorder	Carbon dioxide narcosis
	Cardiac arrhythmia
	Congestive heart failure
	Hypotension
	Myocardial infarction
	Respiratory failure
	Shock
Systemic illness	Infection with fever and sepsis
	Neoplasm
	Postoperative state
	Sensory deprivation
	Severe trauma
	Substance intoxication or withdrawal
	Temperature dysregulation
Drugs of abuse	Alcohol
	Amphetamines
	Cannabis
	Cocaine
	Hallucinogens
	Hypnotics
	Inhalants
	Mushrooms (containing muscimol and ibutinic acid)
	Opioids
	Phencyclidine
	Sedatives
Medications	Analgesics
	Anesthetics
	Antiasthmatic agents
	Anticonvulsants
	Antihistamines
	Antihypertensive and cardiovascular medications

continued

Table 4-6.2. *Continued*

	Antimicrobials
	Antiparkinsonian medications
	Cimetidine
	Corticosteroids
	Disulfiram
	Gastrointestinal medications
	Immunosuppressive agents
	Insulin
	Lithium and psychotropic medications with anticholinergic properties
	MAOIs
	Muscle relaxants
	Salicylates
Toxins	Anticholinesterase
	Carbon dioxide
	Carbon monoxide
	Heavy metal and other industrial poisons
	Organophosphate insecticides
	Volatile substances, such as fuel or organic solvents

MAOI, monoamine oxidase inhibitor.

ods interspersed with periods of confusion. Patients may have associated symptoms of anxiety, sedation or insomnia, restlessness, perceptual disturbances, and either increased or decreased psychomotor activity. Patients may have complete disorientation to time and, in severe cases, may have loss of orientation to place and others. Rarely is orientation to self impaired. Disorganized thinking is manifested by rambling, irrelevant, or incoherent speech and impairment in their ability to understand speech. Patients will have difficulty registering, retaining, and recalling memories, as well as impaired problem-solving abilities. Patients are easily distracted and can become agitated because of their inability to discriminate sensory stimuli adequately. Visual, olfactory, or tactile hallucinations or delusions can be present. Patients can have mood alterations ranging from apathy to anger and irritability, leading to occasional outbursts and aggressivity. Caretakers will complain of changes in the patient's sleep–wake cycle, at times completely reversed, with exacerbation of symptoms at bedtime—this is known as sundowning.

MANAGEMENT
Whether family or workers bring the patient to the ED or the patient is hospitalized, the evaluation will be similar. Gather as much information as possible about the patient's history: medical, surgical, psychiatric, and medication regimen. Inquire about history and current use of drugs or alcohol. Confusion and disorientation should make you think of underlying organic disorders. Determine time and acuity of onset of the confusion and assess if there are fluctuations in the level of consciousness during the day.

Ask about associated symptoms, such as headaches, fever, seizures, changes in motor or sensory activity, changes in gait, speech, daily activities, bowel and bladder functioning, or sleep patterns. A full mental state examination (MSE) and a Mini-Mental Status Exam (MMSE) are essential. Test the patient's orientation carefully; try not to reveal the correct answer. Obtain a full medical and neurologic workup, with the clinically important laboratory workup and a CT or MRI. Basic laboratory tests recommended include electrolytes, glucose, liver-function tests, albumin, complete blood count, ECG, chest radiograph (CXR), arterial blood gases or O_2 saturation, and urinalysis. Additional tests may include urine culture and sensitivity, urine and/or serum toxicology screen, VDRL, heavy-metal screen, B_{12} and folate levels, lupus erythematosus (LE) prep, antinuclear antibody (ANA), urinary porphyrins, ammonia level, human immunodeficiency virus (HIV), erythrocyte sedimentation rate (ESR), medication serum levels, lipoproteins (LPs), and EEG.

Focal neurologic findings may occur in patients with delirium, such as dysphasia, tremors, incoordination, or urinary incontinence. The objective of management and treatment in these cases is to uncover the underlying (and we hope reversible) cause of the confusion/disorientation and to treat quickly. Reversible causes include hypoglycemia, hypoxia or anoxia, hyperthermia, severe hypertension, alcohol or sedative/hypnotic withdrawal, Wernicke encephalopathy, and anticholinergic delirium. Improvement in cognition will occur once the condition is treated.

Delirium is a reversible condition but denotes a severe underlying, untreated medical condition and should be considered a medical emergency. If left undiagnosed and untreated, the condition will worsen and can cause permanent damage and death. Older and young patients and those that have a history of dementia, brain injury, and prior episodes of delirium are more vulnerable. In assessing a patient with delirium, remember that their mental status can change during the course of hours, so a clear and lucid mental examination in the face of contrary reports by family or hospital staff should alert you to the possibility of delirium. If you are called for a consultation, review the chart, speak with nursing staff, and ask family members about the patient's functioning.

Differential can be narrowed, based on associated symptoms, such as, if there is a fluctuating course, think of delirium. If there are psychotic symptoms with flat affect, think of psychotic disorders such as schizophrenia. If there is a global cognitive deficit with amnesia, think of dementias. When prominent mood symptoms are present, think of mood disorders.

Avoid treating with medications until a definitive diagnosis of the underlying cause of the confusion/disorientation or delirium can be determined. For difficult behaviors such as anxiety or agitation (avoid benzodiazepines, as they further cloud the patient's cognition or may paradoxically disinhibit the patient), use low-dose, high-potency neuroleptics or low doses of atypical agents. Haloperidol is the most frequently used agent, because it has few anticholinergic side effects, few active metabolites, and has decreased likelihood of producing hypotension. Additionally, it has the advantage of being able to be used PO, IM, or IV in those that require continuous IV infusion (consider 10 mg IV, and then 5 to

10 mg/hr). Since the introduction of atypical neuroleptics, because of their different receptor blockade, they are less prone to cause EPSs. Remember, as in dosing in geriatric patients or medically ill patients, start with very low doses, and go very slowly.

haloperidol (Haldol), 0.5 to 2 mg, PO, IM, or IV (0.25 to 0.5 mg per 4hr in elderly patients); repeat every 2 to 4 hours, with upward titration
or
fluphenazine (Prolixin), 0.5 to 5 mg, PO or IM
or
risperidone (Risperdal), 0.25 to 2 mg, PO
or
olanzapine (Zyprexa), 2.5 to 10 mg, PO
or
quetiapine (Seroquel), 25 mg, PO.

If several doses of neuroleptic medication are ineffective, or neuroleptics are contraindicated, or if alcohol or sedative/hypnotic withdrawal is the causative etiology, consider:

lorazepam (Ativan), 0.5 to 2 mg, PO, IM, or even IV

If the degree of psychomotor agitation is severe and the patient may become violent, consider the use of restraints in conjunction with sedation, as described earlier.

DISPOSITION

In the ED, admission is generally the norm, because the causative underlying condition of the delirium is usually severe enough to require continued assessment, management, and treatment. Recommendations to the admitting team for behavioral control and other associated disturbances can be quite helpful. Psychiatry consultation-liaison (C-L) follow-up is another recommendation that can have a positive impact on the patient's hospital course and ultimate prognosis.

Recommendations, if the patient is hospitalized, include interventions aimed at improving the environment, such as decreasing over- and understimulation, improving sensory impairments, increasing the familiarity of the surroundings, and providing frequent reorientation and reassurance to both the patient and the family. Once the underlying condition has been diagnosed and treated, symptoms of confusion, disorientation, and delirium will begin to fade within the first week, although some may persist longer. The older the patients and the longer they were delirious, the longer the resolution period will be. Patients who are delirious have much higher morbidity and mortality in the ensuing year; the 3-month mortality rate is about 25%, and the 1-year rate is about 50%. Some patients with delirium are thought to go on to develop dementia, although this is not well substantiated in the literature, but empiric evidence has shown a tendency for some patients after an episode of delirium to develop depression or PTSD.

BIBLIOGRAPHY

American College of Emergency Physicians. Clinical policy for the initial approach to patients presenting with altered mental status exam. *Ann Emerg Med* 1999;33:251–281.

Elie M, Rousseau F, Cole M, et al. Prevalence and detection of delirium in elderly emergency department patients. *CMAJ* 2000;163:977–981.

Hustey FM, Meldon S, Palmer R. Prevalence and documentation of impaired mental status in elderly emergency department patients. *Acad Emerg Med* 2000;7:1166.

Johnson J. Identifying and recognizing delirium. *Dement Geriatr Cogn Disord* 1999;10:353–358.

Lipowski ZJ. Update on delirium. *Psychiatr Clin North Am* 1992;15:335–345.

Samuel SC, Evers MM. Delirium: pragmatic guidance for managing a common, confounding, and sometimes lethal condition. *Geriatrics* 2002;57:33–38.

Schuurmans MJ, Duursma SA, Shortridge-Baggett LM. Early recognition of delirium: review of the literature. *J Clin Nurs* 2001;10:721–729.

Schwartz TL, Masand PS. The role of atypical antipsychotics in the treatment of delirium. *Psychosomatics* 2002;43;171–174.

Chapter 4-7 Delusions

DEFINITION

Delusions are a form of disordered thought content, wherein a patient has a false belief not in keeping with the established cultural framework.

PRESENTATION

Delusions are usually based on incorrect inferences about external events and are not related to a person's level of intelligence. Patients with delusions are rarely able to provide rational and reality-based explanations for their symptoms. Delusions can be bizarre—outside the normal realm of possibilities—or nonbizarre, and be either mood congruent or incongruent. Delusions can be categorized into

- Persecutory or paranoid
- Grandiose
- Jealous
- Guilty
- Somatic
- Nihilistic
- Erotic.

A delusion can

Vary in severity and intensity
Fluctuate in degree of fixedness, certainty, systematization, and structure
Affect the person's life
Influence a person's behavior
Deviate from normal beliefs
Cause significant distress to the person.

People can have an overvalued idea, which may be an unreasonable and sustained false belief, which is generally maintained less

firmly than a delusion. People with overvalued ideas have some reality testing and are able to accept rational arguments against
their belief. Conversely, a delusion is united by a single event or
theme, and it is very hard to alter a person's belief about it.

Delusions can cut across many different medical, substance-
related, and primary psychiatric conditions. Persecutory or
paranoid-themed delusions are the most common presenting
type and should be differentiated from paranoid ideation, which
is a state of heightened suspiciousness but does not reach delusional levels. Patients with paranoid personality disorder may
exhibit chronic distrust and suspiciousness of others, but these
symptoms are hardly ever delusional in nature. Similarly, patients with schizotypal personality disorder may have eccentric
thinking but never of delusional proportions. Patients with
schizophrenia also may have delusions as the primary presenting complaint.

In a delusional disorder, a patient will have a highly system-
atized and congruent, yet circumscribed, delusional belief. DSM-
IV-TR dictates that the delusional beliefs must be of at least
1-month duration and be nonbizarre in nature. The more intelli-
gent a person, the more elaborate the delusional system. These
relatively rare disorders are possibly underreported, because patients do not seek help. The prevalence is thought to be about
0.025% to 0.03%, with an annual incidence of one to three new
cases per 100,000 population or about 4% of all new first admissions to a psychiatry unit. Mean age at onset is 40 years (range,
18 to 90s), with a slight preponderance in women. Family studies
have shown an increased prevalence of delusional disorder and
certain personality traits in relatives of delusional disorder subjects. About 25% ultimately are reclassified as having schizophrenia, and 10% are reclassified as a mood disorders. Several
good prognostic indicators are found for delusional disorders:

- Higher level of premorbid functioning
- Female sex
- Age at onset before 30 years
- Sudden onset and short duration of illness
- Existing precipitating factors
- Persecutory, somatic, and erotic delusions fare better than the
  others.

Persecutory delusions are commonly about being followed or
monitored by a large agency such as the FBI, CIA, or other gov-
ernmental agency. People can be fearful that plots exist against
them or their homes are being monitored and bugged. Others
around the person will be involved in the plot, and their rationale
as to why this is occurring to them is usually not very reasonable.
They may believe they are being cheated, poisoned, maligned,
and conspired against. Some patients become quite litigious and
seek retribution for their perceived wrongs by trying to access the
legal system. They can become agitated and even violent when
feeling cornered and overwhelmed.

Delusions of jealousy are usually directed toward the patient's
spouse. Men are more commonly affected than women, although
it is a rare form of delusional disorder. They feel that their spouse
is being unfaithful and having an affair. The patient will have

growing suspicions about the partner's whereabouts, behaviors, and actions. They read infidelity into common occurrences, and arguments ensue. This delusion can cause significant marital or interpersonal stress on the relationship and can escalate to episodes of violence and danger for the accused partner. The partner is usually unable to persuade the patient otherwise. The delusion may disappear if the couple separates.

In *erotomanic delusions,* a person believes that someone, usually of higher status or social importance, is in love with him or her. This is more common in women than in men and is also known as the Clérembault-Kandinsky complex. These patients can become a source of harassment or even stalk their imagined loved ones; this is extremely troublesome with famous figures. Although women are affected more often, in forensic populations, men are more common because they come into contact with the law more frequently in their attempts to contact or pursue their imagined loved ones.

Grandiose delusions and *megalomania* are commonly focused on the person's perceived special abilities, powers, talents, or other prowess. These patients will believe either that they have special attributes or, because of who they are, that they are special and important. These patients have reports of being famous or possessing special powers or having a lot of money. They will try to impress you with their status and, if pushed, will threaten to sue you or slander you in the press because of who they are. The delusions can take on a religious quality as well, with the belief that they are the messiah or have a special relationship or contact with God. These beliefs are often accompanied with elated or expansive mood and associated manic symptoms.

Delusion of guilt or sin usually can be seen in depressed patients. These delusions center on their perception that they are sinful and need to be punished. Many times they explain their depression as a punishment and that they are deserving of their conditions. The perceived faults or sins are usually minor transgressions or events that are thought to be a truly unpardonable acts or behaviors.

Somatic delusions (monosymptomatic hypochondriacal psychosis) are focused on a person's belief that he or she is sick or has a disease, or that the body is abnormal or has changed. Commonly people will believe that they have an undiagnosed serious condition such as infection, infestation of insects, foul body odor, or have HIV or cancer. They may complain about the size of a body part or that an organ may not be functioning properly. These people will seek care from nonpsychiatrists frequently and undergo multiple testing and even medication trials before a psychiatrist sees them. Evidence to the contrary usually does not shake the delusional belief; that the disease is not yet recognized in them or is different in them can be the usual response.

Delusions of reference, a more severe version of ideas of reference (in which a person feels that people or the media are talking to or about him or her), is more entrenched and of delusional proportions. Everything outside the person carries a referential connotation about them and their behavior.

Delusions of control occur when people have complaints that others or external forces are controlling their thoughts, behaviors, or feelings. They may report that they feel their thoughts are being broadcast outside their head so that others may hear them (thought broadcasting), or that their thoughts are being removed from their head (thought withdrawal). They may feel that these forces are inserting thoughts into their minds (thought insertion) or that their thoughts are being controlled (thought control).

MANAGEMENT

It is important not to challenge a person's delusional belief; this may cause more distress or exacerbate the anxiety and possible agitation. It is important to gather a full history and collateral information; this will help clarify whether other associated conditions are present, and the patient's level of functioning and incapacities. A complete physical, medical workup, and urine toxicology are warranted as well.

Inquire about their thoughts and beliefs. Ask questions in a nonjudgmental and nonaccusatory manner. Be empathic. If asked whether you believe or agree with their beliefs, do not deny their belief, but reply that you understand and believe that they believe what they are thinking. You can further state that even though you might not believe what they are saying or experiencing, it does not mean that it is not happening to them. Barring an outright and nontherapeutic alliance with the patient, the less confrontational and judgmental you are in questioning the patient, the better the relationship you will be able to establish and the more information you will obtain. Engaging the patient is crucial. These delusional beliefs are very entrenched, and a patient's insight is usually quite impaired. It is important to find out how these delusional beliefs affect the patient's everyday existence. Is the ability to function impaired because of their severity and their all-encompassing nature? What other associated symptoms exist, and in what larger contextual framework do these delusions belong?

Differential diagnosis includes psychotic disorders, affective disorders, substance-related disorders (intoxication or withdrawal), medical causes, or medication effects:

- Anticholinergics
- Antihypertensives
- Antituberculosis medications
- Antiparkinsonian medications
- Cimetidine
- Disulfiram.

Delusional disorders must be differentiated from mood disorders (although the delusion may be mood congruent, the mood symptoms are not severe enough) and schizophrenia (usually delusions are more bizarre and impair functioning). Malingering, factitious disorders, somatoform disorders, and paranoid personality disorder are other disorders that must be ruled out to diagnose a patient with a delusional disorder.

When sufficient evidence indicates that the delusions developed as the physiological result of a general medical illness, consider a psychotic disorder due to a general medical condition with delusions. See Table 4-7.1 for medical and neurologic disorders that can occur with delusions.

Trying to convince the patients that they may have a problem can be very difficult. If the patient reports suicidal or homicidal

**Table 4-7.1. Medical and neurologic
disorders that can lead to delusions**

Parkinson disease
Huntington disease
B_{12}, folate, thiamine, or niacin deficiencies
Alzheimer or Pick disease
Adrenal, thyroid, or parathyroid conditions
Seizures
Cerebrovascular diseases
Neoplasms
Metabolic abnormalities (hypoglycemia, porphyria, uremia, hyper-
    calcemia, hepatic encephalopathy)

ideation, hospitalization may be called for. If not, trying to engage
the patient and convince him or her to seek outpatient help is crucial. Short-term management of the anxiety or agitation with
short-acting benzodiazepines may help calm the patient and allow
a more thorough interview.

lorazepam (Ativan), 0.5 to 2 mg, PO or even IM

If agitation is severe and the delusions are intense with associated hallucinations, use an atypical or typical neuroleptic with or
without a benzodiazepine (and anticholinergic medication). If the
patient is neuroleptic naïve, be sure to provide psychoeducation
about the medication and inform the patient of the risks and benefits of taking the medication. Patients will usually refuse to take
anything because they believe they do not have a treatable psychiatric condition. You can help them understand the need for
medication, without confronting their delusions, by explaining
that the medications will help them feel calmer and improve or
straighten out their thinking. You can explain that the medication will decrease the level of anxiety and concern they are feeling over their beliefs. Start at a low dose.

olanzapine (Zyprexa), 2.5 to 5 mg, PO
risperidone (Risperdal), 0.5 to 2 mg, PO
quetiapine (Seroquel), 25 to 100 mg, PO
ziprasidone (Geodon), 20 to 40 mg, PO
aripiprazole (Abilify), 10 to 15 mg, PO
haloperidol (Haldol), 0.5 to 2 mg, PO or IM
+ lorazepam (Ativan), 0.5 to 2 mg, PO or even IM
+ benztropine (Cogentin), 0.5 to 2 mg, PO or IM.

In the ED setting, you will not be initiating medication treatment. Remember: the more you engage the patients by helping
them understand the need for medication, the better their medication adherence will be, and the more likely that they will follow up on discharge from the ED. As outpatients, they will
have to address the other associated conditions simultaneous with
other medications. As delusions are treated, the resolution process
initially starts with the patient feeling that the delusional belief
is less relevant in life, with a decrease in the level of preoccupation. Then the patient may admit to faulty logic in thinking about

the delusional belief, although with much resistance. Only much later will a patient concede that the delusional belief was indeed a delusion and, as such, false. In general, close to 50% of patients will recover over the long term, 20% will have some decrease in their symptoms, and 30% will show no change.

BIBLIOGRAPHY

Appelbaum P, Robbins P, Monahan J. Violence and delusions: data from the MacArthur Violence Risk Assessment Study. *Am J Psych* 2000; 157(4):566–572.

Appelbaum P, Robbins P, Roth L. Dimensional approach to delusions: comparison across types of diagnoses. *Am J Psychiatry* 1999;156: 1938–1943.

Forster PL, Buckley R, Phelps MA. Phenomenology and treatment of psychotic disorders in the psychiatric emergency service. *Psychiatr Clin North Am* 1999;23:735–754.

Garety PA, Hemsley DR. Characteristics of delusional experience. *Eur Arch Psychiatry Neurol Sci* 1987;236:294–298.

Kendler KS, Glazer WM, Morgenstern H. Dimensions of delusional experience. *Am J Psychiatry* 1983;140:466–469.

Richards CF, Gurr DE. Psychosis. *Emerg Med Clin North Am* 2000;18: 253–262.

Sachs MH, Carpenter WT, Strauss JS. Recovery from delusions. *Arch Gen Psychiatry* 1974;30:117–120.

Schneider, K (MW Hamilton, translator). *Clinical psychopathology.* New York: Grune & Stratton, 1959.

Spitzer M. The phenomenology of delusions. *Psych Annu* 1992;22: 252–259.

Chapter 4-8 Depersonalization/ Derealization

DEFINITION

Depersonalization is considered an alteration in the perception of the self, so that the usual sense of one's own reality is lost. It is manifested by the sense of unreality or self-estrangement, changes in body image, or in a feeling that one does not control his or her own actions and speech. Derealization is the loss of the sense of reality of one's surroundings; the feeling that something happened, that the world has been changed and altered, a feeling of being detached from one's environment. Although these are distinct phenomena, many times they are grouped under depersonalization.

PRESENTATION

Depersonalization and derealization can occur in the general population, adults and children, as a response to stress. It is thought that these symptoms are more common in women and are rarely found in people older than 40 years. Depersonalization and derealization, as a symptomatic manifestation, can occur in patients with primary psychiatric disorders or medical/neurologic disorders. See Table 4-8.1 for a list of possible causes of depersonalization.

DSM-IV-TR groups depersonalization as a dissociative disorder; along with depersonalization disorders, included in this group, are

Table 4-8.1. Causes of depersonalization

Metabolic	Hypoglycemia, hypoparathyroidism, hyperventilation, hypothyroidism
Neurologic	Seizure disorders, migraines, neoplasms, cerebrovascular disease, trauma, encephalitis, general paresis, dementia (Alzheimer's), Huntington disease, spinocerebellar degeneration
Psychiatric	Schizophrenia, depression, mania, conversion disorders, anxiety disorders (especially posttraumatic stress disorder), obsessive–compulsive disorder, personality disorders
Toxic	Carbon monoxide poisoning, mescaline intoxication; botulism; cocaine, hallucinogen, and cannabis intoxication; alcohol and sedative–hypnotic withdrawal; β-blockers and anticholinergic medications; steroids

dissociative amnesia, dissociative fugue, dissociative identity disorder, and dissociative disorder not otherwise specified (NOS).

In normal individuals, exhaustion, boredom, sensory deprivation, or a response to emotionally traumatic events can manifest as depersonalization and/or derealization. Epilepsy and migraine appear to be the most commonly associated disorders with depersonalization. Left-sided temporal lobe dysfunction and anxiety are thought to be predisposing factors associated with depersonalization. Other findings implicate certain personality structures as risk factors associated with dissociative disorders, such as depersonalization disorder. These are thought to occur in individuals with avoidant temperament and in those who use immature defenses.

Patients with depersonalization and derealization will report that their feelings started relatively abruptly, at times in the context of a life stressor or with another identifiable precipitant. Usually patients are young adults and report either a stable course with little fluctuation or a more episodic occurrence with asymptomatic intervals.

Patients will complain that they feel unreal and that their internal experiences are different, alien to them. They complain of feeling detached and unreal, experiencing themselves as if from the "outside looking in." In cases in which depersonalization and derealization experiences are transient and mild, these symptoms are worrisome to the patient and are usually in the context of an underlying medical, neurologic, or toxic condition. At other times, they can be a manifestation of a primary psychiatric or substance-related disorder. Whatever the underlying causes, the patient is usually concerned and upset at feeling strange and unconnected.

Symptoms of depersonalization and derealization can vary in intensity and, when severe enough and disabling in their intensity, a primary consideration of depersonalization disorder should be considered. Physical actions, internal states, and even thought processes can seem foreign and unrelated to themselves. Anxiety is a common associated finding, and alterations in perception of time and place can be affected as well. Emotional detachment from their surroundings and bodily alteration (extremities being bigger or smaller) can be experienced as well. Certain neurologic conditions, especially those affecting the parietal lobe, can produce a phenomenon of hemidepersonalization, in which half of the body feels unreal or does not exist. Another reported phenomenon is as if it were an "out-of-body" experience; the patients feel they are outside themselves looking in, almost as if they were two separate entities; commonly called doubling. Another phenomenon is reduplicative paramnesia or double orientation, in which patients report that they feel as if they were in two places at the same time.

MANAGEMENT

Patients rarely will have a depersonalization or derealization experience while being interviewed, but if so, they can appear to be unresponsive or partially responsive to the interview. If experiencing an episode of depersonalization or derealization, they may have a trance-like quality and be aloof and distant from the interviewer. Never challenge them; be supportive, and use direct questioning to obtain information about their experience; this alone may help reduce or eliminate the symptom.

The primary task is to determine the underlying reasons for the depersonalization and derealization and treat them. Inquire about other psychiatric symptoms and prior psychiatric or substance-related disorders and treatments. Determine whether recent events, especially traumatic events, occurred, and their impact on their presentation. A complete medical and neurologic workup, including urine toxicology, EEG, and neuroimaging, is indicated. A detailed history of prior traumatic events and experiences, as well as childhood trauma, can be helpful. It is thought that childhood trauma, especially emotional abuse, is correlated to depersonalization disorder.

Treatment consists of determining the underlying cause and treating it. In cases in which severe anxiety is present, the use of short-acting benzodiazepines can be helpful.

lorazepam (Ativan), 0.5 to 2 mg, PO or IM
alprazolam (Xanax), 0.25 to 1 mg, PO.

Many times the use of benzodiazepines in the ED can help relieve or resolve the symptoms.

DISPOSITION

The disposition is dependent on reaching a diagnosis and treating the underlying cause. Patients with primary psychiatric conditions, such as depersonalization disorder or another primary psychiatric condition, should be referred to an outpatient provider for continued treatment. In cases in which the depersonalization and derealization are secondary to a substance intoxication or withdrawal phenomenon, a referral to either inpatient detoxification or outpatient referral to a drug-treatment program is important. Psychoeducation with the patient and family or friends is crucial in helping the patient and the network better understand and manage the disorder.

Ongoing medical care for those with medical or neurologic causes should be done as per the EDs routine for outside referrals.

BIBLIOGRAPHY

Berrios GE, Sierra M. Depersonalization: a conceptual history. *His Psychiatry* 1997;8:213–229.

Dorland's illustrated medical dictionary. 28th ed. Philadelphia: WB Saunders, 1994.

Lambert MV, Sierra M, Phillips ML, et al. The spectrum of organic depersonalization: a review plus four new cases. *J Neuropsychiatry Clin Neurosci* 2002;14:141–154.

Phillips ML, Medford N, Senior C, et al. Depersonalization disorder: thinking without feeling. *Psychol Res* 2001;108:145–160.

Sierra M, Berrios GE. The phenomenological stability of depersonalization: comparing the old with the new. *J Nerv Ment Disord* 2001; 189:629–636.

Simeon D, Guralnik O, Knutelska M, et al. Personality factors associated with dissociation: temperament, defenses, and cognitive schemata. *Am J Psychiatry* 2002;159:489–491.

Simeon D, Guralnik O, Schmeidler J, et al. The role of childhood interpersonal trauma in depersonalization disorder. *Am J Psychiatry* 2001;158:1027–1033.

Chapter 4-9 Depressed Mood

DEFINITION

A mental state of depressed mood is characterized by feelings of sadness, despair, and discouragement. Depression can range from feelings of "blues" to dysthymia and major depression.

PRESENTATION

As described earlier in the MSE chapter, mood is considered one of the manifestations of a person's emotional state, the other being affect. Emotional states are the complex interplay between mood and affect that have psychological, physical, and even behavioral correlates. A person's mood, in other words, the internal subjective emotional condition, can range from normal to euphoric to depressed, more often on a continuum but within certain parameters. Everyone will have a wide variety of mood states and affective manifestations, normally being fully aware and in control of these states. In mood disorders, the control and insight are lost, and people begin to have difficulty functioning.

Depressed mood or a depressive episode can be a manifestation of bereavement or a more serious unipolar depression or a bipolar depression. It can be related to the use of a substance or can be an associated finding of a medical or neurologic disorder. Additionally, many medications widely used in practice today can cause depressive symptoms in the patients taking them. Depression can be seen under many very confusing guises. See Table 4-9.1 for a list of possible medical and neurologic causes of depression. See Table 4-9.2 for medications and substances that may cause depressive symptoms.

Patients can have a depressed or sad mood, or they may complain of irritability. Not all patients can or will report sadness as their chief complaint. Patients can have vague somatic complaints, or

**Table 4-9.1. List of neurologic
and medical causes of depression**

Endocrine	Addison disease; Cushing disease; hyper- and hypoparathyroidism; hyperaldosteronism; menses related, postpartum, thyroid disorders (hypothyroidism or apathetic hyperthyroidism)
Infectious and inflammatory	AIDS, chronic fatigue syndrome, mononucleosis, pneumonias, (viral or bacterial), rheumatoid arthritis, Sjögren syndrome, SLE, temporal arteritis, tuberculosis
Neurologic	Cerebral neoplasms, cerebral trauma, cerebrovascular disease (especially anterior hemispheric lesions), CNS infections, dementia (Alzheimer's disease), epilepsy, Huntington disease, hydrocephalus, migraine, multiple sclerosis, narcolepsy, neurosyphillis, Parkinson's disease, progressive supranuclear palsy, sleep apnea, Wilson's disease
Other	Cancer, cardiopulmonary disease, Klinefelter syndrome, porphyria, postoperative mood disorders, renal disease and uremia, systemic neoplasms
Vitamin deficiencies	Folate, niacin, thiamine, vitamin B_{12}, vitamin C

AIDS, acquired immunodeficiency syndrome; SLE, systemic lupus erythematosus; CNS, central nervous system.

have other neurovegetative symptoms such as change in appetite, sleep, concentration, energy, or libido. Fatigue or lack of energy is one of the most common presenting complaints in a primary care setting, and between 20% to 40% of those patients are thought to have an underlying depressive disorder. These same patients are high users of medical and ED services, and their depression often goes undiagnosed, causing unnecessary suffering. Some patients may report only memory impairment or forgetfulness, whereas others may have a more classic constellation of symptoms. Other may have had a long-standing low-grade depression, usually no more than mild to moderate in intensity (dysthymia). Patients may complain of diurnal variation in their mood, whereas others may report significant changes in mood during specific periods or seasons (seasonal affective disorder). Women may experience intense mood lability and especially depressed mood around the time of their menses, during the postpartum period, and/or during menopause. Some depressed states may be considered normal reactions to stressors or loss, such as bereavement. The hallmark may be a sad or depressed mood, but usually not so much guilt, self-reproach, helplessness, hopelessness, or unworthiness as commonly seen in depression. These symptoms tend to resolve after a few months; determined individually and as a cultural norm. Grief that is pro-

Table 4-9.2.   List of medications and substances that cause depression

Analgesics and anti-inflammatory drugs	Benzydamine, fenoprofen, ibuprofen, indomethacin, opiates, pentazocine, phenacetin, phenylbutazone
Antibacterial, antiviral, and antifungal drugs	Acyclovir, alfamethoxazole, ampicillin, chloramphenicol, clotrimazole, cycloserine, dapsone, ethionamide, griseofulvin, isoniazid, ketoconazole, metronidazole, nitrofurantoin, streptomycin, sulfonamides, tetracycline, thiocarbanilide, trimethoprim
Antineoplastic drugs	6-Azuridine, azathioprine (AZT), bleomycin, C-asparginase, mithramycin, trimethoprim, vincristine, zidovudine
Cardiac and antihypertensive drugs	Bethanidine, clonidine, digitalis, disopyramide, guanethidine, hydralazine, lidocaine, methoserpidine, methyldopa, oxprenolol, prazosin, procainamide, propranolol, reserpine, veratrum
Miscellaneous	Acetazolamide, anticholinesterases, choline, cimetidine, cyproheptadine, diphenoxylate, disulfram, lysergide, mebeverine, meclizine, metaclopramide, methysergide, pizotifen, salbutamol
Neurologic agents	Amantadine, baclofen, bromocriptine, carbamazepine, levodopa, methosuximide, phenytoin, tetrabenazine
Psychotropic drugs	Butyrophenones, phenothiazines
Sedatives and hypnotics	Barbiturates, benzodiazepines, chloral hydrate
Steroids and hormones	Corticosteroids, danazol, oral contraceptives, prednisone, triamcinolone
Stimulants and appetite suppressants	Amphetamine, fenfluramine, diethylpropion, phenmetrazine

tracted and incapacitating is pathologic grief and may be the focus of attention in an ED. Pathologic bereavement may be hard to assess but should be carefully ruled out and differentiated from a major depressive disorder. Stressors such as the loss of a loved one or other stressors can cause patients to have depressed mood as an adjustment reaction (adjustment disorder with depressed mood). Another group of patients may have low-grade depressive symptoms with a history of hypomanic symptoms, commonly called cyclothymic disorder.

As stated earlier, depression and anxiety are highly comorbid. DSM has a new proposed diagnostic category: Mixed Anxiety-

Depression; although not fully accepted, it describes patients with depressive and anxiety symptoms that do not meet criteria for either a mood disorder or an anxiety disorder because of the severity or presentation of the symptoms. These patients may demonstrate depressed mood, poor concentration, sleep disturbance, fatigue, low energy, irritability, worry, tearfulness, hypervigilance, negativistic outlook, hopelessness, low self-esteem, and worthlessness, which affect their social and occupational functioning. Other types of presentations, categorized as depressive disorders NOS in the DSM-IV-TR, include

Premenstrual dysphoric disorder (During the year, most menstrual cycles have associated depressive symptoms, which occur regularly during the last week of the luteal phase and remit on the onset of menses; they are of sufficient severity to affect the woman's life.)

Minor depressive disorder (2 weeks of depressive symptoms but with fewer than the five items required for a major depressive disorder). These patients are seldom diagnosed, having subsyndromal presentations, are often seen in primary care or in the ED for other conditions, and are often left untreated. This can lead to unfavorable health-related outcomes, increased morbidity, increased social and occupational dysfunction, and overall poorer quality of life.

Recurrent brief depressive disorder (recurrent depressive episode lasting 2 days to 2 weeks, occurring at least once a month for 12 months, not related to the menstrual cycle)

Postpsychotic depressive disorder of schizophrenia (major depressive episode occurring in the residual phase of schizophrenia).

Remember to inquire about concurrent episodes of mania (mixed or depressive episodes as well) and symptoms of psychosis (hallucinations, delusions, disorganized behavior or speech, and negative symptoms). If evidence of concurrent psychosis and prominent affective symptoms is found, with at least a 2-week period during which the patient had no affective symptoms but with continued psychosis, think about schizoaffective disorder.

Adolescents may not express themselves as adults do and may have what are known as "depressive mood-equivalents." These may be acting-out behaviors, poor school performance, truancy, sexual acting out, drug use, etc. See Chapter 6.1.

Most depressive episodes may be further specified by their severity and other characteristics, such as a seasonal component, postpartum onset, and longitudinal course. Anxiety is a common finding in patients with depression as well as psychosis. Patients with rapid cycling—four or more episodes of depressive, mania, mixed or hypomanic episodes in a 12-month period—tend to have more severe and frequent depressive episodes.

MANAGEMENT

Depression is a serious condition with significant associated stigma. Many patients will have difficulty opening up and confiding; you must approach the depressed patient with empathy, reassurance, and a supportive stance. Under no circumstance should you ever minimize a person's complaint of depression or make disparaging or flippant comments such as "cheer up," or "you'll just get over it," or worse yet, "what have you got to be depressed about."

A thorough medical and neurologic workup and a review of medications are indicated. Speak with family and collaterals to gather as much information as possible. Inquire about suicide in ALL patients (see Chapter 4.21). Depression is a risk factor for suicide, and a thorough suicide assessment should be a standard part of every evaluation. The Hamilton Depression Rating Scale can assist in determining symptom severity and baseline functioning if time permits (see Appendix D). In 1983 Paterson et al. developed the SAD PERSONS Scale for assessing the risk of suicide. Although the scale has sensitivity and specificity problems, it is a good guide to make certain all pertinent risk factors for suicide are determined. The higher the number of points scored, the greater the risk; 1 (or 2) point(s) are scored for each factor deemed present: 0, very little risk/10, very high risk.

Sex	male	1
Age	<19 or >45 years old	1
Depression	endorses depressive symptoms	2
Previous attempt	yes (including prior hospitalizations)	1
Ethanol (drug) use	yes (acute or chronic)	1
Rational thinking loss	medical etiology or psychosis	2
Separated, divorced, widowed	recent or anniversary	1
Organized plan	well thought out, lethal plan	2
No social support	no friends, family, or supports	1
Stated future intent	determined or ambivalent	2

Inquire carefully about hypomanic or manic symptoms to rule out bipolar illness (Chapter 4.10). Determine the severity and functional impairment of the depression. Patients with underlying medical disorders should have their medical condition treated first and foremost. Depression in cardiac patients is a strong predictor of higher morbidity and mortality, especially in patients recovering from a myocardial infarction (MI). Depression secondary to medical causes has several characteristics that distinguish it from a primary psychiatric depression:

- Older age at onset
- Better response to electroconvulsive therapy (ECT)
- Improvement at discharge
- More "organic" features on the MSE
- Lower family incidence of alcoholism and depression
- Less likely to have suicidal thoughts or attempts.

Medications that are potentially causative agents should be carefully reviewed and if possible discontinued in consultation with the patient's treating or prescribing physician. If the physician is unavailable, recommendations for medication discontinuation or change should be addressed at some later point. Patients with active substance abuse should be dealt with accordingly. See Chapters 4.14 and 4.24.

Differentiating between normal and pathologic grief can be hard. Consider depression when the grief has persisted for longer than 6 months; has occurred several months after the loss; the patient has alteration in self-esteem, psychomotor functioning, or suicidal ideation; or the grief is so severe that it causes severe social and personal impairments. See Table 4-9.3 for a list of

Table 4-9.3.   Risk factors for pathological bereavement

Young age
Poverty
Low self-esteem
Limited social and familial supports
Multiple prior losses
Overly dependent on deceased
Loss of young child
Loss of parent for adolescent
Ambivalence toward the deceased
Unexpected or untimely death or after long terminal illness
Death by suicide, murder, or manslaughter

several risk factors that may increase the likelihood of developing pathologic bereavement.

Assess patients for co-occurring anxiety symptoms; symptom severity, course, and treatment options/response will be different. Lifetime and 12-month rates of comorbidity of depression and each anxiety disorder range from 10% to 30%, with as high as 50% comorbidity between depression and any anxiety disorder. Patients with rapid cycling should be diagnosed carefully because treatment with antidepressants has been shown to be detrimental, with possible acceleration of cycling, and requiring mood stabilizers instead.

Short-term interventions in the ED will be aimed at relieving the acute anxiety with the use of short-acting benzodiazepines.

lorazepam (Ativan), 0.5 to 2 mg, PO (IM if severely anxious and needing immediate relief)

If the patient is psychotic, consider using neuroleptics, depending on the severity of the psychosis.

haloperidol (Haldol), 1 to 5 mg (PO or IM)
fluphenazine (Prolixin), 2 to 5 mg (PO or IM)
risperidone (Risperdal), 0.5 to 2 mg (PO)
olanzapine (Zyprexa), 5 to 10 mg (PO)
quetiapine (Seroquel), 25 to 100 mg (PO)
ziprasidone (Geodon), 20 to 40 mg (PO)
aripiprazole (Abilify), 10 to 15 mg (PO).

DISPOSITION

Depending on the severity of the depressive symptoms, the presence of psychotic symptoms or suicidality will dictate the outcome. Patients with associated psychotic symptoms or with suicidality may require inpatient hospitalization. Safety consideration is a key factor in determining admission and potentially requiring enhanced observation (one-on-one observation) if the patient is unable to feel safe on the floor. Patients with mild to moderate depression, with good family supports and some level of insight, may benefit solely from outpatient therapy. The decision to admit a patient with mild to moderate depression rests on the willingness to be admitted, psychiatric history, prior response to medications, prior suicide attempts, support systems, and history of compliance with treatment. Psychoeducation that focuses on depression as a medical illness with effective treatment options can be quite useful. Treatment options such as psychotherapy, psychopharmacologic intervention, or ECT should be broached with the patient and family as much as possible. If the patient is severely depressed and requires inpatient hospitalization, the option of ECT should be raised; with several conditions, ECT treatment should be considered first line:

- Psychotic/delusional depression
- Intense suicidality and depression
- Severe malnutrition/dehydration and depression
- Catatonia
- Severe manic excitation
- Treatment failures
- History of positive response
- Medical condition that precludes use of antidepressants.

If the patient is discharged, referral to an outpatient provider should be arranged as soon as possible. Initiation of an SSRI antidepressant should be carefully weighed and determined by the policies and procedures of individual EDs and readily available aftercare referral sources. Many reasons can be listed for not starting a person on an antidepressant agent from the ED, as well as many reasons for initiating an antidepressant medication. This is a controversial area, and different clinicians will feel differently about prescribing medication to ED patients, despite the possible low risk and high benefits. Availability of aftercare, psychoeducation, careful documentation, continuity of care plans from the ED, and patient history of compliance are all factors that may influence this decision one way or another. If initiating an SSRI, psychoeducation must be provided regarding the risks and benefits, and especially those side effects that may affect future adherence, such as weight changes, sexual dysfunction, and discontinuation syndromes. If these can be assured, many clinicians may believe that it is a safe and rational decision and provide the patient with a prescription for an antidepressant with enough medication to get him or her to the first follow-up appointment. Records should be copied and sent to the referring agency or provider, with the patient's release of information signed before discharge, to ensure adequate continuity of care. Patients with medical conditions that need attention or ongoing treatment should be referred to the primary caretaker or referred to one. Medication changes or discontinuation of medications should be discussed if possible with the patient's physician or service. A call or letter with the ED finding can be quite helpful for the treating physician. Patients with substance abuse can be referred to inpatient detoxification units, if clinically warranted, or to specialized dual-diagnosis units if available.

BIBLIOGRAPHY

Banazak DA. Minor depression in primary care. *J Am Osteopath Assoc* 2000;100:783–787.
Brown TM, Stoudemire A. *Psychiatric side effects of prescription and over-the-counter medications: recognition and management.* Washington, DC: American Psychiatric Press, 1998.
Calabrese JR, Shelton MD, Bowden CL, et al. Bipolar rapid cycling: focus on depression as its hallmark. *J Clin Psychiatry* 2001;62 (suppl 14):34–41.

Glick RL. Initiation of antidepressant in the emergency setting. *Psych Annu* 2000;30:251–257.

Hockberger RS, Rothstein RJ. Assessment of suicide potential by nonpsychiatrists using "SAD PERSONS" score. *J Emerg Med* 1988;6:99.

Jacobs S, Kim K. Psychiatric complications of bereavement. *Psych Annu* 1990;20:314–317.

Kessler RC, McGonale KA, Zhao S, et al. Lifetime and 12-month prevalence of DSM-III-R psychiatric disorders in the United States: results from the national comorbidity survey. *Arch Gen Psychiatry* 1994;51:8–19.

Lagomansino I, Daly R, Stoudemire A. Medical assessment of patients presenting with psychiatric symptoms in the emergency setting. *Psychiatr Clin North Am* 1999;22:819–850.

Parkes CM. Risk factors in bereavement: implications for the prevention and treatment of pathological grief. *Psych Annu* 1990;20:308–313.

Paterson WM, Dohn HH, Bird J, et al. Evaluation of suicidal patients: the SAD PERSONS Scale. *Psychosomatics* 1983;24:343–349.

Rosen RC, Lane RM, Menza M. Effects of SSRIs on sexual function: a critical review. *J Clin Psychopharmacol* 1999;19:67–85.

Sampson SM. Treating depression with selective serotonin reuptake inhibitors: a practical approach. *Mayo Clin Proc* 2001;76:739–744.

Stein MB, Kirk P, Prabhu V, et al. Mixed anxiety-depression in a primary-care clinic. *J Affect Disord* 1995;34:79–84.

Zinbarg RE, Barlow DH, Liebowitz M, et al. The DSM-IV field trial for Mixed Anxiety-Depression. *Am J Psychiatry* 1994;151:1153–1162.

Chapter 4-10 Elated/Irritable Mood

DEFINITION

Elation is a state of emotional excitement marked by an increase in mental and physical activity. Irritability is a state that makes an individual more prone to frustration, impatience, annoyance, or excessive anger. Mania is a phase of bipolar disorder characterized by elation or expansiveness, irritability or agitation, hyperexcitability, and increased speed of thought and speech.

PRESENTATION

As discussed earlier, a person's mood can fluctuate widely, especially with a mood disorder. Patients with mood disorders can have moods that range from the unpleasant and low (dysphoric mood) to heightened levels of moods (manic or hypomanic mood). These may take on the form, in order of severity, of

- Elevated mood (a heightened, above-normal cheerful mood)
- Expansive mood (exaggerated expression of feelings with an overestimation of importance or significance)
- Elated mood (feelings of intense euphoria, triumph, optimism, occasionally accompanied by grandiosity)
- Irritable mood (feeling of excessive annoyance and quick to anger).

These increased mood states are commonly seen in primary mood disorders, but also can occur in the context of substance-related disorders, especially intoxication and withdrawal, medical conditions, and medication-related conditions. The most frequent presentation of elated or irritable mood is in the context of a manic episode. Manic episodes can be seen as part of a bipolar disorder, schizoaffective disorder, or mania due to a general medical condition or substance-related condition. See Table 4-10.1 for a list of possible causes of mania.

Patients are commonly brought in by a family member or co-worker because of the lack of insight most patients have when manic. Patients at first may appear quite appealing and charismatic, and then become quite easily and rapidly irritable and intrusive. Patients will have a characteristic elated or expansive mood, which can be very engaging and can be minimized or missed by the inexperienced clinician. These patients are usually poor and unreliable historians. Nonadherence with medication and aftercare is a common reason for a patient's deterioration and exacerbation of symptoms. Although not extensively studied or addressed in the literature (ranging from approximately 18% to 52%), nonadherence with mood stabilizers has a huge impact on exacerbation of symptoms and ED presentations. Additionally, many can appear quite seductive and dressed in inappropriate clothing and makeup, at times trying to seduce the clinician or becoming frankly sexually provocative.

Patients can be very talkative and hyperactive; if psychotic, they can be disorganized and agitated. More than three fourths of patients with mania experience delusions, mostly mood-congruent.

Table 4-10.1. Possible causes of mania

Systemic/Metabolic	Uremia and hemodialysis, dialysis dementia, hyperthyroidism, pellagra, carcinoid syndrome, vitamin B_{12} deficiency, postpartum mania, paraneoplastic syndromes
CNS	Huntington disease, postencephalitic Parkinson disease, encephalitis, neurosyphilis, AIDS encephalopathy, Wilson disease, general paresis, cerebral trauma, thalamotomy, cerebrovascular accidents, multiple sclerosis, frontal and temporal neoplasms, temporal lobe epilepsy, Pick disease, Kleine-Levin syndrome, Klinefelter syndrome
Medications	Baclofen, bromide, bromocriptine, captopril, cimetidine, corticosteroids, cyclosporine, decongestants, disulfram, hydralazine, isoniazid, levodopa, methylphenidate, metrizamide, procarbazide, yohimbine
Drugs	Amphetamines, cocaine, hallucinogens, opiates and opioids, phencyclidine (PCP)

CNS, central nervous system; AIDS, acquired immunodeficiency syndrome.

Patients whose insight is impaired will not see their mood or behavior as problematic, although family and friends will. If patients are irritable, they may have poor frustration tolerance, may be unpredictable and agitated, and can become violent. Patients may be labile in their moods and switch from one mood extreme to the other. Patients will test limits, being demanding and alternating with neediness. Their behavior can cause havoc in an ED by interrupting the clinical care, disrupting the milieu, or demanding increased clinician's time and attention. Patients may be hard to interrupt and difficult to interview, their speech being loud, rapid, and ultimately even disorganized with neologisms, incoherencies, flight of ideas, or loosening of associations. They may be intrusive and disruptive, disinhibited and hypersexual—occasionally disrobing or even fondling themselves in public. Their appearance can often be eccentric: bright-colored clothing, jewelry, and excessive makeup in peculiar colors or combinations. Patients can be preoccupied and perseverate in a rapid and pressured fashion on themes of a religious, political, financial, paranoid, or sexual nature. Patients may be grandiose, feeling an exaggerated sense of self or overly powerful and knowledgeable. Grandiosity can range from mild forms to the severely delusional. Patients may believe they have a special connection to God or are on an important religious quest or mission.

Certain patients may have hypomanic symptoms and no significant degree of impairment. These patients seldom make it to the ED. They have an elated or expansive mood for a period with feelings of inflated self-worth, no need for sleep and feeling energized despite it, talkative or even pressured, with increased distractibility and goal-directed activities. They also may be involved in "pleasurable activities that have a high potential for painful consequences." These symptoms are a change from a patient's normal state and a disruption in their functioning although not severe enough to cause a significant impairment or to require hospitalization.

Hypomanic or manic symptoms also may be seen in patients with rapid cycling, which is a pattern of at least four episodes (in 12 months) of either a major depressive, manic, mixed, or hypomanic episode. These patients usually have a longer course of illness, more often are females, have a history of antidepressant use and thyroid disease; they are older, with less than favorable lithium (and even carbamazepine) responses in the past.

Patients with mania, as with depressive episodes, may develop psychosis, with similarly higher rates of symptom severity and morbidity. Patients being treated for depression with an antidepressant and with an undiagnosed or unrecognized hyperthymic temperament or bipolar diathesis can be "switched" or "flipped" into a manic episode. The rates vary from 5% to 10% during the acute phase of antidepressant treatment, but still high enough to make certain that this must be assessed carefully before SSRI initiation.

Remember to inquire about concurrent episodes of mania (mixed or depressive episodes as well) and symptoms of psychosis (hallucinations, delusions, disorganized behavior or speech, and negative symptoms). If evidence exists of concurrent psychosis and prominent affective symptoms, with at least a 2-week period where the patient had no affective symptoms but continued with psychosis, think about schizoaffective disorder.

MANAGEMENT

The quick and safe symptomatic reduction in an acute manic episode is one of the main goals of the ED intervention. Obtain as much collateral information as possible. Patients have little insight and will minimize or rationalize their behaviors, being quite convincing and charming in the process. Determine the duration, severity, and impairment. Assess for substance use or abuse as well as high-risk behaviors, such as unprotected sex, gambling, or reckless driving.

With such patients, maintain firm limits and follow the ED protocols closely, especially with patients who have a tendency to test, challenge, and try to subvert those limits. Maintain firm boundaries and set limits, especially in those patients who are seductive or overtly sexual with staff. Assess carefully if patient is agitated or violent (see Chapter 4.2). Conduct a full medical and neurologic examination and obtain laboratory tests as clinically indicated, including urine toxicology. Determine patient's history of mania or bipolar illness, as well as prior episodes, functioning, and treatment strategies. Assess psychosis carefully to rule in or out other causes of elated or irritable mood. Determine degree of danger as per poor insight, reckless behavior, unpredictability, and agitation. Assess suicide risk factors and potential for violence. Patients who are hypersexual should be counseled on HIV risk factors and offered HIV testing. Medical workup of sexually transmitted diseases is indicated, as is a pregnancy test in women of childbearing age.

Hypomanic patients with some insight and in established care can be treated immediately with benzodiazepines or even an increase in their dose of mood-stabilizing medication.

Treatment in the ED consists mainly of behavioral control. Consider using

clonazepam (Klonopin), 0.5 to 2 mg, PO; can be repeated every 4 to 6 hours.
lorazepam (Ativan), 1 to 2 mg, PO or IM; can be repeated every 4 to 6 hours.

If the patient is psychotic, consider

haloperidol (Haldol), 2 to 5 mg, PO or IM, every 4 to 6 hours, with or without the use of benzodiazepines or anticholinergics, as clinically determined.
or
olanzapine (Zyprexa), 5 to 15 mg, PO.

Valproate has become a primary choice in the treatment of acute mania because it is relatively safe and it can be given at high doses as an oral loading therapy. Studies have shown that more than half of the patients respond favorably to valproate oral loading, with no significant difference in side effects when compared with regular slow titration of valproate. See Table 4-10.2 for a list of the most common side effects of mood stabilizers.

Some EDs may have protocols for the rapid loading of anticonvulsant medication such as valproate or even lithium, although

Table 4-10.2. Common side effects of mood stabilizers

Lithium	Edema
	Hypothyroidism
	Mental dulling
	Nausea
	Nephrogenic diabetes insipidus
	Polyuria
	Psoriasis
	Tremor
	Weight gain
Carbamazepine	Blurred or double vision
	GI upset
	Hematologic abnormalities
	Impairment of task performance
	Skin rash
	Vertigo
Valproate	GI upset
	Hair loss
	Increased liver-function tests
	Tremor
	Weight gain

GI, gastrointestinal.

the latter is still largely unexamined as an option. Studies reviewed recommended a lithium dose of 20 mg/kg/day, which was well tolerated and effective at improving affective and psychotic symptoms. Make yourself familiar with your institution's policies and protocols on rapid loading. In acutely manic patients, the recommended initial dose of valproate is

valproate (Depakote), 30 mg/kg daily for 2 days, and then 20 mg/kg daily

This strategy of oral loading allows therapeutic serum levels (greater than 50 µg/mL) of valproate to be reached quickly, decreasing the time to reach therapeutic effect. Many of the newer atypical neuroleptics are being studied to determine their efficacy alone or in combination with traditional mood stabilizers or benzodiazepines for use in acute mania. The findings are promising, but their widespread use in the ED is still in the early stages.

DISPOSITION

Most patients who are brought to the ED in a manic state are, by definition, functionally impaired and require hospitalization. Degree of danger to self or others will determine the need for immediate inpatient hospitalization. Consider the need for enhanced supervision, as well as the need for one-on-one observation, if the patient is suicidal, violent, hypersexual, or too uncontrollable. Mood-stabilizer maintenance therapy will be crucial once the patient is stabilized after admission. Traditional mood stabilizers such as lithium are still very effective, although anticonvulsants like carbamazepine, valproate, and the newer agents (lamotrigine, gabapentin, and topiramate) are being widely used with good (but uncontrolled) results.

Once patients with hypomanic symptoms are stabilized in the ED with benzodiazepines or an additional dose of their mood stabilizer, they may be discharged back to their outpatient provider. A call or letter to the provider informing them of the patient's condition and medications provided in the ED is important. Occasionally a prescription for a few days of a benzodiazepine [clonazepam (Klonopin), 1 mg, PO, q12hr] can help keep a patient stable until the psychiatrist sees him or her. In your assessment, you must weigh the risks and benefits of outpatient versus inpatient follow-up and factor in the possibility of dependence, if prescribing a benzodiazepine. Psychoeducation regarding the use of benzodiazepines and their short-term nature is very important. Psychoeducation about safe sex practices and symptom recognition also can help a patient avert an untoward outcome in the future.

BIBLIOGRAPHY

Baldessarini RJ, Tondo L, Hennen J, et al. Is lithium still worth using? An update of selected recent research. *Harv Rev Psychiatry* 2002; 10(2):59–75.

Bowden CL. Novel treatments for bipolar disorder. *Expert Opin Invest Drugs* 2001;10:661–671.

Brown TM, Stoudemire A. *Psychiatric side effects of prescription and over-the-counter medications: recognition and management.* Washington, DC: American Psychiatric Press, 1998.

Calabrese JR, Shelton MD, Rapport DJ, et al. Current research on rapid cycling bipolar disorder and its treatment. *J Affect Disord* 2001;67:241–255.

Chengappa KN, Gershon S, Levine J. The evolving role of topiramate among other mood stabilizers in the management of bipolar disorder. *Bipolar Disord* 2001;3:215–232.

Coryell W, Leon AC, Turvey C, et al. The significance of psychotic features in manic episodes: a report from the NIMH collaborative study. *J Affect Disord* 2001;67:79–88.

Gilmer WS. Anticonvulsants in the treatment of mood disorders: assessing current and future roles. *Expert Opin Pharmacother* 2001;2: 1597–1608.

Grunze H, Erfurth A, Amann B, et al. Intravenous valproate loading in acutely manic and depressed bipolar I patients. *J Clin Psychopharmacol* 1999;19:303–309.

Henry C, Sorbara F, Lacoste J, et al. Antidepressant-induced mania in bipolar patients: identification of risk factors. *J Clin Psychiatry* 2001;62:249–255.

Hirschfeld RM, Allen MH, McEvoy JP, et al. Safety and tolerability of oral loading divalproex sodium in acutely manic bipolar patients. *J Clin Psychiatry* 1999;60:815–818.

Keck PE Jr, McElroy SL, Bennett JA. Pharmacologic loading in the treatment of acute mania. *Bipolar Disord* 2000;2:42–46.

Keck PE Jr, McElroy SL, Tugrul KC, et al. Valproate oral loading in the treatment of acute mania. *J Clin Psych* 1993;54:305–308.

Keck PE Jr, Mendlwicz J, Calabrese JR, et al. A review of randomized, controlled clinical trials in acute mania. *J Affect Disord* 2000; 59(suppl 1):S31–S37.

Keck PE Jr, Strakowski SM, Hawkins JM, et al. A pilot study of rapid lithium administration in the treatment of acute mania. *Bipolar Disord* 2001;3:68–72.

Lagomansino I, Daly R, Stoudemire A. Medical assessment of patients presenting with psychiatric symptoms in the emergency setting. *Psychiatr Clin North Am* 1999;22:819–850.

Lima WJ, Dopheide JA, Kramer BA, et al. A naturalistic comparison of adverse effects between slow titration and loading of divalproex sodium in psychiatric inpatients. *J Affect Disord* 1999;52:261–267.

Macdonald KJ, Young LT. Newer antiepileptic drugs in bipolar disorder: rationale for use and role in therapy. *CNS Drugs* 2002;16: 549–562.

Martinez JM, Russell JM, Hirschfeld RM. Tolerability of oral loading of divalproex sodium in the treatment of acute mania. *Depress Anxiety* 1998;7:83–86.

McElroy SL, Keck PE Jr. Pharmacologic agents for the treatment of acute bipolar mania. *Biol Psychiatry* 2000;48:539–557.

McElroy SL, Keck PE Jr, Tugrul KC, et al. Valproate as a loading treatment in acute mania. *Neuropsychobiology* 1993:27:146–149.

Miller DS, Yatham LN, Lam RW. Comparative efficacy of typical and atypical antipsychotics as add-on therapy to mood stabilizers in the treatment of acute mania. *J Clin Psychiatry* 2001;62:975–980.

Sachs GS, Grossman F, Ghaemi SN, et al. Combination of a mood stabilizer with risperidone or haloperidol for treatment of acute mania: a double-blind, placebo-controlled comparison of efficacy and safety. *Am J Psychiatry* 2002;159:1146–1154.

Scott J, Pope M. Nonadherence with mood stabilizers: prevalence and predictors. *J Clin Psychiatry* 2002;63:384–390.

Thase ME, Sachs GS. Bipolar depression: pharmacotherapy and related therapeutic strategies. *Biol Psychiatry* 2000;48:558–572.

Tohen M, Baker RW, Altshuler LL, et al. Olanzapine versus divalproex in the treatment of acute mania. *Am J Psychiatry* 2002;159: 1011–1017.

Yatham LN. The role of novel antipsychotics in bipolar disorders. *J Clin Psychiatry* 2002;63(suppl 3):10–14.

Chapter 4-11 Exposure to Traumatic Events

DEFINITION

Trauma and the reaction to trauma can be considered a state of psychic or behavioral disorder or dysequilibrium resulting from mental or emotional stress or physical injury.

PRESENTATION

People who have experienced a traumatic event, depending on their injuries and the severity of the event, may seek help in an ED. According to the National Comorbidity Study, the most common traumatic events are

- Witnessing a killing or serious injury
- Sexual molestation, assault, or rape

- Natural or man-made disasters
- Physical attack or abuse
- Being threatened with a weapon
- Life-threatening accident and injuries
- Combat
- Shootings and stabbings
- Unexpected death of relative or friend
- Child diagnosed with life-threatening illness
- Witnessing injury.

Because of the lack of understanding regarding the exposure to traumatic events and the risks of developing acute stress disorder and/or PTSDs, many patients will not be seen by a psychiatrist nor will appropriate treatment be instituted beyond the typical ED care required by the patients and their injuries. Assaults and rapes usually triaged to the general adult ED for management sometimes, but not routinely, will have a psychiatric consultation called if deemed clinically necessary by the ED physician. The events of September 11 increased the awareness about the importance of a person's mental well-being, and now more physicians understand the importance of psychiatric intervention soon after the exposure to a traumatic event. Given our current understanding of PTSD and its severity, poorer prognosis, and increased morbidity and mortality, it is important to assess, especially in the ED, those patients that may be at more risk to develop PTSD and to institute treatment as quickly as possible.

The lifetime incidence of experiencing a traumatic event severe enough to cause PTSD is more than 50%, according to the National Comorbidity Survey. The incidence of experiencing a traumatic event is 51.2% in female and 60.7% in male subjects, and approximately 20% of individuals exposed to a traumatic event may develop PTSD. Given these staggering numbers and the fact that PTSD is the fifth most prevalent major psychiatric illness, after major depression, simple phobia, social phobia, and alcohol dependence, heightened awareness is the key. Additionally, approximately 8% of Americans will experience PTSD in their lifetimes, whereas 4% will experience PTSD during any given year. It is important to keep in mind that the family members and/or friends of victims of trauma (especially murder victims) are at risk and also may have acute stress or PTSD symptoms. Homeless individuals, especially those with psychiatric disorders, are also at significant risk of exposure to traumatic experiences, such as personal violence. Studies have shown that patients with severe traumatic brain injury are more likely to go on to develop PTSD symptoms.

Different risk factors exist not only for exposure to trauma but also for the development of PTSD after the exposure to trauma. For example, studies have shown that being male, early misconduct, low educational levels, and family history of mental illness are strong predictive factors for exposure to trauma. Other studies showed that being female, early childhood losses and separations, history of anxiety or depressive disorders, and family history of anxiety and antisocial personality disorder are highly predictive risk factors for the development of PTSD after exposure to a traumatic event.

Although it is a matter of some debate, women exposed to traumatic events appear to be twice as susceptible as men to develop PTSD. Certain traumatic events are more likely to increase the risk of developing PTSD (being held captive, being tortured, or being kidnapped have the highest risk, although the incidence of these events in the United States is relatively low). Rape and physical (domestic violence) or sexual assaults are associated with higher risk and are more common.

After actual exposure to a traumatic event, in which the patients are exposed to actual or threatened death or serious injury to themselves or someone else, the victims must respond with intense fear, helplessness, or horror. Acute stress disorder shares many of the same symptoms with PTSD, although it also has dissociative symptoms that may be unique predictors of the possible development of PTSD. PTSD symptoms usually develop within the first 3 months after the traumatic event, although much less frequently, the onset can occur months or years later. Symptoms of PTSD can persist for months or years after the traumatic event. It is thought that close to 30% of patients recover completely; 60% will have mild to moderate symptoms; and 10% will remain unchanged or worsen, occasionally becoming chronic, with duration of symptoms greater than 3 months.

In the early stages, the patient may report dissociative symptoms, such as:

- Sense of detachment and emotional unresponsiveness
- Decreased awareness of the surroundings ("being in a daze")
- Derealization (see Chapter 4-8)
- Depersonalization (see Chapter 4-8)
- Dissociative amnesia.

Patients will generally report hyperarousal symptoms, such as:

- Difficulty staying asleep
- Irritability
- Poor concentration
- Hypervigilance
- Exaggerated startle response.

The patients may complain of reexperiencing the event, characterized by:

- Recurrent or intrusive memories
- Recurrent distressing dreams
- Illusions, hallucinations, or dissociative flashback episodes
- Intense distress when exposed to cues
- Intense distress when exposed to internal or external cues.

Most patients also report some avoidance of stimuli associated with the event:

- Avoidance of thoughts
- Avoidance of feelings or conversations about places, people, or activities connected to the event
- Decreased interest or participation in social, occupational, or personal activities
- Feeling detached from others
- Emotional numbing with restricted range of affect
- Sense of a limited and somewhat bleak outlook on the future.

PTSD patients may have somatic symptoms such as gastro-intestinal (GI) problems, cardiovascular problems, or headaches, which can confuse the diagnosis.

MANAGEMENT

Acute stress disorder was introduced in the DSM-IV to identify—early on—trauma survivors who were at risk of developing chronic PTSD 1 month after the exposure to a traumatic event and to distinguish between normative and pathologic acute stress responses. Studies found that dissociative response to a traumatic event, overall severity of acute PTSD symptoms, extent of the exposure to the traumatic event, and preexisting vulnerability factors, for example, assisted in the prediction of and subsequent development of PTSD, as in the following:

Personality disorders
History of psychiatric illness
History of trauma or stress (physical or sexual abuse)
Caretaker dysfunction (neglect or limited social supports)
Genetic liability
Family history of psychological disorders

The diagnosis for acute stress disorder changes to acute PTSD after 1 month duration, and if the symptoms persist for more than 3 months, the diagnosis changes to chronic PTSD. Many patients who have been exposed to a traumatic event and develop symptoms of PTSD that persist for more than 3 months have a harder time recovering, and a growing literature suggests that patients with PTSD have higher rates of anger and impulsivity and a higher risk for suicide. It is therefore very important to identify in the acute trauma phase those individuals who are at risk of developing chronic PTSD to provide an early intervention. Immediate intervention may shorten the course of normal post-traumatic response, reduce PTSD symptoms, prevent development of chronic PTSD and other chronic psychiatric disorders, such as major depressive disorder, help restore functioning, and even prevent functional deterioration. Careful assessment of dissociative response immediately after exposure to a traumatic event and severe reexperience of symptoms can help identify individuals at high risk. Acute reactions to trauma can be less severe, because of both the severity of the actual traumatic crises (loss of job or financial hardship) and a syndromic presentation. These patients may have an adjustment disorder if the symptoms (anxiety, depression, behavioral) commence within 3 months of the stressor and last no more than 6 months after termination of the stressor.

Because emergence of symptoms can occur at any time after the exposure to the traumatic event, it is important always to be on the lookout for these symptoms, even if the traumatic event is not the focus of clinical attention. Asking about traumatic events and exposure to traumatic events is important and necessary. Many times a minor stressor can trigger and exacerbate symptoms of PTSD. Occasionally, because of the increased comorbidity of PTSD, associated symptoms and disorders might be present as well. PTSD is highly comorbid with major depression, substance-related disorders, phobias, dysthymia, agoraphobia, generalized anxiety disorder, panic disorder, psychosis, violence with aggression, and/or impulsivity. Men have more comorbid alcohol abuse and dependence than do women. Because of the many co-occurring and associated comorbid conditions, the overlap of symptoms can confuse the diagnosis and make the differential diagnosis a complex task. Patients with PTSD often exhibit a greater number of health problems and functional impairment. The incidence of suicide attempts in patients with PTSD is approximately 20% and is related to the high comorbidity of PTSD with depression. It is thought that the occurrence of depression shortly after the exposure to a traumatic event is an important predictor and mediator in determining the chronicity of PTSD. Between 79% and 88% of patients diagnosed with PTSD have one or more additional psychiatric disorder, and more than 40% of women and more than 60% of men with PTSD have three or more additional psychiatric disorders. It is thought that premorbid depression is a risk factor for the development of PTSD after a traumatic event and that depression secondary to PTSD commonly occurs in patients with histories of severe childhood trauma.

Risk factors are related to the characteristics of the traumatic event:

- Severity (i.e., impact on person, property, and livelihood)
- Duration
- Physical and emotional proximity to the event.

Moreover, the characteristics of the individuals and their vulnerability factors are important and play a role in predisposing persons to development of PTSD:

- Family history
- Social supports
- Childhood traumatic events
- Preexisting psychiatric disorder
- Personality traits.

Immediate treatment in the ED is limited to dealing with extreme anxiety symptoms or associated psychotic symptoms. Certain hospital EDs have rape units or teams that are especially staffed and trained to deal with patients who are victims of sexual assault or rape. In general, the treatment focus will be based on short-term crisis interventions, which may include:

- Reviewing the events and trying to change patient's distorted perceptions about them
- Normalizing the experience and decreasing anxiety and arousal
- Preventing psychiatric symptom emergence or exacerbation
- Obtaining symptom resolution and reestablishing emotional stability
- Restoring "power" and control and returning to precrises level of functioning.

The overall principles of crisis intervention are that it:

- Be short-term
- Be located close in time and place to the event
- Have focused goals (resolution of crisis)
- Assess the patient's strengths and weaknesses
- Recognize both the harmful and the helpful impacts of a patient's social context (family, work, community)

- Emphasize the understanding of the impact and the ultimate resolution of the crisis
- Be oriented to minimize dependency and maximize mastery
- Be based on active, directive, and flexible therapist behavior.

See Table 4-11.1 for some crisis-intervention techniques.

A complete medical workup, including laboratory tests and a urine toxicology examination, is important. A sympathetic and nonjudgmental approach along with a calm and reassuring environment and demeanor can help to allay a patient's concerns and fears. Providing information, reassurance, and permission for the patient to express self and ventilate are all key components. Setting limits as well as assisting as an advocate or facilitating the patient's empowerment also is crucial. Do not press or pry excessively in obtaining a history for the patient to recall every last

Table 4-11.1. Crisis-intervention techniques

1. Establish rapport:
   a. Convey acceptance and genuine involvement
   b. Reinforce help-seeking behaviors
   c. Invite patient to work on issues
   d. Collaborative/directive (depending on patient's level of functioning)
   e. Provide structure
2. Define the problem:
   a. Define the problem in patient's own terms
   b. Explore depth, implications, changeability of their concerns
   c. Allow open-ended exploration
   d. Focus on NOW and HOW (not THEN and WHY)
   e. Help assign priorities
   f. Make realistic and explicit contract with patient
3. Explore feelings:
   a. Acknowledge
   b. Accept
   c. Explore implications of feelings and why it is important to explore them
   d. When not to deal with feelings
   e. Promote hope
   f. Reduce anxiety, denial, and blame
4. Explore past coping mechanisms:
   a. Transition from problem to problem solving
   b. Take inventory of client's internal and external resources
   c. Avoid tried solutions and reexplore rejected solutions
5. Explore alternatives and develop action plan:
   a. Generate (collaborative) alternatives
   b. Explore consequences
   c. Explore feelings about alternatives
   d. Get commitment to specific plans
   e. Rehearse
   f. Encourage appropriate pacing
   g. Explain problem-solving strategies

detail of the traumatic event. Be supportive and acknowledge the pain or anger at the events. Involve family or friends (if the patient is willing)—they too may require some assistance and reassurances. Psychoeducation for family as well as the patient is important.

For patients with intense discomfort and anxiety or agitation, consider

lorazepam (Ativan), 1 to 2 mg, PO

In cases in which the anxiety and agitation are related to or associated with psychotic symptoms, such as hallucinations or intense paranoia, consider

haloperidol (Haldol), 2.5 to 5 mg, PO or IM
Fluphenazine (Prolixin), 1 mg to 5 mg PO
risperidone (Risperdal), 1 to 2 mg, PO
olanzapine (Zyprexa), 2.5 to 5 mg, PO
Quetiapine (Seroquel), 25 to 100 mg PO
Ziprasidone (Geodon), 10 to 20 mg PO
Aripiprazole (Abilify), 10 to 15 mg PO.

Psychoeducation for the patient and the family/friends regarding the working diagnosis and disposition plans is important.

DISPOSITION
IMPORTANT: Available evidence suggests that early intervention and treatment is the key! Once a determination is made that a person exposed to a traumatic event is symptomatic, depending on the severity of the symptoms and any co-occurring medical or psychiatric disorders, a disposition plan must be formulated. If the person has severe symptoms of flashbacks, nightmares, anxiety, depression, suicidality, substance abuse, irritability, functional impairment, or violence potential, an inpatient psychiatric hospitalization may be indicated. Plans for admission to a psychiatric inpatient unit—for safety, continued evaluation, and initiation of psychopharmacologic/psychotherapeutic interventions—can be very useful. Patients with milder symptoms and fewer functional impairments can be referred to an outpatient provider to initiate treatment as outlined earlier. Psychoeducation with the patient and family/friends is important, and discussion about the medication and treatment options can help improve adherence with aftercare follow-up plans.

Although studied primarily in patients with PTSD, cognitive behavioral therapy (CBT) and prolonged exposure/anxiety-management techniques may be effective for resolving acute trauma responses and minimizing the risk of chronic PTSD. A major consideration for the treatment of acute stress disorder is the timely provision of CBT and prolonged exposure techniques, which studies suggest may be effective in minimizing and even preventing the development of PTSD.

Psychopharmacologic agents, especially the SSRIs, are effective in the treatment of PTSD—at upper-normal ranges of the usual antidepressant dose—either alone or in combination with CBT, although the combination of medication and psychotherapy is recommended and most effective. The FDA has approved the use of sertraline in the treatment of PTSD.

BIBLIOGRAPHY

American Psychiatric Association. *Diagnostic and statistical manual of mental disorders.* 4th ed., 4-TR. Washington, DC: American Psychiatric Association, 1999.

Arana GW, Rosenbaum JF, eds. *Handbook of psychiatric drug therapy.* 4th ed. Philadelphia: Lippincott Williams & Wilkins, 2000.

Ballenger JC, Davidson JRT, Lecrubier Y, et al. Consensus statement on posttraumatic stress disorder from the International Consensus Group on Depression and Anxiety. *J Clin Psychiatry* 2000; 61(suppl 5):60–66.

Beckman JC, et al. Health status, somatization and severity of posttraumatic stress disorder in Vietnam combat veterans with posttraumatic stress disorder. *Am J Psych* 1998;155:1565–1569.

Birmes P, Carreras D, Ducasse JL, et al. Peritraumatic dissociation, acute stress, and early posttraumatic stress disorder in victims of general crime. *Can J Psychiatry* 2001;46:649–651.

Blank AS. Clinical detection, diagnosis and, differential diagnosis of posttraumatic stress disorder. *Psychiatr Clin North Am* 1994;38: 351–383.

Boudreaux ED, McCabe B. Critical incident stress management, I: interventions and effectiveness. *Psychiatr Serv* 2000;51:1095–1097.

Brady KT, et al. Sertraline treatment of comorbid PTSD and alcohol dependence. *J Clin Psych* 1995;56:502–505.

Breslau N. Gender differences in trauma and posttraumatic stress disorder. *J Gend Specif Med* 2002;5:34–40.

Breslau N. The epidemiology of posttraumatic stress disorder: what is the extent of the problem? *J Clin Psychiatry* 2001;62(suppl 17):16–22.

Breslau N, et al. Traumatic events and posttraumatic stress disorder in an urban population of young adults. *Arch Gen Psychiatry* 1991;48:216–222.

Breslau N, et al. Trauma and posttraumatic stress disorder in the community: the 1996 Detroit Area Survey of Trauma. *Arch Gen Psychiatry* 1998;55:626–632.

Bryant RA, et al. Treating acute stress disorder: an evaluation of cognitive behavioral therapy and supportive counseling techniques. *Am J Psych* 1999;56:11.

Bryant RA, et al. Treatment of acute stress disorder: a comparison of cognitive-behavioral therapy and supportive counseling. *J Consult Clin Psychol* 1998;56:862–868.

Cardena E, et al. *Dissociative disorders in DSM-IV sourcebook.* Washington, DC: American Psychiatric Press, 1996.

Carlson EB, Dalenberg C, Armstrong J, et al. Multivariate prediction of posttraumatic symptoms in psychiatric inpatients. *J Trauma Stress* 2001;14:549–567.

Cohen LH, Claiborn WL, Specter GA. *Crisis intervention.* 2nd ed., Vol IV. Community-Clinical Psychology Series. New York: Human Science Press, 1983.

Davidson J. Issues in the diagnosis of posttraumatic stress disorder. In: Oldhan JM, Riba MB, Tasman A, eds. *Review of psychiatry.* Washington, DC: American Psychiatric Press, 1993.

Davidson J, et al. Posttraumatic stress disorder in the community: an epidemiological study. *Psychol Med* 1991;21:713–721.

Forster P, King J. Traumatic stress reactions and the psychiatric emergency. *Psych Ann* 1994;24:603–609.

Freedman SA, Brandes D, Peri T, et al. Predictors of chronic posttraumatic stress disorder: a prospective study. *Br J Psychiatry* 1999;174:353–359.

Giaconia RM, et al. Traumas and posttraumatic stress disorder in a community population of adolescents. *J Am Acad Child Adolesc Psychol* 1995;34:1369–1380.

Holbrook TL, Hoyt DB, Stein MB, et al. Perceived threats to life predicts posttraumatic stress disorder after major trauma: risk factors and functional outcome. *J Trauma* 2001;51:287–292.

Irwin C, et al. Comorbidity of posttraumatic stress disorder and irritable bowel syndrome. *J Clin Psych* 1996;57:576–578.

Jacobsen LK, Southwick SM, Kosten TR. Substance use disorders in patients with posttraumatic stress disorder: a review of the literature. *Am J Psychiatry* 2001;58:1184–1190.

Kaplan HI, Sadock BJ, eds. *Comprehensive textbook of psychiatry.* 8th ed. Baltimore: Williams & Wilkins, 1999.

Kaplan Z, Iancu I, Bodner E. A review of psychological debriefing after extreme stress. *Psychiatr Serv* 2001;52:824–827.

Kessler HS, et al. Past-year use of outpatient services for psychiatric problems in the National Comorbidity Survey. *Am J Psych* 1999;156: 115–123.

Kessler RC, et al. Posttraumatic stress disorder in the National Comorbidity Survey. *Arch Gen Psychiatry* 1995;52:1048–1060.

Kessler RC, McGonale KA, Zhao S, et al. Lifetime and 12-month prevalence of DSM-III-R psychiatric disorders in the United States: results from the national comorbidity survey. *Arch Gen Psychiatry* 1994;51:8–19.

Kotler M, Iancu I, Efroni R, et al. Anger, impulsivity, social supports, and suicide risk in patients with posttraumatic stress disorder. *J Nerv Ment Disord* 2001;189:162–167.

Marshal RD, et al. Pharmacotherapy in the treatment of posttraumatic stress disorder and other trauma-related syndromes. In: Yehuda R, ed. *Psychological trauma.* Washington, DC: American Psychiatric Press, 1998:133–177.

Marshal RD, et al. Review and critique of the new DSM-IV diagnosis of acute stress disorder. *Am J Psych* 1999;56:11.

Martenyi F, Brown EB, Zhang H, et al. Fluoxetine versus placebo in posttraumatic stress disorder. *J Clin Psychiatry* 2002;63:199–206.

McCabe B, Boudreaux ED. Critical incident stress management, II: developing a team. *Psychiatr Serv* 2000;51:1499–1500.

McFarlane AC, et al. Physical symptoms in posttraumatic stress disorder. *J Psychosom Res* 1994;38:715–726.

Mellman TA, David D, Bustamante V, et al. Predictors of posttraumatic stress disorder following severe injury. *Depress Anxiety* 2001;14:226–231.

Morgan CA III, Hazlett G, Wang S, et al. Symptoms of dissociation in humans experiencing acute, uncontrollable stress: a prospective investigation. *Am J Psychiatry* 2001;158:1239–1247.

Mueser KT, Rosenberg SD, Goodman LA, et al. Trauma, PTSD, and the course of severe mental illness: an interactive model. *Schizophr Res* 2002;53:123–143.

Resnick HS, et al. Prevalence of civilian trauma and posttraumatic stress disorder in a representative national sample of women. *J Consult Clin Psychol* 1993;61:984–991.

Rosenberg SD, Mueser KT, Friedman MJ, et al. Developing effective treatments for posttraumatic disorders among people with severe mental illness. *Psychiatr Serv* 2001;52:1453–1461.

Rothbaum BO, et al. Sertraline in the treatment of rape victims with PTSD. *J Trauma Stress* 1996;9:865–871.

Samson AY, et al. Posttraumatic stress disorder in primary care. *J Fam Pract* 1999;48:222–227.

Schatzberg AF. New indication for antidepressants. *J Clin Psychiatry* 2000;61(suppl 11):9–17.

Schuster MA, Stein BD, Jaycox L, et al. A national survey of stress reactions after the September 11, 2001, terrorist attacks. *N Engl J Med* 2001;345:1507–1512.

Shalev A, et al. Posttraumatic stress disorder: somatic comorbidity and effort tolerance. *Psychosomatics* 1990;31:197–203.

Sommerfield TN, et al. Factors associated with outcome of cognitive-behavioral treatment of chronic PTSD. *Behav Res Ther* 2000;38: 191–202.

Stein MB, McQuaid JR, Pedrelli P, et al. Posttraumatic stress disorder in the primary care medical setting. *Gen Hosp Psychiatry* 2000;22: 261–269.

Tucker WM. How to include trauma history in the diagnosis and treatment of psychiatric inpatients. *Psychoanal Q* 2002;73:135–144.

Warshaw MG, et al. Quality of life and dissociation in anxiety disorder patients with histories of trauma. *Am J Psych* 1993;150:1512–1516.

Wilkeson A, Lambert MT, Petty F. Posttraumatic stress disorder, dissociation, and trauma exposure in depressed and nondepressed veterans. *J Nerv Ment Disord* 2000;188:505–509.

Williams WH, Evans JJ, Wilson BA, et al. Brief report: prevalence of posttraumatic stress disorder symptoms after severe traumatic brain injury in a representative community sample. *Brain Inj* 2002;16:673–679.

Chapter 4-12 Homicidal Ideation/Violence

DEFINITION

Violence is defined as the behaviors used by individuals that intentionally threaten to, attempt to, or actually inflict harm on others. It can generally be divided into emotional and cognitive. Emotional violence can be related to fear, anger, frustration, and lack of autonomy. Cognitive violence is usually more motivated by potential profit or personal gain.

Although the U.S. Justice Department data for 2000 indicated that the homicide rate had decreased 1.1% from 1999, violence continues to be a daily occurrence and one that you will be confronted with in the ED. The workplace unfortunately has not been spared this societal malady, and hospitals, especially emergency settings, are prime locations for violence to occur. Any ED or psychiatric emergency room should be considered a high-risk site, given its degree of acuity and potential for being seemingly chaotic. These acute care settings are a prime example of workplaces that can create or exacerbate volatile situations, ultimately ending in violent acts. Based on recent studies, thousands of assaults occur in American hospitals each year. Mental health workers are at significant risk of experiencing some form of patient-related violence. This has created a serious occupational health hazard. Studies conducted on board-certified psychiatrists have shown that they have a 5% to 48% chance of being physically assaulted by a patient during their careers. Surveys conducted on psychiatry residents found that assaults were twice as high among psychiatry residents than among medical residents. Studies have shown that 40% to 50% of psychiatry residents will be attacked physically during their 4-year training program. In a survey of psychiatry residents, two thirds felt either untrained or undertrained in dealing with violent patients.

PRESENTATION

Over the years, an increase has been reported in the number of aggressive and violent patients in the ED. Patients with homicidal ideation can be seen in a variety of ways. Staff in ED settings, including psychiatrists, will be frequently required to assess violent patients. Patients will voice threats of violence, from unspecified, vague threats ("I just feel like I want to hurt or kill someone.") to targeted homicidality of an individual ("I am going to kill my wife."). Violent patients are not a homogeneous group; although some common characteristics and risk factors/correlates are found, each case should be assessed individually. See Table 4-12.1 for factors associated with violence and Table 4-12.2 for common correlates and predictors of violence.

Table 4-12.1.   Factors associated with aggression and violence

Genetic	Possible sex chromosome abnormalities, such as XXX, XXY, or XYY. Genetic metabolic disorders, such as Sanfilipo or Vogt syndrome or phenylketonuria have been associated with aggressive personalities
Hormonal	Certain hormonal changes have been associated with onset of violent acts, such as thyroid storm or Cushing disease. Androgens, estrogens, and progestins and their regulation also have been implicated
Environmental	Unpleasant surroundings, air pollution, loud and irritating noises, and overcrowded situations can enhance the likelihood of violence
Historic	History of early violence, battered or abused as children, poor parental models, limited availability of significant others, poor schooling, and prior violent episodes are linked to violence
Interpersonal	Low frustration tolerance, direct provocation, exposure to violence
Biochemical	GABA and serotonin have been linked with impulsivity and aggression
Neurologic	Brain lesion, such as tumors, trauma, or seizures (complex partial seizures and postictal states, temporal, frontal, or limbic lesions)

GABA, γ-aminobutyric acid.

Table 4-12.2. Common correlates and predictors of violence

History	Childhood abuse or neglect
	History of suicide attempts or self-mutilation
	Prior violence and/or family violence
Age and sex	Young (13 to 25 years)
	Males
Psychiatric factors	Active symptoms of psychiatric disorders (command auditory hallucinations, paranoid delusions, psychotic disorganization of thought, excitability)
	Combination of serious mental illness and substance abuse
	Personality disorders
	Substance-related disorders (intoxication and/or withdrawal)
	IMPORTANT: Chronic alcoholism is more predictive of violence than is immediate alcohol use, and the higher the number of comorbid psychiatric disorders, the greater the rate of violence
Emotional factors	"Acting out" behavior
	Angry or rageful affect
	Emotional lability
	Irritability and/or impulsivity
	Poor frustration tolerance
Social factors	Limited or poor social supports
	Low socioeconomic status
	Medication noncompliance
Neurobiologic factors	Delirium; HIV/AIDS
	Mental retardation
	Neurologic diseases
	Seizures; structural brain abnormalities
	Traumatic brain injury

HIV, human immunodeficiency virus; AIDS, acquired immunodeficiency syndrome.

The most important is a history of violence, regardless of diagnosis, which indicates an increased risk of subsequent violent behavior.
Violence and homicidal threats are not unique symptoms seen only by a psychiatrist; they can be symptoms or findings in many other disorders. See Table 4-12.3 for primary psychiatric and nonpsychiatric disorders associated with violence. Antisocial personality disorders; alcohol or drug intoxication; borderline personality disorder; intermittent explosive disorder; mental retardation; conduct disorder; and personality change due to a general medical condition, aggressive type are just a few possible psychiatric disorders associated with violence.
The signs and symptoms you will encounter in a patient who is agitated and potentially violent are enumerated. I list them on a spectrum of severity from least agitated to outright violence. It is

Table 4-12.3.   Disorders associated with violence

Primary psychiatric disorders (DSM-IV)
 Substance-abuse disorders (alcohol-related disorders, amphetamine intoxication, inhalant intoxication, phencyclidine intoxication), antisocial personality disorders, borderline personality disorders, dementia, delirium, dissociative disorders, intermittent explosive disorders, mental retardation, conduct disorder, oppositional defiant disorder, posttraumatic stress disorders, personality change due to a general medical condition—aggressive type, premenstrual dysphoric disorder, sexual sadism, and schizophrenia, paranoid type.

Other etiologies
 Medications; intracranial pathology causing dementia, delirium, affective or psychotic syndromes, personality changes (trauma, infection, neoplasm, anatomic defect, vascular malformation, cerebrovascular accident, degenerative disease); seizure or seizure-like syndromes including behaviors occurring during ictal, postictal, and interictal periods; systemic disorders causing dementia, delirium, affective or psychotic syndromes, personality changes (metabolic, endocrine, infectious, environmental); and other specific disorders

crucial to be able to assess the patient in the earlier stages of agitation to institute some measure of containment and to deescalate the possibility of violence. The sooner you can respond and resolve the escalating violence, the safer it will be for the patient and the staff. When a patient has crossed the limit of violence and poses a threat to others, it is time to act decisively. Changes or shifts in behavior observed in the ED should be cues that escalation to full-blown violence might occur. The rule in the ED should be **ACT FAST!**

Pacing → Psychomotor agitation → Threatening remarks → Combative posture and stance → Acting-out behavior → *Violent Outcome*
Guardedness → Suspiciousness → Paranoid ideation → Paranoid delusions → Carrying or access to weapons → *Violent Outcome*
Poor impulse control or low frustration tolerance → Emotional lability → Irritability and/or impulsivity → *Violent Outcome*

Violent outcomes can be screaming, cursing, yelling, spitting, biting, throwing objects, hitting or punching at self or others, and/or attacking or assaulting behavior.

MANAGEMENT
The ED is a less than "ideal" evaluation setting, but despite the inherent environmental limitations, this is where the task of managing the violent patient will take place. The most common scenario in the ED is the arrival of a patient who either is already agitated or who becomes progressively more agitated during the wait to be seen. Other typical examples might be a patient, calmly waiting for a bed, who suddenly and surprisingly becomes agitated and combative. Other sources of agitation might be the product of

an irate patient or family member at the multiple loci of stress and apparent disorganization in a busy and loud ED. The priority in the psychiatric emergency room is the safety of patients and staff. See Table 4-12.4 for the American Psychiatric Association Task Force on Clinical Safety Guidelines. For a more thorough description of emergency behavioral management approaches, see Chapter 3.

Although no diagnostic measures are available to determine violence, we know that *past history of violence is the best predictor of future violence.* The prompt recognition of patients with histories of violence (if known to your hospital) at triage or registration is important. Many hospitals have some system to identify those patients at high risk and thus from the start take the necessary safety measures, whether that means enhanced observation status, a thorough search, or a security observation. Recognition of these patients from the outset can raise a clinician's level of awareness and minimize the possibilities of acting out and thus catching people off guard. Security removal of all weapons, whether by a manual search (as outlined earlier) or with a metal detector will vary according to each institution's policies but must be carried out.

It is imperative that the patient should be questioned directly about

- The intent to harm themselves or harm others
- Possession of a weapon
- Formulation of a definitive plan
- Recent violence
- Current alcohol or drug use
- Adherence to aftercare and medication management
- Associated psychiatric or medical conditions.

By asking these questions, the ED staff can preliminarily gather very important information and tentatively establish a relationship with the patient. The actual management of a violent patient was outlined in Chapter 3. Remember that the more aware and the higher the level of suspicion for acting-out, agitated, or violent behavior you have, the less likely it is that an explosive situation

Table 4-12.4. American Psychiatric Association task force on clinical safety guidelines

Sets forth a set of reasonable, minimal clinical standards across institutions and the legal arena for the management of violence

Does not make specific recommendations about techniques of approaching or restraining a violent patient but indicates that seclusion or restraints be considered analogous to cardiopulmonary resuscitation within the institution.

Written specific guidelines and a manual for the use of these procedures.

Approval of the guidelines by the hospital administration, legal department, and the state.

Education of staff regarding the actual policies and procedures as well as frequent in-servicing in the actual rehearsal/implementation of the techniques.

Feedback from staff regarding the guidelines, with subsequent revisions if needed.

will occur. Make certain that your space, your self, and the patient are all in order and safe. Do not be caught off guard or by surprise; keep in mind the following approaches:

- Environmental manipulation
- Deescalation techniques
- Physical restraints/seclusion
- Pharmacologic interventions (PO or IM).

An important task, once safety has been achieved, is the medical workup of the violent patients. This is fundamental to establish a diagnosis and future treatment recommendations. Disorientation, abnormal vital signs, head trauma, alteration in levels of consciousness, and no prior psychiatric history should lead you to think about "organic" causes. Even those patients with a psychiatric history should have a complete medical workup to rule out medical conditions. Consider the following: CBC, SMA-7 (especially important is glucose), calcium, CPK, alcohol and drug screen, and CT/MRI as needed. CXR, arterial blood gases (ABGs), LP, and liver- and thyroid-function tests should be ordered as clinically indicated.

Rapid tranquilization has become a standard of care that has been shown to be safe and effective. Traditional approaches use a typical antipsychotic such as haloperidol with or without the use of benzodiazepines, like lorazepam. The newer atypical agents, widely used in practice, have slower titration schedules and/or dose-limiting adverse effects that keep them from becoming first-line ED options. Newer preparations, such as oral liquid forms, rapidly dissolving tablets, and parenteral (IM) forms of olanzapine (Zyprexa) or ziprasidone (Geodon) are becoming useful alternatives for the management of violence but require more studies and experience to back up their potential use and effectiveness in the ED setting. Preliminary data suggest that these agents are better tolerated, have fewer side effects, and are effective in reducing agitation and psychosis, as well as making the transition from IM to PO easier and better tolerated.

For rapid tranquilization of different types of patients, use "cocktails," as described below—remember always to use sound clinical judgment when making these decisions. Use agents described later all in one syringe, thus avoiding the need to give an agitated or violent patient more than one IM at a time and minimizing needle-stick injuries. Titratability, rapid onset of action, and decreased side effects are important considerations for these cocktails, although strong evidence and studies to support this are limited.

Mild to Moderate Agitation / Cooperative Patient / No Psychosis:

lorazepam (Ativan) 0.5mg to 2mg PO - repeat lorazepam 1mg to 2mg PO every 30 to 60 minutes as needed until sedation.(max dose 10–15mg in 24h period)

Mild to Moderate Agitation / Cooperative Patient / Psychosis:

lorazepam (Ativan) 0.5mg to 2mg PO
or
haloperidol (Haldol) 1mg to 5mg PO
fluphenazine (Prolixin) 1mg to 5mg PO
Repeat above as needed 30 to 60 minutes as needed until sedation. (max dose 25–50mg in 24 h period)

If neuroleptic naïve add: anticholinergic agent (benztropine 0.5 to 2mg PO) to each dosing.
or
risperidone (Risperdal) 0.5 to 2mg PO
Repeat in 60 minutes as needed until sedation (max dose 6–10mg in 24h period)
or
olanzapine (Zyprexa) 2.5 to 10mg PO
Repeat in 60minutes as needed until sedation (max dose 20–30mg in 24h period)
or
quetiapine (Seroquel) 25 to 100mg PO
Repeat in 60minutes as needed until sedation (max dose 300–575mg in 24h period)
or
ziprasidone (Geodon) 10 to 20mg PO
Repeat as needed 2 to 4 hours until sedation (max dose 40mg in 24h period)
or
aripiprazole (Abilify) 10 to 15mg PO (max dose 30mg in 24 hour period)

Moderate to Severe Agitation/Cooperative/With or without psychosis:

lorazepam (Ativan) 1mg to 2mg PO or IM
[either alone or in combination]
haloperidol (Haldol) 5mg to 10mg PO or IM
or
fluphenazine (Prolixin) 5mg to 10mg PO or IM
Repeat above as needed 30 to 60minutes as needed until sedation.
If neuroleptic naïve add: anticholinergic agent (benztropine 0.5 to 2mg PO) to each dosing.
or
ziprasidone (Geodon) 10mg to 20mg PO or IM
Repeat as needed 2 to 4 hours until sedation

Moderate to Severe Agitation/Uncooperative/With or without psychosis:

lorazepam (Ativan) 1mg to 2mg IM
+
haloperidol (Haldol) 5mg to 10mg IM
or
fluphenazine (Prolixin) 5mg to 10mg IM
Repeat above as needed 30 to 60minutes as needed until sedation.
If neuroleptic naïve add: anticholinergic agent (benztropine 0.5 to 2mg PO) to each dosing.
or
ziprasidone (Geodon) 10mg to 20mg IM
Repeat as needed 2 to 4 hours until sedation

Recent studies also showed that valproate can be effective in the management of violence, with significant decreases in the violent behaviors, especially in patients with "organic" causes, dementias, mental retardation, and/or bipolar disorder, manic type.

DISPOSITION

Once behavioral control has been established, whether through verbal techniques or more-restrictive measures like acute psychopharmacologic intervention or physical restraints, a plan for aftercare must be developed. Most often, if a person has expressed homicidality or demonstrated agitation to the point of assaultive or violent behavior and has a primary psychiatric disorder, inpatient hospitalization is usually the best option. Most psychiatrists, despite the legal pressures, will admit someone with violence only if they deem that the patient will benefit from an established treatment modality. Most states have laws that allow a physician to admit, voluntarily or involuntarily, for stabilization and treatment anyone who is an imminent risk to others. Occasionally, overnight or more extended ED stays can help, especially when drugs and/or alcohol are part of the precipitating triggers. In cases of actual criminality and police custody, the patient should be transferred to a forensic psychiatric service for further assessment and subsequent management in the correctional setting. Certain patients will be deemed safe for discharge but only after careful assessment, evaluation, and monitoring, with input from the patient's family/friends. This decision should be carefully weighed and very carefully documented. Plans and strategies must be worked out with the family and patient to ensure safety and monitoring and to deal with any possible recurrence of violence.

Inefficiently managed violence, whether because of inappropriate psychopharmacologic intervention or improper implementation of physical restraints or seclusion and poor documentation, can have negative consequences and outcomes for the patient and the staff.

Remember these thoughts:

- When in doubt, admit.
- Better to be safe than sorry.
- Always be cautious.

BIBLIOGRAPHY

Allen MH, Currier GW, Hughes DH, et al. The expert consensus guideline series: treatment of behavioral emergencies. *Postgrad Med* 2001;1–90.

American Psychiatric Association Task Force on Clinician Safety, American Psychiatric Association, Tardiff K. Management of the violent patient in an emergency situation. *Psychiatr Clin North Am* 1988;11:539–549.

American Psychiatric Association. *Diagnostic and statistical manual of mental disorders.* 4th ed. Washington, DC: American Psychiatric Association, 1999.

Arana GW, Rosenbaum JF, eds. *Handbook of psychiatric drug therapy.* 4th ed. Philadelphia: Lippincott Williams & Wilkins, 2000.

Ayd FJ. Haloperidol: twenty years clinical experience. *J Clin Psych* 1978;39:807.

Bienek SA, Ownby RL, Penalver A, et al. A double-blind study of lorazepam versus the combination of haloperidol and lorazepam in managing agitation. *Pharmacotherapy* 1998;18:57–62.

Black KJ, et al. Assaults by patients on psychiatric residents at three training sites. *Hosp Community Psychiatry* 1994;45:706–710.

Bodkin JA. Emerging uses for high potency benzodiazapines in psychotic disorders. *J Clin Psych* 1990;51(suppl):41.

Braunwald E, et al., eds. *Harrison's principle of internal medicine.* 15th ed. New York: McGraw-Hill, 2001.

Breier A, Meehan K, Birkett M, et al. A double-blind, placebo-controlled dose-response comparison of intramuscular olanzapine and haloperidol in the treatment of acute agitation in schizophrenia. *Arch Gen Psychiatry* 2002;59:441–448.

Brook S, Lucey JV, Gunn KP. Intramuscular ziprasidone compared with intramuscular haloperidol in the treatment of acute psychosis: Ziprasidone I.M. Study Group. *J Clin Psychiatry* 2000;61:933–941.

Citrome L, Volvaka J. Violent patients in the emergency setting. *Psychiatr Clin North Am* 1999;23:789–801.

Clinton JE, Sterner S, Steimacheers Z, et al. Haloperidol for sedation of disruptive emergency patients. *Ann Emerg Med* 1987;16:319.

Cressman WA, Plostnieks J, Johnson PC. Absorption, metabolism, and excretion of droperidol in human subjects following IM and intravenous administration. *Anesthesiology* 1973;38:363.

Currier GW. Atypical antipsychotic medications in the psychiatric emergency service. *J Clin Psychiatry* 2000;61(suppl 14):21–26.

Currier GW, Simpson GM. Risperidone liquid concentrate and oral lorazepam versus intramuscular haloperidol and intramuscular lorazepam for treatment of psychotic agitation. *J Clin Psychiatry* 2001;62:153–157.

Currier GW, Trenton A. Pharmacological treatment of psychotic agitation. *CNS Drugs* 2002;16:219–228.

Daniel DG, Potkin SG, Reeves KR, et al. Intramuscular (IM) ziprasidone 20 mg is effective in reducing acute agitation associated with psychosis: a double-blind, randomized trial. *Psychopharmacology* 2001;155:128–134.

Donlon PT, Hopkin J, Tupin JP: Overview: safety and efficacy of rapid neuroleptization method with injectable haloperidol. *Am J Psych* 1979;136:273.

Dorland's illustrated medical dictionary. 28th ed. Philadelphia: WB Saunders, 1994.

Dubin WR, Feld JA. Rapid tranquilization of the violent patient. *Am J Emerg Med* 1989;7:313.

Harwood-Nuss AL, et al., eds. *The clinical practice of emergency medicine.* 2nd ed. Lippincott-Raven, 1996.

Hill S, Petit J. The violent patient. *Emerg Med Clin North Am* 2000;18:301–315.

Hughes DH. Acute psychopharmacological management of the aggressive psychotic patient. *Psychiatr Serv* 1999;50:1135–1137.

Hughes DH. Assessment of the potential for violence. *Psych Ann* 1994;24:579–583.

JCAHO. *Comprehensive accreditation manual for hospitals.* Oakbrook Terrace, IL: JCAHO, 1996.

Kao LW, Moore GP. The violent patient: clinical management, use of physical and chemical restraints, and medicolegal concerns. *Emerg Med Pract* 1999;1:1–23.

Kaplan HI, Sadock BJ, eds. *Comprehensive textbook of psychiatry.* 8th ed. Baltimore: Williams & Wilkins, 1999.

Kinon BJ, Roychowdhury SM, Milton DR, et al. Effective resolution with olanzapine of acute presentation of behavioral agitation and positive psychotic symptoms in schizophrenia. *J Clin Psychiatry* 2001;62(suppl 2):17–21.

Lavoi FW. Consent, involuntary treatment, and the use of force in an urban emergency department. *Ann Emerg Med* 1992;21:25–32.

Lindenmayer JP, Kotsaftis A. Use of sodium valproate in violent and aggressive behaviors: a critical review. *J Clin Psych* 2000;61:123–128.

Marx JA, Hockberger RS, Walls RM. *Rosen's emergency medicine: concepts and clinical practice.* 5th ed. St. Louis: Mosby, 2002.

Mcneil DE, et al. The role of violence in decisions about hospitalizations from the psychiatric emergency room. *Am J Psych* 1984;141:1232–1235.

Mendoza R, Djenderedjian AH, Adams J, et al. Midazolam in acute psychotic patients with hyperarousal. *J Clin Psych* 1987;48:291.

Modell JG, Lenox RH, Weiner S. Inpatient clinical trail of lorazepam for the management of manic agitation. *J Clin Psychopharmacol* 1985;5:109.

National Crime Victimization Survey (NCVS), U.S. Census Bureau, Bureau of Justice Statistics (http://www.icpsr.umich.edu/NACJD/SDA/ncvs.html).

Presley D, Robinson G. Violence in the emergency department: nurses contend with prevention in the healthcare arena. *Nurs Clin North Am* 2002;37:161–169.

Salzman C, Green A, Rodriguez-Villa F, et al. Benzodiazepines combined with neuroleptics for management of severe disruptive behavior. *Psychosomatics* 1986;27(suppl 1):17–22.

Schatzberg AF, Nemeroff CB, eds. *Textbook of psychopharmacology.* Washington, DC: American Psychiatric Press, 1995.

Schwartz TL, Park TL. Assaults by patients on psychiatric residents: a survey and training recommendations. *Psychiatr Serv* 1999;50:381–383.

Snyder W. Hospital downsizing and increased frequency of assaults on staff. *Hosp Community Psychiatry* 1994;45:378–380.

Tardiff K. Prediction of violence. *J Pract Psych Behav Health* 1998;xx:12–19.

Tintinalli JE, Kelen GD, Stapczynski JS. *Emergency medicine: a comprehensive study guide.* New York: McGraw-Hill, 2000.

Wright P, Birkett M, David SR, et al. Double-blind, placebo-controlled comparison of intramuscular olanzapine and intramuscular haloperidol in the treatment of acute agitation in schizophrenia. *Am J Psychiatry* 2001;158:1149–1151.

Chapter 4-13 Impulsivity

DEFINITION

Impulsivity is characterized by sudden spontaneous inclination or incitement to an unpremeditated or irrational action. It lies on the behavioral spectrum of aggression and violence behaviors and can be considered the outward behavioral manifestation of this emotional state.

PRESENTATION

Impulsivity, like aggression and violence, is diagnostically nonspecific and can be a manifestation of many different disorders, both psychiatric and medical. Because it lies on the spectrum of aggression/violence, it shares many of the possible associated diagnoses for those conditions. See Table 4-13.1 for a list of common psychiatric, medical, and medication- and drug-related disorders associated with impulsivity. Impulsivity can range from inappropriate acting-out behaviors such as tantrums or unprovoked fits of rage, like those seen in patients with mental retardation, to impulsive self-mutilatory behavior, as seen in patients with borderline personality disorders, to paraphilias and other types of

Table 4-13.1. Disorders associated with impulsivity

AIDS
Akathisia
Alcohol intoxication or withdrawal
Alzheimer disease
Amphetamine intoxication or amphetamine-induced psychotic disorder
Analgesics
Anticholinergic delirium
Antisocial personality disorder
Anxiolytic disinhibition
Attention deficit/hyperactivity disorder
Bipolar disorder
Borderline personality disorder
Brain tumors
Brief psychotic disorder
Cerebrovascular disease/stroke
Cocaine intoxication or cocaine-induced psychotic disorder
Conduct disorder
Delirium
Delirium, dementia, and other cognitive disorders
Delusional disorder
Encephalitis
Huntington disease
Hyper- or hypothyroidism
Hypoglycemia
Intermittent explosive disorder
Meningitis
Mental retardation
Multiple sclerosis
Oppositional defiant disorder
Parkinson disease
Porphyria
Posttraumatic stress disorder
Schizoaffective disorder
Sexual sadism
SLE
Steroid induced mood disorder (mania) or delirium
Substance-related disorders
TBI
Vitamin deficiencies
Wilson disease

AIDS, acquired immunodeficiency syndrome; SLE, systemic lupus erythematosus; TBI, traumatic brain injury.

impulse-control disorders. Additionally, impulsive behaviors can be seen in patients with hypomanic or manic episodes, oppositional defiant, conduct, attention-deficit/hyperactivity, substance-related, and antisocial personality disorders.

Most patients, when questioned, will report an increasing need to act on the impulse; the tension and pressure to do so tend to increase steadily. An inability to resist the behavior is felt, and then the patient feels relief and gratification after satisfying the impulse. Patients with these types of disorders seldom make it to the ED on their own, because their insight into and awareness of their behaviors is frequently missing. Generally, the overlap with other psychiatric disorders makes impulsivity a common symptom and one that may occasionally precipitate an ED visit, but most often, family/friends or the police/court bring these patients to the ED for an evaluation. Substance use, such as alcohol and other drugs, can increase impulsivity and get the patients into trouble and ultimately the ED. In certain people, with small amounts of alcohol, a pathologic intoxication may develop, and they become impulsive and even violent. This occurs in persons who otherwise have good impulse control and with just a small amount of alcohol become very intoxicated and act out their impulses and aggression. This is called *alcohol pathological intoxication* and can occur with confusion, disorientation, and possibly diminished recall for the event. Concerned family or friends or the police/emergency medicine service (EMS) will bring in patients after they have been in a brawl or other altercation after drinking. The patient may report transient hallucinations or illusions and the characteristic acting-out behaviors because of impulsivity. This disorder usually resolves with a deep and heavy sleep.

Individuals with *intermittent explosive disorder* recurrently fail to resist acting on their impulsive or aggressive behaviors and will, after the precipitating event or just unprovoked, destroy property or assault people. Other patients in the impulse-control disorder NOS category with kleptomania, pyromania, trichotillomania, or pathologic gambling, may, depending on the severity of their symptoms and external support network's level of concern, appear in the ED. Patients with *kleptomania* will repeatedly be unable to resist impulsive stealing of objects with no other motivation than the relief or pleasure resulting from the act of stealing. Patients with *pathologic gambling* will continue to gamble to the point that it leads to serious interference in their life. *Pyromaniacs* are unable to resist their impulses to start fires deliberately, having a fascination with fire, its consequences, and related activities, and subsequent relief or gratification. The triad of bedwetting after age 6 years, fire setting, and torturing of animals is a pathologic sign associated with future behavioral dyscontrol and violence. Patients with *trichotillomania* have the impulse to pull out their own hair, which also is followed by relief.

Paraphilias are characterized by sexual fantasies, impulses, or behaviors that involve either nonhuman objects, suffering or humiliation, children, or other nonconsenting person. These too are frequently impulsive acts, which have serious consequences for the patient and others. They are:

- Exhibitionism, surprise exposure of the person's genitals to a stranger

- Fetishism, the use of nonhuman objects to produce or enhance sexual arousal with or in the absence of a partner
- Frotteurism, touching or rubbing one's genitals against the body of a nonconsenting person
- Pedophilia, sexual activity with a child, usually age 13 or younger, or in the case of an adolescent, a child 5 years younger than the perpetrator
- Masochism, being beaten, humiliated, bound, or tortured to enhance or achieve sexual excitement
- Sadism, infliction of pain, suffering, or humiliation to enhance or achieve sexual excitement
- Transvestic fetishism, heterosexual men dressing in women's clothes (cross-dressing) to produce or enhance sexual arousal, usually without a real partner, but occasionally with the fantasy that the man is the female partner
- Voyeurism, the observing of an unknowing and nonconsenting person, usually unclothed and/or engaged in sexual activity, to produce sexual excitement.

Borderline personality disorder is the most common personality disorder in the clinical setting and often goes either incorrectly diagnosed or underdiagnosed. It affects close to 2% of the general population, 3 times more women than men, and causes significant interpersonal distress and functional impairment in addition to being associated with self-destructive behaviors and suicides—8% to 10% of patients with borderline personality disorder go on to commit suicide. These patients exhibit extreme instability in their relationships, emotional state, and self-image; having marked impulsivity that places them at serious risk of harm. These impulsive or behavioral dyscontrolled symptoms, which may be chronic, include:

- Impulsive aggression
- Self-mutilation
- Self-damaging behavior (i.e., risky sexual activities, such as unprotected sex, promiscuity, substance abuse, shoplifting, and reckless driving and spending)
- Bingeing and purging
- Frequent suicide attempt/gestures
- Provocative behaviors that may incite assaults.

These behaviors and affect states can be easily precipitated by a change or a stressor; these may include things such as a disruption in the patient's relationships, feeling abandoned, change in clinician, feeling betrayed, feeling unjustly accused, or feeling seriously misunderstood or blamed. These situations can drive a patient into a rage and may precipitate an ED visit, usually in the context of intense suicidality or even a gesture.

Violence can be seen as well, usually hurling objects, breaking things, physical assaults, especially common and with worse outcomes if there are associated antisocial traits.

Patients with borderline personality disorder and substance abuse have poorer outcomes, with higher risks of suicide and death or injury from accidents. Substance abuse actually lowers their threshold for impulsive behaviors, and these patients tend to minimize or hide substance abuse.

Some patients who are neither mentally retarded, borderline, nor psychotic repeatedly and impulsively self-mutilate. Although mainly seen in women, self-mutilation can be seen in men in prison. A sense of relief results after the cutting, burning, head or limb banging, biting or chewing self, and picking at wounds, all of which seem to provide a self-soothing outlet for the patient.

Patients with *antisocial personality disorder* regularly disregard and violate the rights of others; they may be aggressive or destructive, usually impulsive, with frequent breaking of laws or rules, being deceitful, stealing, and showing little or no remorse for their behaviors.

Adults as well as adolescents with *attention-deficit/hyperactivity disorder* (ADHD) can, because of the hyperactivity, be very impulsive. This impulsivity can have a motor component as well as a cognitive component; the lack of self-control and subsequent acting-out behaviors are a hallmark and may prompt an ED visit. Close to 60% of childhood ADHD persists into adulthood and must be assessed carefully. These children or adults have a very hard time regulating their impulses and motor behavior. Adults with ADHD have many other comorbid psychiatric disorders, such as depression, anxiety, and personality and substance-abuse disorders, which can confound the clinical picture at times. Adults with ADHD will have motor hyperactivity, difficulties concentration and paying attention, mood lability (often being labeled temperamental or hot tempered), emotionally overreactive, disorganized and unable to complete tasks, and impulsive. They also exhibit stubbornness, conflicts with authority, interpersonal problems, employment instability, poor frustration tolerance, and overall, a feeling of being overwhelmed. Misdiagnosis in these cases is quite common, negatively affecting outcomes and prognosis.

Closely related to this disorder are those children/adolescents with *oppositional defiant disorder* or *conduct disorder* (CD), who may be brought to the ED by a parent or other caretaker/agency. These patients are impulsive and act out, thus getting themselves into trouble and precipitating an ED visit. The families of these patients come seeking a solution to the problematic behaviors and impulsivity, often unrealistically hoping for a quick solution. These visits are commonly precipitated by major crises in the life of the family because of these behaviors. Families often request hospitalization or placement because they feel overwhelmed and unable to control their children. Some known factors are strongly predictive of future delinquency in adolescents with CD; these include past offenses, antisocial peers, limited social network, early substance use, male sex, early aggression, low socioeconomic status (SES), risk-taking behaviors, impulsivity, poor academic performance, early medical traumas, large family size, severe family stressors, dysfunctional home life, abusive parents, and parents with antisocial features.

Patients with hypomania or mania are characteristically more impulsive, and if they are grandiose and have elated mood can frequently engage in "pleasurable activities that have a high potential for painful consequences," such as reckless driving, sexual promiscuity, or spending sprees. This impulsiveness is usually accompanied by many other signs and symptoms of bipolar illness and is a common reason for a psychiatry ED visit.

MANAGEMENT

Every patient's ability to remain in control of his or her behavior and impulses should be assessed. Impulse control is part of the

MSE and a critical component in the ED. It is a gauge of a person's ability to understand the established societal parameters and limitations, as well as a direct indication of dangerousness to self or others. Determining a person's impulse control is done through indirect and direct observation of the patient's current and past behaviors. History of their actions and behaviors can help in the assessment. Can the patient control the sexual or aggressive impulses without acting on them? If the patient acted on them, what precipitated the impulse? What were some contributing factors? Could anything have stopped them from acting on the impulses? Can the patients control themselves while in the ED or if necessary in the hospital? These important questions must be answered to assure safety for the staff and the patient. **Impulsivity is a harbinger of possible violence—internally or externally directed—and must be assessed and addressed quickly to decrease the likelihood of its occurring.**

A complete medical, psychiatric, and neurologic workup is fundamental to rule out other underlying causes for these behaviors. Seizures (preictal, ictal, or postictal states) can be accompanied by impulsive behavior and mistaken for a primary psychiatric disorder. For example, pathologic intoxication may occur more often in elderly patients taking sedative/hypnotics, patients that are more tired or anxious when they drink, and those with a history of poor impulse control. Intermittent explosive disorder is more common in younger males, with serious current and past psychosocial stressors as well as a history of prior impulsive behaviors. These patients may report an aura-like sensation before their loss of control.

In general, the approach to any of these patients remains similar, in that a calm and reassuring manner is the key, taking into account safety precautions that you would take when confronted with someone who may be potentially explosive or violent. Restraints, seclusion, and psychopharmacologic interventions are all viable if the behavior continues to escalate. Consider the use of benzodiazepines PO/IM for the management of the impulsivity; neuroleptics can be tried in conjunction as well, if the benzodiazepines do not provide the desired effect. Self-destructive and impulsive behaviors may be a way for certain patients to contain their intense emotional upheavals, which is why it is important to maintain very firm limits in the ED.

We know that an important immediate and serious risk factor for suicide is impulsivity (along with anxiety, panic, and depression). It is quite important to inquire about self-mutilatory or wrist-cutting behavior. This can point in the direction of the spectrum of mood, anxiety, dissociative, or personality disorder illnesses, thus indicating a treatment option. A history of trauma or abuse also can be an important clue. More commonly, self-mutilatory or wrist-cutting behaviors are self-soothing acts with little or no intent to die, although these patients can eventually kill themselves. Ask the patients with self-mutilatory or wrist-cutting behavior if this helps calm them or relieve their anxiety. Look for scars in places that are not exposed, such as the inner arms or thighs or abdomen.

Accurate and thorough evaluation of comorbid conditions is crucial, especially in adults with impulsive behaviors. In adults with ADHD and because of the high levels of comorbid conditions, it is imperative to address all these factors and recommend a course of action, providing psychoeducation about the disorders and treatment alternatives. Treatment will be outpatient and consists of stimulant medications, as in children, and occasionally with SSRI antidepressants as well. Mixed amphetamine salts (Adderall), methylphenidate (Ritalin or Concerta), and pemoline (Cylert) are all useful in the outpatient treatment of ADHD.

In patients with paraphilias, care must be taken to assess that no one is imminently at risk, especially children. In these cases, thought must be given to appropriate management and notification; legal counsel may be needed to advise on how best to deal with these patients. Patients with impulse-control disorders might benefit form short-acting benzodiazepines in the ED, and a referral to a specialized center/clinic or psychiatrist can be of great benefit.

Family psychoeducation and meetings in the ED are helpful when dealing with difficult adolescents and may help set priorities for the issues and empower the family to make necessary (often quite difficult) decisions pertaining to their child/adolescent. Recommendations for aftercare are important, as well as for local agencies (even judicial) that deal with these types of adolescents or give parents recourse in dealing with them.

DISPOSITION

As stated earlier, safety assessment is crucial when dealing with patients with poor impulse control. In general, many of these patients with serious psychiatric conditions may require inpatient psychiatric hospitalization. Several factors may assist in making that determination:

- Behaviors that are considered too impulsive and dangerous and cannot be managed at the outpatient level
- Nonadherence with aftercare plans and medications, resulting in deterioration of the patient's clinical condition
- Serious psychiatric or medical comorbidities that require further evaluation and treatment, which cannot be performed or sustained at the outpatient level
- Significant social, occupational, or interpersonal functional impairments
- Imminent danger to self or others, with increased suicidal ideation or serious suicide attempts
- Other variables, such as associated psychosis, substance abuse or dependence, or others that would impair their judgment.

BIBLIOGRAPHY

American Psychiatric Association Clinical Resources. *Practice guidelines for the treatment of patients with borderline PD.* Washington, DC: American Psychiatric Association, 1999.

American Psychiatric Association. *Diagnostic and statistical manual of mental disorders.* 4th ed, 4-TR. Washington, DC: American Psychiatric Association, 1999.

Arana GW, Rosenbaum JF, eds. *Handbook of psychiatric drug therapy.* 4th ed. Philadelphia: Lippincott Williams & Wilkins, 2000.

Bassarath L. Conduct disorder: a biopsychosocial review. *Can J Psych* 2001;46:609–616.

Dorland's illustrated medical dictionary. 28th ed. Philadelphia: WB Saunders, 1994.

Elliott H. Attention deficit hyperactivity disorder in adults: a guide for the primary care physician. *South Med J* 2002;95:736–742.

Fawcett J. Treating impulsivity and anxiety in the suicidal patient. *Ann N Y Acad Sci* 2001;932:94–102.

Gallagher R, Blader J. The diagnosis and neuropsychological assessment of adult attention deficit/hyperactivity disorder: scientific study and practical guidelines. *Ann N Y Acad Sci* 2001;931:148–171.

Hollander E, Buchalter AJ, DeCaria CM. Pathological gambling. *Psychiatr Clin North Am* 2000;23:629–642.

Horrigan J, Barnhill J. Low-dose amphetamine salts and adult attention deficit hyperactivity disorder. *J Clin Psych* 2000;61:414–417.

Kaplan HI, Sadock BJ, eds. *Comprehensive textbook of psychiatry.* 8th ed. Baltimore: Williams & Wilkins, 1999.

Murphy KR, Barkley RA, Bush T. Young adults with attention deficit hyperactivity disorder: subtype differences in comorbidity, educational, and clinical history. *J Nerv Ment Disord* 2002;190:147–157.

O'Sullivan RL, Mansueto CS, Lerner EA, et al. Characterization of trichotillomania: a phenomenological model with clinical relevance to obsessive-compulsive spectrum disorders. *Psychiatr Clin North Am* 2000;23:587–604.

Paterson R, Douglas C, Hallmayer J, et al. A randomized double-blind, placebo controlled trial of dextroamphetamine in adults with attention deficit hyperactivity disorder. *Aust N Z J Psychiatry* 1999;33:494–502.

Rouse JD. Borderline and other dramatic personality disorders in the psychiatric emergency services. *Psych Ann* 1994;24:598–602.

Santosh PJ, Taylor E. Stimulant drugs. *Eur Child Adolesc Psychiatry* 2000;(suppl 1):27–43.

Schatzberg AF, Nemeroff CB, eds. *Textbook of psychopharmacology.* Washington, DC: American Psychiatric Press, 1995.

Spencer T, Wilens TE, Biederman J, et al. A double-blind, crossover comparison of methylphenidate and placebo in adults with childhood-onset attention deficit hyperactivity disorder. *Arch Gen Psychiatry* 1995;52:434–443.

Spencer T, Biederman J, Wilens T, et al. Adults with attention-deficit/hyperactivity disorder: a controversial diagnosis. *J Clin Psych* 1998;59(suppl):59–68.

Ward MF, Wender PH, Reimherr FW. The Wender Utah Rating Scale: an aid in the retrospective diagnosis of attention deficit hyperactivity disorder. *Am J Psych* 1993;150:885–890.

Chapter 4-14 Intoxication Phenomenon

DEFINITION

Intoxication phenomena are the changes in physiological and psychological functioning, mood state, cognitive process, behavioral, social and occupational functioning, or all of these, as a consequence of short-term ingestion of a substance or drug (to be used interchangeably) or psychoactive or psychotropic medications. These changes are directly related to the substance's effect on the CNS.

Drugs are considered nonfood chemical substances or preparations that are used for therapeutic purposes (medications) or for pleasure (recreational drug); many drugs (e.g., morphine, diazepam, amphetamine, nitrous oxide) can be used for either of these two purposes. The Drug Enforcement Agency (DEA) has classified, according to schedules, some drugs judged as having abuse potential. These "controlled substances" are drugs judged to have potential for abuse and are restricted under the law; they are divided into five schedules according to their potential for abuse, their accepted medical uses, their safety, and their potential for dependence. See Appendix B for a partial list of some DEA Controlled Substances by Schedule.

PRESENTATION

A large number of patients seen in the ED either have a history of substance abuse or dependence or may be intoxicated—estimates range from 30% to 90%. Even before a full interview, if it is suspected or obvious that a patient is under the influence of a drug, the patient must be questioned so that appropriate care can commence even before the workup. This is necessary to anticipate any untoward events that can occur from drug intoxication such as delirium, withdrawal phenomenon, or violent behavior. Additionally, the patient must be questioned about the amount of use in the event that an overdose may have occurred. In this instance, the patient may require immediate medical attention. Patients can have an alteration in their level of consciousness and cognition that developed rapidly, either during substance intoxication or related to a particular medication use. These patients need immediate medical attention as well.

Of the varying substances of abuse, each has a unique and characteristic intoxication phenomenon and presentations. Most patients that are acutely intoxicated, either brought to the ED by others—including the police or EMT—or walk in on their own, have chief complaints that focus on a manifestation of their intoxication phenomenon, such as psychomotor activation with cocaine intoxication or hallucinations with lysergic acid diethylamide (LSD) or phencyclidine (PCP) intoxication. Keep in mind that many patients may use more than one substance or use other substances to enhance or mitigate the "bad" effects of their "drug of choice."

Chronic alcohol and drug users are known to use ED services repeatedly, primarily because of their lack of adequate access to primary care, as well as the inherent medical complications they have, often exacerbated by intoxication and related injuries and accidents. These patients stretch the ED resources, dramatically increase healthcare costs, contribute to overcrowding, and tax the staff, creating a less than conducive environment for their bona fide needs to be addressed and managed adequately.

Intoxicated children and adolescents coming to an ED are commonly inadequately assessed, managed, documented, and properly referred. Education of staff about these presentations can assist in improving the detection and management of these patients.

All drug-intoxication states must be preceded by recent ingestion or exposure to the specified drug with consequent maladaptive behavioral or psychological changes with a series of characteristic signs and symptoms that develop shortly afterward. See Table 4-14.1 for a list of drugs classified as psychedelics or "mind-altering" drugs—a group of drugs that produce perceptual alterations with intact reality testing. Following the DSM classification of substances into 11 classes, these are the common acute intoxication presentations for each class (except for nicotine, which does not have a reported specific intoxication phenomenon). Although the agents are not listed, psychiatric patients frequently abuse anticholinergic agents. These medications cause a stimulating effect, which may help to alleviate feelings of depression, negative symptoms of the illness, or just cause a high. Many times these agents are used in combination with alcohol and drugs of abuse.

Alcohol Intoxication

Alcohol use and abuse is a serious public health problem, with high rates of morbidity and mortality—more than 100,000 deaths/year. Alcohol remains the most common substance used by patients who use the ED for services. Patients may have symptoms of alcohol use anywhere on the spectrum, from drinkers "at risk" for injury and illness (driving while intoxicated) all the way through patients with serious alcohol-related problems and dependence. Patients with alcohol intoxication may exhibit inappropriate sexual or aggressive behavior, mood lability, impaired judgment, impaired social or occupational functioning, with the following signs developing during or shortly after alcohol use:

1. Slurred speech
2. Incoordination
3. Unsteady gait
4. Nystagmus
5. Impairment in attention or memory
6. Stupor or coma.

Amphetamine or Similarly Acting Sympathomimetic Intoxication

After recent use of amphetamines or a related substance (e.g., methylphenidate), patients can have euphoria or affective blunting; changes in sociability; hypervigilance; interpersonal sensitivity; anxiety, tension, or anger; stereotyped behaviors; impaired judgment; perceptual disturbances; or impaired social or occupational functioning, with two (or more) of the following signs, developing during or shortly after use of an amphetamine or a related substance:

1. Tachycardia or bradycardia
2. Pupillary dilation
3. Elevated or reduced blood pressure
4. Perspiration or chills
5. Nausea or vomiting
6. Evidence of weight loss
7. Psychomotor agitation or retardation
8. Muscular weakness, respiratory depression, chest pain, or cardiac arrhythmias
9. Confusion, seizures, dyskinesias, dystonias, or coma.

Table 4-14.1.   Psychedelic drugs

Category	Drug(s)
Anticholinergics	Antihistamines Cyclic antidepressants Phenothiazines Belladonna alkaloids (jimson weed, mandrake, henbane, deadly nightshade, matrimony vine)
Arylhexylamines	Phencyclidine (PCP) and congeners Ketamine
Cocaine	Cocaine
Ergot-based compounds	D-Lysergic acid diethylamide Convolvulaceae (morning glory family) Argyreia (wood rose)
Indolealkylamines	Peyote (cactus) Psilocybin (mushroom) Psilocin (mushroom)
Miscellaneous plants	Yohimbine Catnip Juniper Kava kava Nutmeg Periwinkle Maté
Mushrooms	Psilocybin/psilocin Muscarine Ibotenic acid/muscimol
Opioids	Pentazocine Meperidine analogues
Phenylethylamines	Mescaline Methamphetamine TMA-2 (2,4,5-trimethoxyamphetamine) DOM/STP (dimethoxyamphetamine) PMA (*para*-methoxyamphetamine) DOB (4-bromo-2,5-dimethoxyamphetamine) 2CB/MFT (4-bromo-2,5-methoxyphenyl-ethylamine) MDA (methylenedioxyamphetamine) MDMA (methylenedioxymethamphetamine) MDEA (methylenedioxyethamphetamine) MMDA (methoxymethylenedioxyamphetamine)
Tetrahydro-cannabinols (THCs)	Marijuana Hashish

Caffeine Intoxication

Rarely is someone seen in an ED with complaints of caffeine intoxication, although they may have some of the following signs and symptoms that may be confused for another medical condition. Patients with caffeine intoxication have had a recent consumption of caffeine, in excess of 250 mg (e.g., more than 2 to 3 cups of brewed coffee) and five (or more) of the following signs, developing during, or shortly after, caffeine use:

1. Restlessness
2. Nervousness
3. Excitement
4. Insomnia
5. Flushed face
6. Diuresis
7. GI disturbance
8. Muscle twitching
9. Rambling flow of thought and speech
10. Tachycardia or cardiac arrhythmia
11. Periods of inexhaustibility
12. Psychomotor agitation.

Cannabis Intoxication

Marijuana is the second most used drug in the United States. Patients will exhibit impaired motor coordination, euphoria, anxiety, sensation of slowed time, impaired judgment, social withdrawal, with two (or more) of the following signs, developing within 2 hours of cannabis use:

1. Conjunctival injection
2. Increased appetite
3. Dry mouth
4. Tachycardia.

Cocaine Intoxication

Patients with cocaine intoxication will usually be chronic users and have euphoria or affective blunting; changes in sociability; hypervigilance; perceptual disturbances; interpersonal sensitivity; anxiety, tension, or anger; stereotyped behaviors; impaired judgment; or impaired social or occupational functioning; with two (or more) of the symptoms listed developing during, or shortly after, cocaine use. They are often overwhelmed, irritable, feeling panicky, paranoid with occasional auditory and visual hallucinations, and very dysphoric. This state of desperation can precipitate intense suicidal ideation and even violence. Symptoms of intoxication include:

1. Tachycardia or bradycardia
2. Pupillary dilation
3. Elevated or reduced blood pressure
4. Perspiration or chills
5. Nausea or vomiting
6. Evidence of weight loss
7. Psychomotor agitation or retardation
8. Muscular weakness, respiratory depression, chest pain, or cardiac arrhythmias
9. Confusion, seizures, dyskinesias, dystonias, or coma.

Hallucinogen Intoxication

Hallucinogens are still widely used and popular drugs, especially among adolescents and young adults. LSD or "acid" is one of the major drugs that make up this class and a potent mood-altering chemical. LSD comes in tablets, capsules, and liquid form, added to absorbent blotter paper and divided into small squares with colorful, cartoon-like (Beavis and Butthead, Bart Simpson, etc.) designs. The patients' response is rather variable and idiosyncratic and dependent on the amount taken. They may have marked anxiety or depression, ideas of reference, fear of losing one's mind, paranoid ideation, impaired judgment, or impaired social or occupational functioning. These experiences are called "trips," and an adverse reaction is called a "bad trip," which usually resolves after 12 hours. They also complain of perceptual changes occurring in a state of full wakefulness and alertness (e.g., subjective intensification of perceptions, depersonalization, derealization, illusions, hallucinations, or synesthesias) that developed during, or shortly after, hallucinogen use. Patients also may complain, days or even years after LSD use, of flashback experiences, which are sudden in onset and very frightening. Additionally, these patients will have two (or more) of the following signs:

1. Pupillary dilation
2. Tachycardia
3. Sweating
4. Palpitations
5. Blurring of vision
6. Tremors
7. Incoordination.

Inhalant Intoxication

Inhalants can cause irreversible physical and mental damage, including loss of sense of smell; nausea and nosebleeds; and liver, lung, and kidney problems. Inhalants can cause tachycardia and arrhythmias by starving the body of oxygen. Prolonged use can develop muscle wasting and reduced muscle tone and strength. Inhalants can be deadly, even with the first-time use, causing death by suffocation, choking on vomit, or heart attack. Inhalants include numerous household and commercial products (glue, paint thinner) that can be abused by sniffing or "huffing" (inhaling through one's mouth) for an intoxicating effect. Patients will exhibit belligerence, assaultiveness, apathy, impaired judgment, or impaired social or occupational functioning that developed during, or shortly after, use of or exposure to volatile inhalants—excluding anesthetic gases and short-acting vasodilators—and two (or more) of the following signs, developing during, or shortly after, inhalant use or exposure:

1. Dizziness
2. Nystagmus
3. Incoordination
4. Slurred speech
5. Unsteady gait
6. Lethargy
7. Depressed reflexes

8. Psychomotor retardation
9. Tremor
10. Generalized muscle weakness
11. Blurred vision or diplopia
12. Stupor or coma
13. Euphoria

Opioids

After an initial opioid rush, users experience alternately wakeful and drowsy states, often feeling drowsy for several hours. Because of the depression of the CNS, mental functioning becomes clouded, and breathing may become slowed to the point of respiratory failure. Traditionally these patients have initial euphoria followed by apathy, dysphoria, psychomotor agitation or retardation, impaired judgment, or impaired social or occupational functioning, as well as pupillary constriction (or pupillary dilation due to anoxia from severe overdose) and one (or more) of the following signs, developing during or shortly after opioid use:

1. Drowsiness or coma
2. Slurred speech
3. Impairment in attention or memory.

Phencyclidine or Similar-Acting Arylcyclohexylamines

Patients may show belligerence, assaultiveness, impulsiveness, unpredictability, psychomotor agitation, impaired judgment, or impaired social or occupational functioning that developed within an hour (less when smoked, "snorted," or used IV), and two (or more) of the following signs:

1. Vertical or horizontal nystagmus
2. Hypertension or tachycardia
3. Numbness or diminished responsiveness to pain
4. Ataxia
5. Dysarthria
6. Muscle rigidity
7. Seizures or coma
8. Hyperacusis.

Sedatives, Hypnotics, and Anxiolytics

Patients may experience inappropriate sexual or aggressive behavior, mood lability, impaired judgment, impaired social or occupational functioning, with one (or more) of the following signs, developing during or shortly after sedative, hypnotic, or anxiolytic use:

1. Slurred speech
2. Incoordination
3. Unsteady gait
4. Nystagmus
5. Impairment in attention or memory
6. Stupor or coma.

These are the commonly ascribed signs and symptoms of intoxicated persons. Pure intoxication with one substance is harder to see now, and patients will typically have intoxication from multiple substances, making the presentation confusing and more complex. An additionally confounding problem in certain EDs is the increase in abuse of "club drugs" and their impact on patients' immediate presentations. "Club drugs" is a general term used for certain illicit substances, primarily synthetic, that are usually found at nightclubs, bars, and raves (all-night dance parties). The number of ecstasy or methylenedioxymethamphetamine (MDMA) ED mentions reported to the Drug Abuse Warning Network (DAWN) increased 58% from 1999 to 2000. The number of γ-hydroxybutyrate-related (GHB) ED mentions totaled 4,969, and the number of ketamine mentions totaled 263 in 2000. These both represent significant increases since 1994, when 56 GHB mentions and 19 ketamine mentions were recorded. The pharmacokinetics of MDMA and GHB are considered nonlinear, making any estimate of a dose–response very difficult to gauge in the ED.

Club drugs:

MDMA/MDA (X, Ecstasy, E, hug drug, M&M, XTC, Adam, Clarity, Lover's Speed.)

GHB (Georgia home boy, liquid ecstasy, somatomax, scoop, liquid X, soap, easy lay, cherry meth, salty water, organic quaalude, grievous bodily harm)

Rohypnol (Roofies, rophies, roach, rope or date rape drug)

Ketamine (K, Special K, vitamin K, ketaset, super K, jet, super acid, special LA coke)

Methamphetamine (ice, speed, crank, crystal, glass, meth, chalk)

Numerous dangers are associated with the use of club drugs.

- MDMA has hallucinogenic and amphetamine-like properties, and MDA is the parent compound, which also is abused. Evidence exists that it can cause confusion, depression, insomnia, cravings, anxiety, and paranoia. Psychosis has been reported as well. Muscle tension, involuntary teeth clenching (lollipops are used to counter this effect), nausea, blurred vision, faintness, chills, and sweating are commonly reported. It can cause tachycardia and hypertension, which can lead to heart or kidney failure. It can cause severe hyperthermia from the combination of the drug's stimulant effect with the often hot, crowded atmosphere of a rave. Ecstasy users also may have long-term brain injury. Research has shown that MDMA/MDA can cause damage to the parts of the brain that are critical to thought and memory and can cause long-lasting brain serotonin depletion in rats, apparently as a result of terminal degeneration of serotonin neurons. Coma, profound hyperpyrexia, disseminated intravascular coagulopathy, rhabdomyolysis, and acute renal failure have occurred in young adults who use ecstasy. Acne-like rash in people who use MDMA may be a harbinger of underlying liver damage. Such a presentation can resemble neuroleptic malignant syndrome (NMS) or serotonin syndrome.
- GHB and Rohypnol are CNS depressants that are often connected with drug-facilitated sexual assault, rape, and robbery. These drugs cause muscle relaxation, loss of consciousness, and an inability to remember what happened during the hours after ingesting the drug. Rohypnol's trade name is flunitrazepam, a benzodiazepine that is banned in the United States (Rivotril in Mexico). The sedative/hypnotic effect, muscle relaxation, and

amnesia can be exacerbated with the use of alcohol and even can be lethal, because of withdrawal seizures. Additionally, they can cause physical and psychological dependence. Recently more reports have been noted of clonazepam (Klonopin) being sold as a substitute or as an aid to enhance the effects of heroin or other opiates. GHB is a popular dietary supplement and recreational drug and has euphoric, sedative, and anabolic effects. GHB is used in nightclubs for similar effects, although being a liquid, it is harder for the individual to gauge the amount used or the amount required to reach the desired effect, so overdoses are common. When it is mixed with alcohol, nausea and difficulty breathing can occur; seizure and coma have been reported, especially when it is combined with methamphetamines. ED presentations for intoxication with these substances are increasing. Several congeners of GHB have emerged on the scene; these include γ-butyrolactobe and 1,4-butanediol. These substances are being abused and show intoxication phenomena similar to those of GHB.

- Ketamine, a PCP derivative, is a dissociative anesthetic, used in animals and for conscious sedation; its abuse has increased dramatically. Ketamine is used in venues similar to those of MDMA or GHB and can cause impaired motor function, high blood pressure, amnesia, seizures, and respiratory depression. It is taken most often in a powdered form, smoked, mixed in drinks, or snorted, but can be used IM and even IV. The effects are rapid and have a short duration. Patients have nystagmus, mydriasis, agitation, slurred speech, floating-like sensation, rigidity, anxiety, vivid dreams or hallucinations, and even seizures. The dissociative-like or out-of-body experiences are called "K-holes" or "K-land." Several days after ingestion, patients may experience persisting memory impairments.
- Methamphetamine is a powerfully addictive stimulant that dramatically affects the CNS. It is a white, odorless, bitter-tasting powder that is easily dissolved in liquids or easily snorted, smoked, taken orally, or injected. An initial brief but pleasurable "rush" or "flash" is followed by agitation, and in some individuals, this can lead to violence. Because of this, a binge/crash pattern of use results, and tolerance develops almost immediately. Increased energy and alertness, decreased appetite, convulsions, high body temperature, shaking, stroke, seizures, and cardiac arrhythmia are all symptomatic of methamphetamine abuse. Its use is a substantial problem in many areas of the United States and a frequent ED complaint. Illegal production of methamphetamine with lead acetate as a reagent and other contaminants has the potential risk of acute lead poisoning. Many IV users of methamphetamine will have similar risk factors for HIV/AIDS and hepatitis B and C because of needle sharing.

Because club drugs are illegal and are often produced in unsanitary laboratories, it is impossible for the users to know exactly what they are taking; quality and potency can vary significantly from batch to batch. Additionally, substitute drugs are sometimes sold in place of club drugs without the user's knowledge. For example, PMA (*para*-methoxyamphetamine) has been used as a substitute for MDMA. When users take PMA thinking they are really ingesting MDMA, they often think they have taken weak ecstasy because PMA's effects take longer to appear. They then ingest more of the substance to attain a better high, which can result in overdose death.

MANAGEMENT

Priorities are to determine the patient's stability, to identify the drugs used, to treat toxic effects as they manifest, and to institute behavioral management as needed. It is always important to gauge the patient's level of use; do they meet criteria for abuse or dependence for a particular substance(s). Assessing this will facilitate not only the management but also the treatment and disposition.

Substance Abuse Criteria: Use resulting in a failure to fulfill major role obligations at work, school, or home; use in physically hazardous situations; use resulting in recurrent legal problems; and use despite persistent or recurrent social or interpersonal problems.

Substance Dependence Criteria: Tolerance (need for markedly increased amounts of substance to achieve intoxication or desired effect, or markedly diminished effect with continued use of same amount of substance) and withdrawal (substance-specific syndrome details); substance taken in larger amounts or over longer periods than intended; persistent desire or unsuccessful effort to reduce or control substance use; too much time spent in activities obtaining, using, or recovering from substance effects; important social, occupational, or recreational activities given up or reduced; use despite persistent or recurrent physical or psychological problems caused or exacerbated by substance.

Gather history on types of alcohol or drugs used, amounts used, route of use, age at onset of first use, means of obtaining the drugs, setting used, consequences of use, family history of drug use, prior drug treatments, and medical and psychiatric history. Ask about abuse or misuse of anticholinergic or other prescribed medication. Remember that many prescription drugs have a resale value on the street, and a black market exists for these agents. It is important to gauge the longest period of sobriety ever obtained; this will assist in making a determination for the aftercare level of services required. Remember to ask specifically about the amount, especially of alcohol; "three beers" might not sound like a lot until you inquire about the actual size of the beer, which may be 40 ounces, making 120 ounces of alcohol, a lot of alcohol. The number of bags of heroin or cocaine is important to inquire about as well.

Most alcohol and drug users will rarely make use of established medical services, relying on EDs as *de facto* primary care settings and most often a major entry point into the healthcare system. Additionally, many physicians are not too familiar with the significant morbidity and mortality of alcohol and drugs and their roles as an etiologic factor in accidents and crimes. Alcohol dependence and intoxication are important risk factors for suicide—25% of alcoholics commit suicide—usually as part of the alcohol's effects on increasing a patient's level of distress, increasing aggressivity, and limited and/or impaired cognition and judgment. Violence and acute alcohol intoxication can be related, and more than 50% of those convicted of homicides are alcoholics. This is why the diagnosis, management, and prevention through treatment of these disorders are so crucial in the ED. Despite much evidence on the high prevalence of alcohol and drug abuse in ED samples, the appropriate assessments and referrals are seldom achieved. In a recent study, fewer than 5% of patients admitted to an ED with alcohol intoxication were referred for ongoing treatment. Contrary to what many ED physicians may believe, screening and brief interventions in the ED can be effective. The ED must be seen as an opportunity to intervene—a "teachable moment"— and make a difference in the patient's life and drinking habits. Some reports indicate that making an effort and linking patients to aftercare plans is effective from the ED (see Table 4-14.4 for a summary of ED brief interventions).

Monitor vital signs, assess for changes in level of consciousness, evidence of head trauma, needle tracks and abscess, and other physical signs of intoxication. Complete a physical examination; obtain laboratory and alcohol levels, urine or serum toxicology examination, and other diagnostic tests as clinically warranted. Blood alcohol levels (BALs) are usually reliable indicators of serum alcohol concentration (in milligrams per deciliter) but are greatly affected by individual variables, such as weight, amount and speed of alcohol consumption, time since last drink, metabolic clearance of alcohol, and presence of food. See Table 4-14.2 for a chart on BAL and clinical findings. An average person will be able to reduce their BAL by 15 mg/dL/hr, whereas a chronic alcohol drinker can metabolize about 30 mg/dL/hour. Women usually have higher alcohol levels and lower thresholds for intoxication. In patients who are tolerant, BALs of greater than 250 can have minimal clinical findings, and patients with BAL of greater than 150 and no intoxication phenomenon indicate alcoholism.

Barring serious medical complications and need for support- ive or resuscitative measure, a thorough and orderly history with physical and laboratory examinations is indicated. A reli- able history is oftentimes difficult, and reliance on collateral sources of information might be the key. Determining the quan- tity and frequency of substance use will assist in determining

Table 4-14.2.   Blood alcohol levels

Blood Alcohol Level		Clinical Findings (Nontolerant Patient)
%	mg/dl	
0.03	30	None (one drink)
0.05	50	Mild coordination problems Inattention Unsteadiness (two drinks)
0.10	100	Impaired memory Romberg + (eyes open) (four to five drinks)
0.20	200	Stupor
0.25	250	Anesthesia
>0.35	350	Respiratory arrest

abuse or dependence and other possible dysfunctional behaviors. Many questionnaires and screening tools are available for detection of alcoholism and abuse, including certain laboratory results and urine toxicology. See Table 4-14.3 for urine toxicology screen and detectability. Screening for alcohol problems in the ED might include these easy, simple-to-use questionnaires:

• *NIAAA Quantity and Frequency Questions*
On average, how many days per week do you drink alcohol?
On a typical day when you drink, how many drinks do you have?
What is the maximum number of drinks you had on any given occasion during the last month?

• *CAGE* Have you ever . . .
. . . thought you should **C**UT back on your drinking? (C)
. . . felt **A**NNOYED by people criticizing your drinking? (A)
. . . felt **G**UILTY or bad about your drinking? (G)
. . . had a morning **E**YE-OPENER to relieve hangover or nerves? (E)

Screen as positive if there is an affirmative response to one or more CAGE questions and/or consumption in men is more than 14 drinks/week or more than four drinks/occasion; in women, more than seven drinks/week or more than three drinks/occasion, and in patients older than 65 years, more than seven drinks/week or more than three drinks/occasion.

Alcohol intoxication, when serious, will require more than just a bed and periodic monitoring. Remember to lay the patient face down or on the side to avoid aspiration of vomitus. Consider the need for IM folate and thiamine while in the ED, and recommendations for the continuation of such on the inpatient unit if admitted or a prescription if discharged. Vitals signs should be monitored frequently, while the patient is awake, to monitor for any signs and/or symptoms of alcohol withdrawal. Alcohol serum levels are to be done when clinically indicated. Always remember to do a thorough neurologic examination; patients with alcohol intoxication have frequent falls, and subdural hematomas are a common finding.

Table 4-14.3. Urine drug screen and detectability after last use

Drugs	Detectability after Last Use (days)
Amphetamines	1–2
Short-acting barbiturates	3–5
Long-acting barbiturates	10–14
Benzodiazepines	2–9
Cocaine	$\frac{1}{2}$ to 4
Methaqualone	7–14
Opiates	1–2
PCP	2–8
Cannabinoids	2–8 (acute)
	14–42 (chronic)

PCP, phencyclidine.

Table 4-14.4. ED DIRECT: brief intervention

E—Empathy
Adopt a warm, reflective and understanding style. Avoid a blaming, confrontational, or coercive style

D—Directness
Maintain eye contact, and raise the subject, "I would like to take a few minutes to talk about your alcohol use"

D—Data
Feedback: "I am concerned about your drinking." Our screening indicates that (a) you are above what we consider the safe limits of drinking; and (b) you are at risk for alcohol-related illness, injury, and death. Offer comparison with national norms

I—Identify willingness to change
"On a scale from 1 to 10, how ready are you to change your drinking patterns?" If the response is ≤6, then ask, "Why not less?" If the response is ≥7, then the patient is ready; move on to recommendations. The response will help the physician to identify discrepancies and assist the patient to move along the continuum from ambivalence to change

R—Recommend action/advice
All patients: "We recommend that you never drive after drinking."
At-risk/harmful drinkers: Statement of recommended drinking limits. Follow up with your primary care physician
Screen positive, but unsure if dependent drinker: Abstain from drinking, and refer for further assessment to social work, psychiatry, or a specialized treatment facility or alcohol counselor.
Dependent drinkers: Abstain from drinking and refer to a detoxification center, specialized alcohol-treatment facility, Alcoholics Anonymous (AA), and primary care

E—Elicit response
"How does this sound to you?" or "Where does this leave you?"

C—Clarify and confirm action
Possible clarification: "We have just completed a screening test for a whole spectrum of alcohol problems that may lead to an increase risk of illness and injury. We are not attempting to label you as an 'alcoholic.' We are recommending what we know to be safe drinking limits. We want you to follow up with your primary care physician, just as we would with any patient who has screened positively for other health problems such as high blood pressure or a high sugar level."
Possible confirmation: "We are very concerned about your drinking. In the interest of your health (and family), we recommend immediate referral for further assessment and treatment. We know that cutting back or abstaining from alcohol is very difficult to do on your own. We would like to offer you help."

T—Telephone referral
"Would you be willing to speak with a counselor, social worker, etc., now?" "I'd like to call right now for an appointment or referral. What do you think?"

Reference: Alcohol screening and brief intervention in the medical setting. DOT HS 809 467, July 2002; http://www.nhtsa.dot.gov/people/injury/alcohol/alcohol-screening/alcohol-index.html

Treatment will consist of managing the excitement, anxiety, or agitation; consider

lorazepam (Ativan), 1 to 2 mg, PO or IM

Initially cocaine and amphetamine intoxication are characterized by increased psychomotoric activity, restlessness, mood lability, and transient psychosis, which can then dramatically turn into depression, dysphoria, and stupor or coma. Chest pain in cocaine intoxication is not uncommon and warrants a thorough workup.

Agitation may respond to

lorazepam (Ativan), 1 to 2 mg, PO or IM

For psychosis and agitation, consider

haloperidol (Haldol), 2 to 5 mg, PO or IM
or
fluphenazine (Prolixin), 1 mg to 5 mg PO or IM
ziprasidone (Geodon), 10 mg to 20 mg PO or IM

Marijuana and hallucinogens typically will not be seen in the ED unless an adverse reaction to the drug occurs, such as a panic attack, delirium, psychosis, or flashbacks. Management usually requires observation in a calming and reassuring environment. The management of PCP intoxication, often intense agitation, is best with benzodiazepines, because low-potency neuroleptics can exacerbate the intoxication, cause hypotension, and decrease the seizure threshold, by accentuation of anticholinergic effect. Marijuana contains toxins and cancer-causing chemicals, which are stored in fat cells for as long as several months. Users experience the same health problems as tobacco smokers, such as bronchitis, emphysema, and bronchial asthma.

Consider

lorazepam (Ativan), 1 to 2 mg, PO/IM or IV; repeat if necessary. If, after several doses, no effect or signs of benzodiazepine toxicity are seen, consider adding
haloperidol (Haldol), 2 to 5 mg, PO or IM
or
fluphenazine (Prolixin), 2 to 5 mg, PO or IM
or
ziprasidone (Geodon), 10 mg to 20 mg PO or IM

In chronic opioid users, collapsed veins, infection of the heart lining and valves, abscesses, and liver disease may develop. Opioid intoxication can lead to opioid overdose, which is a medical emergency and will be handled primarily in the general ED with supportive measures and opiate antagonists such as naloxone (Narcan). Sedative, hypnotics, and anxiolytic intoxication is similar to alcohol intoxication, and the management is comparable.

It is important to assess carefully risk factors for HIV/AIDS and hepatitis B or C, because many drug abusers may be injecting drugs, alone or in a group, with possible needle sharing. Underlying medical conditions should be explored and treated as clinically indicated in the ED setting.

Psychiatric disorders, whether substance induced or exacerbated by the drug intoxication, must be assessed carefully. If suicidality, homicidality, psychosis, or other dangerous behaviors exist, or inability to care for self because of impaired judgment, these must be factored into the decision for hospitalization.

DISPOSITION

Patients with substance-related intoxication phenomenon, once medically cleared and stabilized, must be referred for ongoing treatment of their abuse/dependence and any co-occurring psychiatric illness. One option is a referral to an inpatient, medically supervised detoxification program or a general medical unit where detoxification can occur and be supervised. Other options are outpatient-based detoxification programs. Severity of abuse/dependence, willingness to change and comply with treatment plans, and medical or psychiatric comorbidity will determine the appropriate level of care for each patient. Those with more serious psychiatric comorbidities, such as depression, anxiety, psychosis, or other psychiatric manifestations, and requiring inpatient hospitalization for treatment, should be admitted into a dual-diagnosis unit or a mentally ill and chemical abuser (M.I.C.A.) unit, where the focus on mental illness and substance-related disorders is integrated and parallel. These specialized units with a therapeutic milieu are run by specialists in addiction psychiatry. Substance-abuse outpatient programs can run the gamut from 12-step recovery groups (AA or NA) to halfway houses, rehabilitations programs (28 days to 18 months), or therapeutic communities. Consultation with the patients, who may have a better sense of the community-based resources, either from personal experience or through that of others, can assist in making a more individualized referral. Patients usually have a sense of where they want to go and what level of treatment works best for them. Social work services should have a list of local community-based programs in your area as well. Adherence with aftercare is an important factor in determining outcomes; more than three fourths of patients who attended 12 months of an aftercare program remained abstinent, with subsequent decrease in medical utilization, improved employment performance, and fewer legal problems. These are important reasons that an adequate assessment and appropriate referral can make such a huge impact from an ED setting.

Other important treatment options, especially with patients who have opioid abuse or dependence, are methadone maintenance programs and even needle-exchange programs, two examples of harm-reduction programs that, for the right individual, can be very effective.

Given the increased medical morbidity and mortality of this patient population, a referral to a primary care clinic or physician is important as well. Referral to social services for assistance with entitlements also should be part of a comprehensive and multidisciplinary disposition plan.

The *Patient Placement Criteria* of the American Society of Addiction Medicine enumerates six goals and criteria for determining levels of intensity for aftercare. These include

- Determination of level of intoxication or potential for withdrawal
- Determination of medical comorbidity
- Determination of emotional and psychiatric comorbidity
- Determination of patient's acceptance or rejection of treatment
- Determination of relapse potential
- Determination of availability of supportive environment.

Depending on the circumstances and possibilities, different outpatient or residential alternatives must be discussed with the patient.

In the United States, adolescents can consent to substance-abuse treatment, but each state has its own local interpretation of this, and staff should be aware of the limitations and rules in their area. The adolescent's capacity to consent and parental notification are critical issues that must be dealt with. Confidentiality should be maintained when possible, and limitations to confidentiality explained to the patient. Confidentiality of drug testing, records, results, and so on must be handled delicately in terms of parental involvement and patient's confidentiality. It is preferable that a family be involved in this process, but at times it may be in the patient's interest they not be included. These are all issues for which an ED must have clear policies in accordance with the local and state legislation.

BIBLIOGRAPHY

Bernstein E, Bernstein J, Levenson S. Project ASSERT: an ED based intervention to increase access to primary care, preventive services, and the substance abuse treatment system. *Ann Emerg Med* 1997;30: 181–189.

Bialer PA. Designer drugs in the general hospital. *Psychiatr Clin North Am* 2002;25:231–243.

Bowen OR, Sammons JH. The alcohol abusing patient: a challenge to the profession. *JAMA* 1988;260:2267–2270.

Buhrich N, Weller A, Kevans P. Misuse of anticholinergic drugs by people with serious mental illness. *Psychiatr Serv* 2000;51:928–929.

Curran HV, Monaghan L. In and out of K-hole: a comparison of the acute and residual effects of ketamine in frequent and infrequent ketamine users. *Addiction* 2001;96:749–760.

D'Onofrio G, Bernstein E, Bernstein J, et al. Patients with alcohol problems in the emergency department, Part 1: Improving detection. *Acad Emerg Med* 1998;5:1200–1209; Part 2: Intervention and referral. *Acad Emerg Med* 1998;5:1210–1217.

D'Onofrio G, Mascia R, Razzak J, et al. Utilizing health promotion advocates form selected health risk screening and intervention [Abstract]. *Acad Emerg Med* 2001;8:543.

Ewing JA. Detecting alcoholism: the CAGE questionnaire. *JAMA* 1984;252:1905–1907.

Goldsmith RJ. Overview of psychiatric comorbidity. *Psychiatr Clin North Am* 1999;22:331–349.

Graeme KA. Pharmacologic advances in emergency medicine. *Emerg Med Clin North Am* 2000;18(4):625–636.

Harwood HJ. *Updating Estimates of the Economic Costs of Alcohol, Abuse in the United States: Estimates, Update Methods and Data: report prepared by the Lewin Group for the National Institute of Alcohol Abuse and Alcoholism, 2000.*

Hoffman NG, Miller RB, Keskinen BA. Treatment outcomes for abstinence based programs. *Psychiatr Ann* 1992;22:402–408.

Hufford MR. Alcohol and suicidal behavior. *Clin Psychol Rev* 2001;21:797–811.

Kameron DB, Pincus HA, MacDonald DJ. Alcohol abuse, other drug abuse, and mental disorders in medical practice. *JAMA* 1986;255: 2054–2057.

Kaminer Y. Addictive disorders in adolescents. *Psychiatr Clin North Am* 1999;22:275–288.

Lindenbaum GA, et al. Patterns of alcohol and drug abuse in an urban trauma center: the increasing role of cocaine abuse. *J Trauma* 1989;29:1654–1658.

Mason PE, Kerns WP II. Gamma hydroxybutyric acid (GHB) intoxication. *Acad Emerg Med* 2002;9:730–739.

Miller NS, Owley T, Eriksen A. Working with drug/alcohol addicted patients in crisis. *Psych Ann* 1994;24:592–597.

Miro O, Nogue S, Espinosa G, et al. Trends in illicit drug emergencies: the emerging role of gamma-hydroxybutyrate. *J Toxicol Clin Toxicol* 2002;40:129–135.

Reynaud M, Schwan R, Loiseaux-Meunier MN, et al. Patients admitted to emergency services for drunkenness: moderate alcohol user or harmful drinkers? *Am J Psych* 2001;158:96–99.

Substance Abuse and Mental Health Services Administration, Office of Applied Studies. *Emergency department trends from the Drug Abuse Warning Network (DAWN): preliminary estimates from January-June, 2001 and revised estimates from 1994 to 2000.* Rockville, MD: DAWN Series D-20. Publication No. (SMA) 02-3634, 2002.

Taliafero EH, et al. Substance abuse education in residency training programs in emergency medicine. *Ann Emerg Med* 1989;18:127–130.

Teter CJ, Guthrie SK. A comprehensive review of MDMA and GHB: two common club drugs. *Pharmacotherapy* 2001;21:1486–1513.

Thornquist L, Biros M, Olander R, et al. Healthcare utilization of chronic inebriates. *Acad Emerg Med* 2002;9:300–308.

Ungar JR. Current drugs of abuse. In: Schwartz GR, Bucker N, Hanke BK, et al., eds. *Emergency medicine: the essential update.* Philadelphia: WB Saunders, 1989:210–224.

Weddle M, Kokotailo P. Adolescent substance abuse: confidentiality and consent. *Pediatr Clin North Am* 2002;49:301–315.

Wilk AI, Jensen NM, Havinhurst TC. Meta-analysis of randomized control trials addressing brief interventions in heavy alcohol drinkers. *J Gen Intern Med* 1997;12:274–283.

Zealberg JJ, Brady KT. Substance abuse and emergency psychiatry. *Psychiatr Clin North Am* 1999;23:803–817.

Chapter 4-15 Malingering

DEFINITION

Malingering is considered the willful, deliberate, fraudulent feigning or exaggeration of the physical and psychological symptoms of an illness or injury for the purpose of a consciously desired end. **Always remember: there must be a clear and ulterior motive to the malingerers behavior.**

PRESENTATION

Malingering is different from factitious disorder or conversion disorder in that its purpose is to avoid punishment, conscription, or other responsibilities; reap financial gain; or obtain drugs, safe haven, or room and board. Malingering is seen predominantly in male-only settings—prisons, military, factories—with an approximate 1% incidence among mental health patients in the general population. This increases to about 5% in the military population and can be as high as 10% to 20% in litigious contexts such as in interviews with criminal defendants. Patients who are malingering will often have vague, ill-defined, and extremely subjective accounts of their symptoms. These symptoms—often back- or headaches, anxiety, depression—are often difficult to diagnose, with no clear underlying medical cause. Malingerers will complain about their symptoms and the functional impairment they may cause with little objective evidence to back their complaints. A patient who is malingering will have many more discrepancies between the complaint and any objective findings. Usually inconsistency is found in what a malingerer will report, what the physician observes, and what is known to be the actual symptom pattern. Discrepancy exists between the findings and the alleged history or impairment. At times, the symptoms or even the physical findings can appear to be self-inflicted. Such patients may be less cooperative with diagnostic testing and not comply as readily with recommended treatments. Patients will tend to become upset and uncooperative if mention is made of no significant findings or of a good prognosis.

MANAGEMENT

Suspicion of malingering should be high when the patient is seen in the context of a medicolegal situation, referred by an attorney for an examination. If available, prior records will reveal frequent visits or hospitalizations with differing diagnoses, injuries, or complaints. A review of these records can heighten the level of suspicion about malingering. The main objective in determining whether a patient is malingering is to avoid the implementation of unnecessary treatments. Physicians, including psychiatrists, are not very good at detecting malingering. The more familiar you are with psychiatric phenomena and diagnostic criteria, the easier it will be to pick up on fake or feigned symptoms. Malingerers will often choose depression or paranoid disorders. Malingerers will complain about visual hallucinations more often than will genuinely psychotic patients. Studies have shown that as malingerers grow tired, their replies tend to become more normal. MSE results are exaggerated, with more approximate answers than those in control groups. A higher incidence of visual hallucinations and hallucinations is found with atypical content. Unlike genuinely psychotic patients, malingerers will often call attention to their delusions.

Once a level of suspicion has been aroused, you should conduct the interview and evaluation in the same manner that you would for anyone else. Try to be neutral and avoid confronting the patient, because this may lead to a potentially unpleasant situation if the malingerer feels revealed or unable to get his or her way. Always consider that the symptoms may be genuine, and perform a thorough clinical evaluation truly to rule out any psychiatric or medical conditions. Order laboratory and other diagnostic tests as indicated to reach a conclusion. Make a thorough psychiatric assessment, and look for common personality and substance-abuse disorders that are associated with malingering. Several factors can assist you in determining when someone is feigning emotional distress after a traumatic event. The malingerer will usually report a significant inability to work in the face of unimpaired abilities to carry out other activities. These patients have a spotty vocational history, with many short-lived jobs or changes and even grievances or lawsuits against former employers. The patient will be evasive during the interview about details of his disability and usually is non-compliant with aftercare plans and recommended treatment. These patients will commonly have cluster B personality traits and be very motivated and active about pursuing legal or disability claims.

The differential diagnoses include factitious disorder, somatization, pain disorder, and conversion disorder, but a defining factor is that in malingering, an *intentional* feigning or production of symptoms occurs with a clear external objective. A motivation and a volitional component are always associated with malingering.

In conversion disorder, an unconscious feigning of illness also is different from the conscious nonpathologic feigning of illness, where the normal behaviors associated with illness are part of avoidance or attention-seeking ploys with no true malicious intent. Conversion disorder can be confused with a physical illness that affects sensory (e.g., anesthesia, blindness) or voluntary motor functioning (e.g., astasia-abasia, paralysis). Usually the deficit fails to conform to known anatomic or physiologic characteristics. A thorough neurologic examination can assist in differentiating conversion symptoms from a true neurologic deficit in many cases. The conscious, pathologic feigning of illness, or factitious disorder, also exists, wherein intentional disease production is found for emotional satisfaction through varied and complex psychological or physical symptoms. Patients with factitious disorder seek to assume the sick role rather than seeking external gain. Munchhausen syndrome is an example of a chronic factitious disorder with feigning illness as the patient's primary life focus, which is often carried out until discovered. Factitious disorder by proxy is the production of illness in the patient's children to elicit sympathy from others and portray an outward semblance of nurturance and caretaking. Factitious disorder by adult proxy is the production of illness in an adult to receive support and sympathy as the primary caretaker.

The actual diagnosis of factitious disorder is hard to make, especially in the ED or other acute care setting. Often the fortuitous discovery is made of a patient engaged in factitious illness behavior (for example, injecting self with pathogens or other noxious substances, finding incriminating paraphernalia among the belongings, receiving inconsistent laboratory findings, as well as ultimately excluding all other possibilities once explored and ruled out).

If the patient's predominant complaint is of physical pain that is not intentionally produced or faked, and it is thought that psychological factors have played a significant role in the onset, severity, exacerbation, or maintenance of the pain, the patient may have a pain disorder. This is a type of somatoform disorder and is further divided based on the categories of factors that are thought to predominate:

- Pain disorder associated with psychological factors
- Pain disorder associated with both psychological factors and a general medical condition
- Pain disorder associated with a general medical condition (only): Psychological factors, if present, are judged to play no more than a minimal role. This is not considered a mental disorder, so it is coded on Axis III with general medical conditions.

Somatization disorder should be thought of and diagnosed when a pattern of medically unexplained complaints and of multiple physical symptoms begins before age 30 years and persists despite evidence to the contrary. Hypochondriasis, conversely, occurs when a patient remains preoccupied with the fear that he or she has a serious medical illness, although medical evaluation has ruled out such an illness. This belief is not of delusional intensity, and attempts at reassurance normally fail.

Adult malingerers often have associated antisocial personality disorder, borderline personality disorder, and/or substance-abuse disorders. Children will often have conduct disorders and anxiety disorders. See the following tables to help in differentiating real from suggestive malingered disorders.

Real vs. Suspicious Auditory Hallucinations (AH)

Real	Suspicious
Intermittent	Continuous
Distinct words or sentences	Vague or inaudible
Commonly associated with delusions	Not associated with delusions
Employ strategies to diminish AH	No strategies to diminish AH
Try to avoid and not obey CAH	Claims that all CAH are obeyed
AH as questions posed about their behavior	AH as questions seeking information
More natural language used to describe	Unnatural or stiff language used to describe

Real vs. Suspicious Visual Hallucinations (VH)

Real	Suspicious
Often associated with AH	Visual alone
Usually seen in color	Black and white
Usually of people, animals, or objects	Dramatic, atypical
Do not change with eyes open or closed	Change with eyes closed
Normal-sized people are the norm	Miniature or giant figures
Related to AH and delusions	Unrelated to AH or delusions

Real vs. Suspicious Delusions

Real	Suspicious
Gradual onset and resolution	Abrupt onset or termination
Tend to keep delusions from others	Eager to call attention to delusion
Conduct consistent with delusion	Conduct inconsistent with delusion

Bizarre delusions accompanied by disorganization behavior	Bizarre content with no apparent accompanying disorganization
No apparent cognitive deficits	Exaggerated cognitive deficit

Real vs. Suspicious Conversion Disorder

Real	Suspicious
Patients are usually friendly, cooperative, and can be dependent and even clingy.	Patients are usually uncooperative, aloof, unfriendly, and more suspicious of your motives.
Patients will welcome evaluations and tests	Avoid or refuse evaluations or tests
Willingly follow recommended treatments	Refuse to follow recommended treatments
Accept and welcome employment options that may address their disability	Refuse any employment opportunities that might address their reported disability
Usually more vague and inaccurate when describing their disability or injury	Extremely detailed in their description of the injury/disability.

Clues to malingered psychosis:

- Malingerers will overact and are eager to call attention to their illness.
- The symptoms may not fit a diagnostic entity.
- In malingering, the behavior usually does not conform to the alleged delusions: no agitation, changes in behavior, barricading room, carrying weapons, etc.
- Contradictions may be found in their accounts.
- Malingerers will try to take control of the interview and try to be intimidating.
- Malingerers are more evasive; repeat questions more often, or usually answer slowly to give themselves more time to think.
- Malingerers are unlikely to show residual or negative symptoms of schizophrenia.
- Malingerers will pretend to have cognitive deficits with psychosis by giving approximate responses.
- Symptoms will be present only when observed.
- Collateral sources will often provide different observations of the patient's functioning, history, and symptoms.

Other clues can help differentiate malingering from other common psychiatric disorders. In cases of malingered mental retardation (very hard to do successfully in this country, given the standardization of testing and evaluations conducted on people suspected of having mental retardation or other developmental disability), usually a significant difference is noted between the level of education reported by the malingerer and the test scores. A difference is seen between their observed and self-reported behaviors and the test scores. On such tests, the malingerer will commonly fail on easy test items while answering difficult items positively. A marked discrepancy may be noted between their reported skills level and their observed behavior. In cases of malingered cognitive disorders, the malingerer will have a hard time mimicking perseveration, will have inconsistent symptoms as related to the reported injury or trauma, and will commonly mix psychotic symptoms with cognitive impairments. A marked discrepancy is found between the individual's self-reported level of social functioning and the reported disability. In cases of malingered amnestic disorder, usually no history of amnestic disorders is found, with a spotty memory loss instead of more global amnesia, as is commonly seen in patients with amnesia. The timing and recovery of their memory may be inconsistent and suggestive, and a high-profile case of amnesia may be reported in the news or local media.

DISPOSITION

If malingering is determined to be the case, you should tell the patient that no medical or psychiatric intervention is warranted. You do not need to confront and tell the patient that he or she is lying. Pointing out discrepancies in the history and presentation and the clinical conundrum these pose for the treatment team may also be a gentle way of presenting the issue of malingering to them. A nonconfrontational and nonadversarial approach may prompt a patient to leave abruptly against medical advice (AMA) and to seek help elsewhere. Usually patients at that point will either leave without a hassle—seeking treatment elsewhere—or will escalate and become more provocative to get their way. Confrontation in a firm and noncondemning manner with offers to assist in getting appropriate psychiatric care might help, although these seldom are accepted.

Psychiatrists are loath to diagnose people with malingering; if the clinical evaluation, history, and documentation are supportive of this diagnosis, then it is important to deal appropriately with the patient. Never treat a condition that does not exist or provide any type of treatment that is not called for. An inpatient admission should be avoided if possible, as it may reinforce the malingerer's behavior. Admission is indicated only if the threats of self-harm are serious enough to be concerned about. If admitted, careful signout to the inpatient team about the clinical suspicion of malingering can help to orient and focus the staff in dealing with the malingerer more effectively—behavioral contracts and predetermined discharge date with appropriate disposition plans being quite helpful.

If factitious disorder or malingering is suspected, involve hospital administrators from the start, seek legal advice, and consult with risk management/ethics committee if necessary.

ED teams should be consistent and firm in their approach to the malingerer, and the documentation should support any decision made. Consistent policies about carfare, access to meals, and sleeping arrangements in the ED are important when dealing with malingerers. Occasionally, when decided by the ED team, a patient seeking a bed and a meal can be allowed to remain in the ED overnight to satisfy this need. A firm discussion about the inappropriate use of an ED setting for these needs and an appropriate referral to social services can also be helpful.

BIBLIOGRAPHY

Harwood-Nuss AL, et al., eds. *The clinical practice of emergency medicine.* 2nd ed. Philadelphia: Lippincott-Raven, 1996.

Nayani TH, David AS. The auditory hallucination: a phenomenological survey. *Psychol Med* 1996;26:177–189.

Resnick PJ. The detection of malingered psychosis. *Psychiatr Clin North Am* 1999;22:159–172.

Resnick PJ. Malingering and posttraumatic disorders. *J Pract Psychiatry Behav Health* 1998;4:329–339.

Resnick PJ. The detection of malingered mental illness. *Behav Sci Law* 1984;2:21–28.

Rogers R, ed. *Clinical assessment of malingering and deception.* 2nd ed. New York: Guilford Press, 1997.

Rundell JR, Wise MG, eds. *Textbook of consultation-liaison psychiatry.* Washington, DC: American Psychiatric Press, 1996.

Simon RI. *Concise guide to psychiatry and law for clinicians.* Washington, DC: American Psychiatric Press, 1992.

Swartz MS, McCracken J. Emergency room management of conversion disorders. *Hosp Community Psychiatry* 1986;37:828–832.

Chapter 4-16 Memory Impairments

DEFINITION

Memory is the process of storing and reproducing or retrieving learned and retained information into consciousness. Memory can be divided into

- Immediate (seconds)
- Recent (minutes to days)
- Remote (months to years).

Amnesia is the partial or total loss of ability to recall past information or experiences, with otherwise preserved intellectual functioning. Amnesia can be divided into anterograde (ability to learn new information) and retrograde (ability to remember previously learned knowledge).

Patients that falsify their memories by distortion in their recall are considered to have paramnesias, which include: *déjà vu* (a novel experience is perceived as being a repetition of a previous memory), *déjà entendu* (an auditory memory is misperceived as if it were recognizable), *déjà pensé* (a new thought is perceived as being previously felt or thought), *jamais vu* (feeling as if a known experience is unfamiliar), and false memories [recollection of an event(s) that did not occur]. Confabulations, another paramnesia, are inaccurate or false reports by patients in an attempt to convey information about their surroundings or themselves. They are made up by the patient in the hopes of "covering up" for the memory deficit. Confabulation can be seen in cases of amnesia, embarrassment, frontal lobe damage, or certain personality disorders.

PRESENTATION

Impairments in memory can be seen in dementia, amnestic disorders, and many other medical and primary psychiatric disorders. Memory disturbances can be commonly encountered in the ED setting as an associated finding in many disorders and even in normal aging. It is a frightening symptom for patients and families, and one that is fraught with concerns about aging and the specter of dementia.

Memory impairment is a common manifestation of a broader cognitive deficit, which requires a specific approach in assessment, management, and treatment. Delirium, amnestic disorders, and dementia are considered cognitive disorders; all have impairments in memory, language, or attention as a characteristic finding.

Memory loss alone does not necessarily mean dementia!

Elderly patients may appear in an ED setting because of age-related medical complications or difficulties, especially falls, but seldom with a primary complaint of memory loss or disturbance. See Chapter 6.3.

An amnestic disorder is characterized by memory loss that causes significant functional impairment, with intact executive functioning and sensorium. Most patients are aware that they have memory loss, but some will respond with indifference or apathy, whereas others will be quite upset and frightened. The memory disturbance affects the ability to learn new information (anterograde) and also may impair the retrieval (retrograde) of previously learned information. See Table 4-16.1 for possible causes of amnestic disorders.

Medications most commonly associated with amnesia are the benzodiazepines—thought to be dose related—as well as certain anticonvulsants, methotrexate, and toxins (mercury, lead, and solvents). Alcohol-induced persisting amnestic disorder is caused by vitamin deficiency from chronic alcohol use and includes peripheral neuropathy, cerebellar ataxia, and myopathy; when resulting from thiamine deficiency it is called Korsakoff syndrome. Another alcohol-related cause of temporary memory loss is blackouts.

Transient amnesia is commonly seen in healthy adults with a sudden onset and a variable but short duration (hours). The most frequently cited causes are head trauma, hypoxia, herpes simplex encephalitis, medications, partial complex seizures, and transient global amnesia. When seen in cases of head trauma or cerebrovascular accidents, the memory loss usually begins at or slightly

Table 4-16.1.   Causes of amnestic disorders

Systemic/Metabolic	Korsakoff syndrome (thiamine deficiency), hypoglycemia
Neurologic	Seizures, head trauma, tumors (especially thalamic and temporal lobe), paraneoplastic limbic encephalitis, postsurgical, herpes simplex encephalitis, hypoxia, transient global amnesia, ECT, multiple sclerosis
Toxic	Alcohol, neurotoxins, sedative–hypnotic medications, certain over-the-counter preparations

ECT, electroconvulsive therapy.

before the moment of trauma, with sudden onset, with short-term and recent memory being most affected. Memory disturbance can occur gradually, especially in cases of vitamin deficiencies or tumors. Patients will complain they cannot remember what they did last evening or even what they had for breakfast. If it is severe enough, they may even have amnesia for place and time, although hardly ever is orientation to person or remote past memory lost. Patients can have associated apathy, lack of motivation, agitation, depression, confusion, and poor insight.

Transient global amnesia is characterized by sudden loss of ability to recall recent events or remember new information, occurring most frequently in middle-aged or older persons. These episodes can last from 6 to 24 hours on average, and patients usually have lack of insight, intact sensorium, confusion, intense anxiety, and no difficulty in performing complex tasks. In almost all cases of acute, sudden, persistent amnesia, the cause can be determined, with ischemic stroke, hypoglycemia, syncope, and seizure being the most likely causes.

Occasionally amnesia can be psychogenic and must be ruled out. Patients with dissociative amnesia experience marked but reversible impairment of recall of important personal information or experience, usually involving emotional trauma.

Dementia is characterized by serious cognitive impairments, especially progressive memory loss and other higher executive-functioning skills, such as abstract thinking, intelligence, learning, language, problem solving, personality structure, orientation, perception, concentration, attention, judgment, and social skills, with no impairment in levels of consciousness. As is apparent, these changes are quite broad and affect many aspects of the person's life, causing social and occupational functional impairments, and are a significant change from the person's prior level of functioning.

Dementia is a condition that affects the elderly, and as age increases, so does the risk of dementia. In patients with HIV, dementia or minor cognitive motor disorders may occur at earlier ages and in about 20% of HIV patients. Generally a cognitive decline is reported by patient and family or collaterals, which is severe enough to cause impairment in the patient's life. This cognitive decline can be alteration in attention, concentration, abstraction, memory, and even speech or language skills, with intact sensorium. Some degree of abnormal motor functioning is present with reduced motivation and behavioral/emotional changes—apathy, irritability, emotional lability, impaired judgment, or inappropriate behaviors. In HIV-associated minor cognitive/motor disorder, the degree of cognitive and motor findings is milder with less impairment in daily living.

Because dementias involve deterioration in mental, behavioral, and emotional functioning and are caused by physical disease, trauma, or drug effects, they are classified according to the probable underlying disease state. See Table 4-16.2 for common causes of dementia. Patients with dementia are usually brought to the ED because of behavioral disturbances, such as wandering, inappropriate sexual or personal behavior, potentially dangerous behaviors like leaving the stove on or the door open, or psychiatric manifestations such as psychosis, depression, paranoia, agitation,

Table 4-16.2. Causes of dementia

Most common causes	Alzheimer disease
	Vascular: multiinfarct, diffuse white-matter disease (Biswanger)
	Alcoholism[a]
	Parkinson disease
	Drug/medication intoxication[a]
Infectious	HIV-related disorders[a]
	Neurosyphilis[a]
	Papovavirus (progressive multifocal leukoencephalopathy)
	Prion (Creutzfeldt-Jakob disease)
	Tuberculosis fungal or protozoan[a]
	Sarcoidosis[a]
	Whipple disease
	Cryptococcal meningitis[a]
CNS	Head trauma and diffuse brain damage:
	Dementia pugilistica
	Chronic subdural hematoma[a]
	Postanoxia
	Postenecephalitis
	Normal-pressure hydrocephalus[a]
	Primary and metastatic tumors
	Paraneoplastic limbic encephalitis
Metabolic/ Systemic	Chronic hepatic encephalopathy[a]
	Chronic uremic encephalopathy[a]
	Progressive uremic encephalopathy (dialysis dementia)[a]
	Hypothyroidism[a]
	Adrenal insufficiency/Cushing disease[a]
	Hypo- and hyperparathyroidism
	Pituitary–adrenal disorders
	Hypoxia or anoxia[a]
	Cardiac arrhythmias[a]
	Respiratory encephalopathy[a]
Toxic	Drug, medication, narcotic poisoning[a]
	Heavy metal intoxication[a]
	Organic toxins
Degenerative	Huntington disease
	Pick disease
	Diffuse Lewy body disease
	Progressive supranuclear palsy (Steel-Richardson syndrome)
	Multisystem degeneration (Shy-Drager syndrome)
	Hereditary ataxias
	Amyotrophic lateral sclerosis
	Frontotemporal dementia
	Cortical basal degeneration
	Multiple sclerosis
	Adult Down syndrome with Alzheimer disease
	Hepatolenticular degeneration
Other	Vasculitis[a]
	Acute intermittent porphyria[a]
	Recurrent nonconvulsive seizures[a]
Psychiatric	Depression (pseudodementia)[a]
	Schizophrenia[a]
	Conversion reaction[a]

[a] Possible reversible causes of dementia
CNS, central nervous system; HIV, human immunodeficiency virus.

mood lability, and sleep or appetite disturbances. Abrupt changes in behavior or personality also can precipitate an ED visit in patients with a diagnosis of dementia.

Because dementia is a slow and progressive illness, patients can manifest a wide array of symptoms from the early stages through profound deterioration in all areas of functioning. Early behavioral signs of dementia include disengagement and apathy, which can progress to agitation. The restless and oppositional aggressive behavior can be the product of delusion (30% to 50% of patients). Patients with delusions will have a more accelerated decline in functioning. The symptoms can range from mild forgetfulness of recent events to loss of earlier learned information such as birth date or name of elementary school. Although orientation is affected in these patients, no matter how severe their dementia, they will not have impairment in their level of consciousness. Language abilities can progressively become affected, characterized by vague or imprecise speech, with difficulties in naming. The hardest part for family and friends is the progressive change in the person's personality: social withdrawal, introversion, hostility, and even paranoia and irritability can be common. In many patients, hallucinations—especially visual— and delusions are associated findings and a common reason for an ED visit. Anxiety, depression, and mood lability also are frequently seen in patients with dementia.

Elderly patients that have depression may have memory impairment that can lead a clinician to think that the patient has a dementing process. This is commonly known as pseudodementia or depression-related cognitive dysfunction, and these patients have a history of depression, a fluctuating course in their memory problems, as well as intact orientation, attention, and concentration. These patients will have flat or depressed affect, positive neurovegetative signs, and a history of psychiatric problems. Often the onset can be timed, and the symptoms are of a more recent occurrence. The family will often be aware of the sudden change, and the patient will also be distressed about the memory problems, with severe recent and remote memory loss.

MANAGEMENT

Because many causes are found for memory impairments, it is important to conduct a thorough medical/neurologic evaluation and approximate diagnosis to institute some disposition plan while in the ED. About 5% to 20% of dementias have reversible causes, so early diagnosis and treatment is the key. Obtain collateral information because these patients are at times bewildered, confused, and upset and may not be able to provide a detailed history. Do not pressure them to remember things or point out their memory loss; be reassuring and supportive.

Memory disturbances must always be taken seriously and not minimized or explained away as part of an age-related phenomenon or a symptom of depression. Instead, these complaints deserve to be taken seriously, at least as a possible early sign of dementia. In the elderly, special care must be taken to perform thorough evaluations and screening, given the possibility of serious comorbid medical conditions. Recent research has identified a transitional state between the cognitive changes of normal aging and Alzheimer disease (AD), known as mild cognitive impairment. Mild cognitive impairment can be seen in patients who experience memory loss to a greater extent than expected for age, yet do not meet criteria for AD. Screening is important because longitudinally, these patients seem to progress to probable AD at a faster rate than do healthy age-matched individuals. Mild cognitive impairment is believed to be a high-risk condition for the development of AD. See Chapter 6.3.

Amnestic disorders require a complete history and physical, thorough neurologic and medical examination, laboratory tests, and neuroimaging. See Table 4-16.3 for a list of differential diagnoses. It is important to determine the underlying cause of the amnesia and possible risk factors: history of head trauma or seizures, infections or tumors, and so on. It can be distinguished from delirium and dementia in that the memory loss is not accompanied by any other prominent cognitive impairment.

Dementia requires a similarly exhaustive and comprehensive medical and neurologic (ask about parkinsonian symptoms, focal motor or sensory deficits, gait abnormalities) evaluation and workup. An important clinical consideration is ruling out delirium, depression, and any reversible causes of dementia before concluding that a patient has dementia. Besides the standard laboratory tests, consider VDRL, B_{12}, folate, thyroid tests, and urinalysis. Chest radiograph, HIV testing, EEG, psychometric testing, parathyroid tests, Lyme titer, angiogram, apolipoprotein E (ApoE) genotyping, and single-photon emission CT (SPECT) or positron emission tomography (PET) scan might be optional focused tests that can help as well, although not necessarily needing to be done in the ED.

Collateral sources of information are crucial, as well as a careful review of medications prescribed, taken, and adhered to. Possible adverse drug–drug interactions in elderly patients, usually with polypharmacy as a common occurrence, are very important to take into account during your assessment. Remember to ask about over-the-counter medication and herbal or traditional remedies that may affect the current presentation as well. No matter how old the patient is, consider drugs and alcohol in your workup: you can be surprised! Superimposed delirium is important to diagnose and manage, as well as any underlying medical condition—acute or chronic—that needs attention. Look for signs of falls or abuse, and ask about recent changes in the person's life and structure; elderly patients are quite susceptible to changes.

A calm, soothing, and reassuring approach works the best, with frequent reorientation and as few stimuli as possible while in the ED.

In patients with pseudodementia, the aim is a timely diagnosis and the ultimate initiation of an antidepressant agent. Short-term treatment will be reserved for psychosis and/or agitation. Remind the caretaker and family that the agitation is not the patient's fault nor is it done on purpose. Low-dose, high-potency typical antipsychotics or atypical agents are the treatment of choice for agitation, although they should be used cautiously and judiciously. See Table 4-16.4 for a comparison of signs of agitation in the elderly. Stay away from low-potency agents such as chlorpromazine (Thorazine), and avoid combining medications as much as

Table 4-16.3. Differential diagnosis for amnestic disorders

Dementia
Delirium
Normal aging
Dissociative disorders
Factitious disorder
Posttraumatic stress disorder
Anoxia
Cerebral infections (herpes simplex)
Frontal and limbic neoplasms or cerebrovascular accidents
Drug induced
ECT
Seizure disorders
Sleep-related amnesia
Wernicke-Korsakoff syndrome
Metabolic (uremia, hypoglycemia, hypertensive encephalopathy,
    porphyria)
Postconcussion amnesia

ECT, electroconvulsive therapy.

**Table 4-16.4. Comparison of severity of
signs of agitation in the elderly**

Severity	Signs
Mild	Whining
	Grunting
	Moaning and crying
	Tapping fingers or feet
	Fidgeting
	Hand wringing
	Extending or flexing limbs
Moderate	Smacking lips
	Clenching fists or jaw
	Rocking or banging head
	Task perseveration
	Shaking
	Slapping knees or thighs
	Stomping feet
	Rocking or bobbing
	Pacing or wandering
Severe	Perseveration
	Cursing
	Wailing or screaming
	Threatening
	Slapping or swatting
	Hitting objects or people
	Throwing objects
	Thrashing
	Kicking objects or people

possible. The cognitive deficits, depression, behavioral disturbances, and sleep disorders are to be dealt with either in an inpatient unit or as an outpatient. Sleep disorders, incredibly trying for the family and caretakers, must be resolved with behavioral and environmental approaches and last with psychopharmacologic agents. In patients with dementia and, as a rule of thumb in elderly patients in general, remember: start LOW and go SLOW.

For acute psychosis and agitation

haloperidol (Haldol), 0.25 to 1 mg, PO
risperidone (Risperdal), 0.25 to 1 mg, PO
olanzapine (Zyprexa), 2.5 to 5 mg, PO

Be very careful with benzodiazepines to avoid oversedation, falls, or even disinhibition.

DISPOSITION

In elderly people with normal aging-related problems, adequate referral to specialized geriatric care is usually sufficient, except if the underlying medical disorders require inpatient hospitalization. Always consult with the patient and the family/friends or guardian about advance directives, such as do-not-resuscitate order, living wills, powers of attorney, or guardianships.

In patients with amnestic disorders, the key is to determine the underlying cause and to treat it accordingly. If memory loss is severe and social supports are lacking, an inpatient psychiatric hospitalization might be indicated until a safe outpatient disposition can be arranged.

In patients with dementia, the determination of any reversible cause and its treatment are the goal. Severe anxiety, suicidality, depression, delusions, hallucinations, and possible self-harming behaviors (wandering) must be dealt with immediately, warranting in most cases a psychiatric, and if possible, a geropsychiatric inpatient hospitalization. Psychoeducation with family and caretakers is quite important, and offering caretakers community-based resources, such as caretaker groups, might help alleviate the burden of caring for someone with dementia. In cases of HIV-associated dementia or associated minor cognitive/motor disorders, the treatment will consist of antiretrovirals and nutritional and neuroprotective therapies. Referral to the outpatient provider or a specialized clinic is indicated.

BIBLIOGRAPHY

American Psychiatric Association. *Diagnostic and statistical manual of mental disorders.* 4th ed, TR. Washington, DC: American Psychiatric Association, 1999.

American Psychiatric Association. Practice guidelines for the treatment of patients with Alzheimer's disease and other dementias of late life.

American Psychiatric Association. Practice guidelines for the treatment of patients with HIV/AIDS. *Am J Psychiatry* 2000;157:1–62.

Arana GW, Rosenbaum JF, eds. *Handbook of psychiatric drug therapy.* 4th ed. Philadelphia: Lippincott Williams & Wilkins, 2000.

Berrios GE. Confabulations: a conceptual history. *J Hist Neurosci* 1998;7:225–241.

Braunwald E, et al., eds. *Harrison's principles of internal medicine.* 15th ed. New York: McGraw-Hill, 2001.

Dorland's illustrated medical dictionary. 28th ed. Philadelphia: WB Saunders, 1994.

Farcnik K, Persyko MS. Assessment, measures and approaches to easing caregiver burden in Alzheimer's disease. *Drugs Aging* 2002;19(3): 203–215.

Fisher CM. Unexplained sudden amnesia. *Arch Neurol* 2002;59: 1310–1313.

Herrmann N. Recommendations for the management of behavioral and psychological symptoms of dementia. *Can J Neurol Sci* 2001; 28(suppl 1):S96–S107.

Honig LS, Mayeux R. Natural history of Alzheimer's disease. *Aging* 2001;13:171–182.

Jonker C, Geerlings MI, Schmand B. Are memory complaints predictive for dementia? A review of clinical and population-based studies. *Int J Geriatr Psychiatry* 2000;15:983–991.

Kahn DA, Alexopoulos GS, Silver JM, et al. Treatment of agitation in elderly persons with dementia: a summary of the expert consensus guidelines. *J Pract Psychol Behav Health* 1998;5:265–276.

Kaplan HI, Sadock BJ, eds. *Comprehensive textbook of psychiatry.* 8th ed. Baltimore: Williams & Wilkins, 1999.

Kaufman DM, ed. *Clinical neurology for psychiatrists.* 4th ed. Philadelphia: WB Saunders, 1995.

Kindermann SS, Dolder CR, Bailey A, et al. Pharmacological treatment of psychosis and agitation in elderly patients with dementia: four decades of experience. *Drugs Aging* 2002;19:257–276.

Lantz MS, Marin D. Pharmacologic treatment of agitation in dementia: a comprehensive review. *J Geriatr Psychiatry Neurol* 1996;9: 107–119.

Lonergan E, Luxenberg J, Colford J. Haloperidol for agitation in dementia. *Cochrane Database Syst Rev* 2002;2:CD002852.

Mega MS. Differential diagnosis of dementia: clinical examination and laboratory assessment. *Clin Cornerstone* 2002;4:53–65.

Montgomery P, Dennis J. Cognitive behavioural interventions for sleep problems in adults aged 60+. *Cochrane Database Syst Rev* 2002;2:CD003161.

Neugroschl J. Agitation: how to manage behavior disturbances in the older patient with dementia. *Geriatrics* 2002;57:33–37.

Patterson CJ, Gass DA. Screening for cognitive impairment and dementia in the elderly. *Can J Neurol Sci* 2001;28(suppl 1):S42–S51.

Petersen RC, Doody R, Kurz A, et al. Current concepts in mild cognitive impairment. *Arch Neurol* 2001;58:1985–1992.

Robinson MJ, Qaqish RB. Practical psychopharmacology in HIV-1 and acquired immunodeficiency syndrome. *Psychiatr Clin North Am* 2002;25:149–175.

Santacruz KS, Swagerty D. Early diagnosis of dementia. *Am Fam Physician* 2001;63(4):703–713.

Schatzberg AF, Nemeroff CB, eds. *Textbook of psychopharmacology.* Washington, DC: American Psychiatric Press, 1995.

Tintinalli JE, Kelen GD, Stapczynski JS. *Emergency medicine: a comprehensive study guide.* New York: McGraw-Hill, 2000.

Vitiello MV, Borson S. Sleep disturbances in patients with Alzheimer's disease: epidemiology, pathophysiology and treatment. *CNS Drugs* 2001;15:777–796.

Watson JD. Disorders of memory and intellect. *Med J Aust* 2001;175: 433–439.

Chapter 4-17 Obsessive/ Compulsive Behavior

DEFINITION

Obsessions are recurrent, persistent thoughts, images, or impulses that are ego-dystonic (in other words, these are unacceptable to and incompatible with the ego or self) and distressing. Obsessions will involuntarily come to mind despite attempts to ignore or suppress them. Compulsions are persistent and irresistible impulses to perform an irrational or apparently useless act—a repetitive and stereotypical action that is performed for an unconscious or unknown purpose.

PRESENTATION

Patients with obsessions and/or compulsions have certain commonalities:

- Intrusive ideas or impulses
- Associated anxiety or dread (can be also feelings of shame, guilt, or disgust)
- They use countermeasures to ward off the anxiety
- They are ego-dystonic; seen by the patient as irrational.

An estimated lifetime prevalence of 2% to 3% is seen for obsessive–compulsive disorder (OCD), making it the fourth most common psychiatric diagnosis. Despite the high prevalence rates, most patients will not willingly come to the ED because of obsessions or compulsions. They are usually brought in by family or friends or because of associated depressive or substance-use disorders. These patients most often seek help outside the context of an ED—usually from nonpsychiatric professionals. It is important to assess every patient for obsessions or compulsions because these are often embarrassing. The patient may not willingly volunteer the information about the obsessions or compulsions. Additionally, because obsessions and compulsions can be associated findings in other primary psychiatric disorders, it is important to inquire about them, even if they are not the primary focus of the immediate presentation.

The most common obsessions and compulsions are as follows.

- The fear of contamination is the most common form of obsessional thinking, usually followed by a compulsive need to wash or avoidance of the feared contaminated object.
- Intrusive thoughts, which may not be accompanied by a compulsion, include sexual or aggressive acts that are usually reprehensible to the patient and cause significant stress and guilt. This obsession at times brings about a compulsion to confess or report the thoughts to the police or others.
- The need for symmetry in the environment makes for compulsive behavior. The urge to keep things precise and organized causes significant impairment in the patient's daily functioning.
- Irrational doubt about certain feared dangers, such as leaving the door unlocked or the stove turned on, requiring frequent checks.

More than half of all patients with obsessions and compulsions have a sudden onset, usually around a stressful event. Many patients will have had symptoms for more than 5 years before seeing a psychiatrist. In adults, OCD has a course that is usually chronic, although mounting evidence indicates that an episodic course also may be possible. Patients with OCD usually have varying insight into their condition.

MANAGEMENT

The most important aspect of the management is to ask the patients if they have any obsessive or compulsive behavior. The patients are usually very embarrassed and often appear depressed and sad—more than 50% have associated depression. These are some questions that should be asked when making an assessment:

Have you ever had any thoughts that bother you or make you anxious?

Do these thoughts stay with you, and are they difficult to get rid of, no matter how hard you try?

Do you ever feel as if you need to keep things extremely clean or have to wash your hands frequently, more than others?

Do you check things over and over in an excessive fashion?

Do you feel as if you have to fix, organize, straighten, or tidy things so much that it takes up a lot of your time and interferes with other things you'd like to do?

Do you worry about acting or speaking more aggressively that you should?

Do you have a hard time getting rid of things, even if they have no practical value?

It is thought that a large number of patients with OCD have other comorbid primary psychiatric disorders, the majority being depressive and anxiety disorders. These comorbid associations tend to increase a patient's level of anxiety and depression as well as occasionally worsening the underlying obsessions and compulsions. It is important, in light of these findings, that a clinician asks questions about obsessive and compulsive behavior. When psychosis or schizophrenia is associated with obsessive–compulsive symptoms, the psychosis tends to be more severe and to have a worse prognosis. Studies have shown a prevalence of obsessive–compulsive phenomena in 1% to 60% of schizophrenic or schizoaffective patients. In these patients, the illness severity seems to be greater, with a poorer prognosis.

Compulsive worry and checking can be part of a generalized anxiety disorder, thus making a thorough assessment important in adequately diagnosing and differentiating these disorders.

Approaching the patient in an empathic, nonjudgmental, and caring fashion when asking about the symptoms can help alleviate the patient's fear and embarrassment. Helping the patient to understand that the behaviors are part of a larger disorder, from which many people suffer, can help normalize the symptoms and allow the patient to open up more.

Conduct a thorough and comprehensive medical workup as well as a psychiatric evaluation. See Table 4-17.1 for a list of differential psychiatric and medical conditions. Tourette disorder, characterized by motor and vocal tics, has a similar age at onset and

Table 4-17.1. Differential diagnosis

Psychiatric	Medical
Generalized anxiety disorder	Temporal lobe epilepsy
Phobias	Tic disorders
Depressive disorders	Postencephalitic complications
Schizophrenia	
Obsessive–compulsive personality disorder	
Tourette disorder	
Hypochondriasis	
Body dysmorphic disorder	
Impulse-control disorders	

symptoms, and a large percentage will meet criteria for OCD. These patients will rarely come to the ED, unless there is symptomatic worsening or they have another acute psychiatric complaint.

As with other psychiatric rating scales mentioned before, the Yale-Brown Obsessive Compulsive Scale (Y-BOCS) Symptom Checklist (see Appendix D) can be useful to assist in establishing a diagnosis of OCD or in determining a baseline severity of symptoms and symptom profile. This 10-item scale may allow either the inpatient team or the outpatient therapist a cross-sectional assessment of the patient's current status while in the ED and provide a score of severity for patients who have both obsessions and compulsions.

For those patients who have severe anxiety, in the ED you can use

lorazepam (Ativan), 0.5 to 2 mg, PO; repeat dose if needed
alprazolam (Xanax), 0.25 to 1 mg PO; repeat dose if needed.

DISPOSITION

In most cases, the patients with OCD will not be admitted unless they have significant suicidal ideation or other debilitating findings that would warrant an inpatient hospitalization. Psychoeducation and referral to psychiatric aftercare are indicated.

The initiation of medication, such as an SSRI, is usually best left for the outpatient psychiatry team to determine, but if your ED and outpatient service are closely linked and you are guaranteed a follow-up appointment, you may start the patient on a low dose of an SSRI, providing a limited supply. Provide the patient with psychoeducation about the medication, side effects, discontinuation syndrome, and issues related to adherence. In patients with schizophrenia or schizoaffective disorder, the addition of an SSRI to their standard medication regimen can be quite beneficial.

The following medications all have FDA approval for the use in OCD: fluoxetine (Prozac), paroxetine (Paxil), fluvoxamine (Luvox), and sertraline (Zoloft). Clomipramine (Anafranil) was the first drug approved by the FDA for OCD and is still considered a standard first-line treatment for OCD.

Outpatient treatment for patients with OCD is not just limited to psychopharmacology; cognitive behavioral therapy (CBT) (exposure, response prevention, flooding, cognitive restructur-

Table 4-17.2.   Prognostic indicators

Good	Bad
Good premorbid social and occupational functioning	Yielding to compulsions instead of resisting
Presence of a precipitating event	Childhood onset
	Bizarre compulsions
Episodic nature of symptoms	Need for hospitalization
	Coexisting major depressive disorder
	Delusional beliefs
	Presence of overvalued ideas
	Personality disorder, especially schizotypal personality disorder

ing), group therapy, and other types of insight-oriented or supportive therapy are usually part of the treatment plan. Psychoeducation for the family and even a referral to family therapy or a family-support group can be helpful.

Some prognostic indicators can help in assessing and coming up with an adequate treatment plan. See Table 4-17.2 for prognostic indicators.

BIBLIOGRAPHY

Abramowitz JS, Foa EB. Does comorbid major depressive disorder influence outcome of exposure and response prevention for OCD? *Behav Ther* 2000;31:795–800.

Abramowitz JS, Franklin ME, Street GP, et al. Effects of comorbid depression on response to treatment for obsessive-compulsive disorder. *Behav Ther* 2000;31:517–528.

Attiullah N, Eisen JL, Rasmussen SA. Clinical features of obsessive-compulsive disorder. *Psychiatr Clin North Am* 2000;23:469–491.

Cath DC, Spinhoven P, Hoogduin CA, et al. Repetitive behaviors in Tourette's syndrome and OCD with and without tics: what are the differences? *Psychiatry Res* 2001;101:171–185.

Chambless DL, Ollendick TH. Empirically supported psychological interventions: controversies and evidence. *Annu Rev Psychol* 2001;52:685–716.

Den Boer JA. Psychopharmacology of comorbid obsessive-compulsive disorder and depression. *J Clin Psychiatry* 1997;58(suppl 8):17–19.

Fabisch K, Fabisch H, Langs G, et al. Incidence of obsessive-compulsive phenomena in the course of acute schizophrenia and schizoaffective disorder. *Eur Psychiatry* 2001;16:336–341.

Fava M, Rankin MA, Wright EC, et al. Anxiety disorders in major depression. *Comp Psychiatry* 2000;41:97–102.

Hoehn-Saric R, Ninan P, Black DW, et al. Multicenter double-blind comparison of sertraline and desipramine for concurrent obsessive-compulsive and major depressive disorders. *Arch Gen Psychiatry* 2000;57:76–82.

Hohagen F, Winkelmann G, Rasche-Rauchle H, et al. Combination of behaviour therapy with fluvoxamine in comparison with behaviour therapy and placebo. *Br J Psychiatry* 1998;173(suppl 35):71–78.

Hollander E, Kaplan A, Allen A, et al. Pharmacotherapy for obsessive-compulsive disorder. *Psychiatr Clin North Am* 2000;23:643–656.

Koran LM. Quality of life in obsessive-compulsive disorder. *Psychiatr Clin North Am* 2000;23:509–517.

Mancini C, Ameringen MV, Farvolen P. Does SSRI augmentation with antidepressants that influence noradrenergic function resolve depression in obsessive-compulsive disorder? *J Affect Disord* 2002;68: 59–65.

Milfranchini A, Marazziti, Pfanner C, et al. Comorbidity in obsessive-compulsive disorder: focus on depression. *Eur Psychiatry* 1995;10: 379–382.

O'Sullivan RL, Mansueto CS, Lerner EA, et al. Characterization of trichotillomania: a phenomenological model with clinical relevance to obsessive-compulsive spectrum disorders. *Psychiatr Clin North Am* 2000;23:587–604.

Reznik I, Sirota P. Obsessive and compulsive symptoms in schizophrenia: a randomized controlled trial with fluvoxamine and neuroleptics. *J Clin Psychopharmacol* 2000;20:410–416.

Schatzberg AF. New indication for antidepressants. *J Clin Psychiatry* 2000:61(suppl 11):9–17.

Schut AJ, Castonguay LG, Borkovec TD. Compulsive checking behaviors in generalized anxiety disorder. *J Clin Psychol* 2001;57: 705–715.

Tek C, Ulug B. Religiosity and religious obsessions in obsessive-compulsive disorder. *Psychiatry Res* 2001;104:99–108.

Tukel R, Polat A, Zdemir O, et al. Comorbid conditions in obsessive-compulsive disorder. *Comp Psychiatry* 2002;43:204–209.

Yale-Brown Obsessive Compulsive Scale (Y-BOCS) Symptom Checklist, adapted from Goodman WK et al. *Arch Gen Psychiatry* 1989;46: 1006–1011.

Chapter 4-18 Overdose

DEFINITION

Overdose is considered either an excessive dose of a therapeutic agent, the ingestion of a lethal or toxic amount of a drug or therapeutic agent, or changes in metabolism or excretion producing a toxic serum level. Overdoses can be intentional, unintentional, or accidental.

PRESENTATION

The most common type of toxicologic emergency in the ED is the adult with an acute, intentional oral drug overdose; however, accidental poisonings in children, parenteral drug abuse, chronic poisoning, industrial and agricultural accidents, and medication reactions or interactions can be seen as well. The most common types of toxic syndromes in the ED can be grouped into four large categories, based on their physical findings, which can help to orient a clinician: anticholinergic antihistamine, sympathomimetic, opiate/sedative/hypnotic alcohol, and cholinergic syndromes. It is important to add lithium toxicity, which can be a problem for psychiatric patients taking this medication. Serotonin syndrome is discussed fully in Chapter 4-22.

See Table 4-18.1 for a list of the common signs and causes of these syndromes.

Table 4-18.1.   Common signs and causes of toxic syndromes

Syndrome	Signs	Causes

Anticholinergic	Altered mental status
	Anxiety
	Arrhythmias
	Ataxia
	Confusion
	Decreased salivation
	Delirium
	Dilated pupils
	Disorientation
	Dry, flushed skin
	Hallucinations
	Hypotension
	Increased temperature
	Lethargy
	Myoclonus
	Seizures
	Tachycardia
	Urinary retention
	Death
		Amantadine
		Antidepressants
		  (Elavil, Norpramin,
		  Sinequan, Tofranil,
		  Surmontil,
		  Ludiomil, Ascendin)
		Antihistamines
		  (Dramamine,
		  Benadryl, Antivert,
		  Phenergan)
		Antiparkinsonian
		  agents (Cogentin,
		  Akineton, Artane)
		Antipsychotic agents
		  (Thorazine,
		  Trilafon, Mellaril,
		  Moban, Loxitane)
		Atropine
		Antispasmodics
		Over-the-counter
		  (analgesics, hyp-
		  notics, menstrual
		  products)
		Muscle relaxants
		  (Flexeril, Norflex)

Sympathomimetic	Altered mental status
	Delusions
	Diaphoresis
	Hyperreflexia
	Hypertension
	Hyperthermia
	Nystagmus
	Arrhythmias
	Rapid and irregular
	  breathing
	Pneumothorax
	Anorexia
	Nausea and vomiting
	Diarrhea
	GI upset
	Hallucinations
	  ("cocaine bugs")
	Anxiety
	Restlessness ("crack
	  dance")
	Suicidal ideation
	Mydriasis
	Paranoia
	Seizures
	Tachycardia (brady-
	  cardia)
		Amphetamine
		Caffeine
		Cocaine
		Methamphetamine
		Over-the-counter
		  decongestants
		Theophylline

continued

Table 4-18.1.   *Continued*

Syndrome	Signs	Causes
Sedative	Altered mental status	Alcohol
	Sedation	Barbiturates
	Analgesia	Benzodiazepines
	Nausea and vomiting	Clonidine
	Bradycardia	Meprobamate
	Coma	Opiates
	Hyporeflexia	
	Hypotension	
	Hypothermia	
	Miosis	
	Respiratory depression	
	Seizures	
	Track marks	
Cholinergic	Altered mental status	Insecticides
	Bowel/bladder	Mushrooms
	incontinence	Organophosphates
	Bradycardia or	Physostigmine
	tachycardia	Pyridostigmine
	Confusion	
	Cramps	
	Emesis	
	Lacrimation	
	Miosis	
	Salivation	
	Seizures	
	Weakness	
	Bronchospasm	

GI, gastrointestinal.

Not all patients will have clear-cut symptoms, as outlined in these categories; great overlap exists, and many patients take multiple drugs, making an accurate diagnosis even more complex. Patients may not have clear-cut, "classic" signs and symptoms as described here, but may have fewer signs, mixed signs, or even partial symptomatic presentations. It is important to always keep in mind that you must treat the individual patient—their vital signs and other relevant clinical findings—not just treat the toxidrome/poison or drug level per se.

Anticholinergic Syndrome
Because many of the medications used in psychiatry and other specialties have high anticholinergic properties, anticholinergic syndrome, especially in the elderly, can be commonly seen. See Table 4-18.2 for a list of anticholinergic substances. In an anticholinergic toxidrome, which is one cause of delirium, remember the following:

Hot as Hades (hyperthermia)
Blind as a bat (visual disturbances)

Table 4-18.2. Anticholinergic agents

Anticholinergic Agents	Generic Name	Brand Name
Antihistamines	Dimenhydrinate	Dramamine
	Diphenhydramine	Benadryl
	Tripelennamine	Pyribenzamine
	Chlorpheniramine	Teldrin, Chlortrimeton
	Cyclizine	Merzine
	Meclizine	Antivert
	Promethazine	Phenergan
Antiparkinsonian agents	Benztropine	Cogentin
	Biperiden	Akineton
	Ethopropazine	Parasidol
	Trihexyphenidyl	Artane
	Procyclidine	Kemadrin
Antipsychotics	Chlorpromazine	Thorazine
	Thioridazine	Mellaril
	Perphenazine	Trilafon
	Molindone	Moban
	Loxapine	Loxitane
Antispasmodics	Clidinium bromide	Librax, Quazan
	Dicyclomine	Bentyl
	Methantheline	Banthine
	Propantheline	Pro-Banthine
	Tridihexethyl	Pathilon
Belladonna alkaloids and synthetic congeners	Atropine	Hyoscyamine
	Belladona alkaloid mixtures	
	Glycopyrrolate	Robinul
	Homatropine	Dia-Quel, Malcotran
	Methscopolamine	Pamine
	Scopolamine	Hyoscine
Cyclic anti-depressants	Amitriptyline	Elavil, Amitril, Endep
	Desipramine	Norpramin, Pertofrane
	Doxepin	Sinequan, Adapin
	Imipramine	Tofranil, Pramine
	Nortriptyline	Aventyl, Pamelor
	Protriptyline	Vivactil
	Trimapramine	Surmontil
	Maprotiline	Ludiomil
	Zimelidine	
	Amoxapine	Ascendin
Ophthalmic agents	Atropine and scopolamine solutions	
	Cyclopentolate	Cyclogyl
	Tropicamide	Mydriacyl

continued

Table 4-18.2. *Continued*

Anticholinergic Agents	Generic Name	Brand Name
OTC products	Analgesics	Excedrin PM, Percogesic
	Cold remedies	Actifed, Allerest, Coricidin, Dristan, Flavihist, Romex, Sine-off
	Hypnotics	Compoz, Sleep-Eze, Sominex, Unisom
	Menstrual products	Pamprim, Premesyn PMS
Skeletal muscle relaxants	Orphenadrine	Norflex
	Cyclobenzaprine	Flexeril

OTC, over the counter.

Dry as a bone (decreased salivation and sweating)
Red as a beet (flushing)
Mad as a hatter (mental-status changes).

Anticholinergic toxicity affects both central and peripheral cholinergic properties as well as nicotinic and muscarinic receptors and produces symptoms consistent with delirium. These include agitation, amnesia, ataxia, confusion, disorientation, hallucinations, typical "picking movements" of the fingers, lethargy, tachycardia, decreased bronchial secretions, dysphagia, hyperythemia, hypo- or hypertension, decreased salivation and sweating, urinary retention, seizures, circulatory collapse, coma, and respiratory failure.

Sympathomimetic Syndrome
These patients have acute overdose or long-term use of cocaine, amphetamines, or decongestants (phenylpropanolamine). See Table 4-18.3 for a list of sympathomimetic agents. The patients will have hypertension, tachycardia, hyperthermia, dilated pupils, piloerection, altered mental status with psychomotor agitation, aggressivity, impulsivity, violence, anxiety, psychosis at times, diaphoresis, tremors, hyperreflexia, seizures, and occasionally shock and dysrhythmias.

Opiate/sedative/alcohol Syndrome
This is the most common toxic syndrome seen in the ED. The syndrome is characterized by a depressed sensorium, with respiratory depression, miosis, hypotension, bradycardia, hypothermia, pulmonary edema, decreased bowel sounds, altered mental-status examination, obtundation, and coma.

Cholinergic Syndrome
Cholinergic syndrome is a fairly uncommon ED presentation but an important syndrome to keep in mind because diagnosis can

4. Acute Psychiatric Presentations 163

Table 4-18.3. Sympathomimetic agents

Category	Name
Amphetamine and derivatives	Amphetamine
	Methamphetamine
	Benzphetamine
	Mephentermine
	Fenfluramine
	Diethylpropion
	Phenmetrazine
	Phendimetrazine
	Methylphenidate
Hallucinogenic amphetamines	PMA (*para*-methoxyamphetamine)
	Bromo-DOB (bromo-dimethoxyamphetamine)
	MDA (methylenedioxyamphetamine)
	MDMA (methylenedioxymethamphetamine)
	MDEA (methylenedioxyethamphetamine)
	MMDA (methoxymethylenedioxy-amphetamine)
	DMA (dimethoxyamphetamine)
Over-the-counter products	Phenylpropanolamine
	Phenylephrine
	Ephedrine
	Pseudoephedrine
	Propylhexadrine
	Caffeine
	Desoxyephedrine
Plants	Ma huang (ephedrine)
	Khat
	Yerba mate (caffeine)
	Coal nuts (caffeine)
	Cacao (caffeine)
	Taxus (ephedrine)
	Acacia spp. (tyramine)
	Cohoba (tryptamine)
	Coca (cocaine)

lead to an effective treatment intervention. This syndrome is caused by organophosphates or pesticide exposure. In contrast to the anticholinergic toxicity (dry), these patients are "wet," with excessive sweating, lacrimation, salivation, bronchorrhea, vomiting, diarrhea, incontinence, cramping, confusion, weakness, altered mental status, fasciculations, miosis, bradycardia or tachycardia, and seizures.

Lithium Toxicity

Lithium for mania is known to be effective at a serum level of 1 to 1.5 mEq/L, with a maintenance level of 0.6 to 1.2 mEq/L. Although these therapeutic levels are still being debated, at levels greater than 1.5 mEq/L, the risks of toxicity increase greatly. Lithium toxicity can have an acute or gradual onset and is normally seen in patients who have intentionally overdosed on their lithium or because of prolonged use have developed a toxic serum level. Lithium toxicity will demonstrate hypotension; altered mental-status examination, ranging from confusion to lethargy to coma; diarrhea; light-headedness and weakness; tremors; localized edema; dermatitis; ataxia; fasciculations; hyperreflexia; myoclonus; and even seizures. Laboratory findings may include leukocytosis and aplastic anemia, ECG abnormalities [arrhythmias, bundle branch block (BBB), prolonged QT interval, ST-T wave abnormalities], and renal-function tests abnormalities. Toxicity can lead to death or permanent neurologic, cardiovascular (myocarditis or cardiovascular collapse), and renal damage (sodium diuresis, nephrogenic diabetes insipidus)—the higher the level and longer the exposure, the greater the intoxication. Several factors may increase the risk of toxicity: intentional or accidental overdose, reduced excretion because of kidney disease or low-sodium diet, dehydration, drug interactions, or individual sensitivity. See Table 4-18.4 for common symptoms of lithium toxicity. See Table 4-18.5 for medications that can affect lithium levels. See Table 4-18.6 for a list of available preparations of lithium, valproic acid, and carbamazepine. See Table 4-18.7 for a list of common side effects and toxicities of valproic acid and carbamazepine.

Other commonly seen overdoses are *acetaminophen* and *tricyclic antidepressant* overdoses. These are the number one and two causes of overdose-related deaths from overdoses. Acetaminophen overdose may present early with very mild nausea, vomiting, diaphoresis, pallor, and progress on to signs of hepatotoxicity, oliguria, protracted nausea and vomiting, and right upper quadrant pain. Then jaundice, coagulation defects, hypoglycemia, and encephalopathy, as well as hepatic and renal failure, will develop.

Table 4-18.4.   Progression of symptoms of lithium toxicity

Polyuria
Nausea
Vomiting
Diarrhea
Slurred speech
Blurred vision
Tinnitus
Tremor
Vertigo
Weakness
Confusion
Drowsiness
Oliguria→anuria
Ataxia
Hyperreflexia
Muscular fasciculations
Nystagmus
Seizures
Impaired consciousness
Coma

Table 4-18.5. Drug interactions with lithium

Drug	Effect
α-Methyl DOPA	↑ Li⁺ toxicity
ACE inhibitors	↑ Li⁺ levels
Acetazolamide	↓ Li⁺ levels
Aminophylline	↓ Li⁺ levels
Antibiotics	↑ Li⁺ levels
Caffeine	↓ Li⁺ levels
Calcium channel blockers	↓ or ↑ Li⁺ levels
Clonazepam	↑ Li⁺ levels
Enalapril	↑ Li⁺ levels
Fluoxetine	↑ Li⁺ toxicity
Mannitol	↓ Li⁺ levels
Metronidazole	↑ Li⁺ levels
NSAIDs	↑ Li⁺ levels
Phenothiazines	↑ intracellular uptake of Li⁺
Phenytoin	↑ Li⁺ levels (?)
Sodium bicarbonate	↓ Li⁺ levels
Sodium chloride	↓ Li⁺ levels
Spirinolactone	↑ Li⁺ levels
Tetracycline	↑ Li⁺ levels
Theophylline	↓ Li⁺ levels
Thiazides	↑ Li⁺ levels
Triamterene	↑ Li⁺ levels
Urea	↓ Li⁺ levels

ACE, angiotensin-converting enzyme; NSAID, nonsteroidal antiinflammatory drug.

Table 4-18.6. Available preparations of lithium, valproic acid, and carbamazepine

Drug	Brand Name	Dosage
Lithium carbonate	Eskalith	300-mg capsules, tablets
	Lithium carbonate	300-mg capsules, tablets
	Lithonate	300-mg capsules
	Lithotabs	300-mg tablets
Lithium carbonate, slow release	Lithobid	300-mg tablets
	Eskalith CR	450-mg tablets
Lithium citrate syrup	Cibalith-S	8 mEq/5 mL (300 mg)
	Lithium citrate syrup	8 mEq/5 mL (300 mg)
Valproic acid	Depakene	250-mg capsules
	Depakene	250 mg/5 mL syrup
	Valproic acid	250-mg capsules
Divalproex sodium	Depakote	125-, 250-, 500-mg tablets
	Depakote	125-mg sprinkle capsules
Carbamazepine	Atretol	200-mg tablets
	Tegretol	100-, 200-mg tablets
	Tegretol	100 mg/5 mL suspension
	Carbamazepine	200-mg tablets
	Carbamazepine	100-mg chewable tablets

Table 4-18.7. Common side effects and toxicities of valproic acid and carbamazepine

Valproic acid	Common	Nausea, vomiting, anorexia, heartburn, diarrhea, thrombocytopenia, platelet dysfunction, ↑ transaminases, sedation, tremor, ataxia, alopecia, weight gain
	Less common	Bleeding tendency, hyperammonemia, incoordination, asterixis, stupor, coma
	Serious	Hepatitis, hepatic failure, pancreatitis, drug rashes (including erythema multiforme)
Carbamazepine	Common	Dizziness, ataxia, clumsiness, sedation, dysarthria, diplopia, nausea, GI upset, reversible mild leukopenia, reversible mild ↑ in LFTs
	Less common	Tremor, memory disturbance, confusional state (esp. elderly and in combination with other meds), cardiac conduction delay, SIADHS
	Serious	Rash (including exfoliation), lenticular opacities, hepatitis, blood dyscrasias (aplastic anemia, leukopenia, thrombocytopenia)

LFT, liver-function test; SIADHS, syndrome of inappropriate antidiuretic hormone secretion.

Tricyclic antidepressant overdose characteristically will cause

- Sodium channel blockade (quinidine-like effect)
- α_1-Adrenoreceptor blockade
- Anticholinergic effects (as described earlier)
- Serotonin and norepinephrine reuptake blockade.

This will manifest as tachycardia, hyperthermia, mydriasis, anhydrosis, red skin, decreased bowel sounds, urinary retention, distended bladder, ileus, agitation, delirium, myoclonus, hyperreflexia, seizures, sedation, and coma.

MANAGEMENT
Any patient for whom a suspicion of an intentional overdose exists must be evaluated and managed in a general ED for monitoring and appropriate care. The immediate medical management of an overdose is outside the scope of this handbook; for more information, refer to a textbook on this subject. See Table 4-18.8 for some general management guidelines.

In general and with any suspected overdose always remember:

- ABC's (airway/breathing/circulation)
- symptomatic and supportive care (individualized to each patient's presentation and not the probable drug/poison overdose

Table 4-18.8. General management guidelines

Acetaminophen	Symptomatic and supportive:
	Emesis, gastric lavage, and/or charcoal
	Within 18 hr, administer acetylcysteine (Mucomyst) 140 mg/kg to start and 70 mg/kg q4h for four to 18 doses
	Monitor serum drug levels for prognosis
	>160–200 µg/mL at 4h, hepatic damage may occur
	>300 µg/mL at 4h, certain hepatic damage
Anticholinergics/ antihistamine	Emesis (avoid if seizures are imminent)
	Gut decontamination with 40F orogastric lavage tube, activated charcoal, sorbitol
	Sodium bicarbonate, 0.5–2 mEq/L as rapid IV injection and repeat as needed to keep blood pH >7.45
	Consider oxygen, D50W, naloxone, thiamine
	Manage cardiac complication and seizures with benzodiazepines, barbiturates, physostygmine salicylate
	In patients with high tricyclic antidepressant drug levels and worsening clinical condition, consider extracorporeal detoxification with sorbent
Sympathomimetics	Emesis, lavage, or charcoal
	Hemodialysis if cerebral edema
	Sedation, reduced external stimuli
	β-blockers
	Manage hypothermia, respiratory and circulatory support
Opiate/sedative/alcohol/ hypnotic	Opiates: Do not give emetics
	Gastric lavage, charcoal
	Respiratory support
	Naloxone, 2-mg IV bolus to awaken and improve respiration, if no response, 2–4 mg IV bolus (repeat as needed to 10 to 20 mg) in both adults and children; if effective response, continuous infusion or repeated boluses every 20 to 60 min (calculated at ⅔ the initial bolus dose that caused reversal, administered qh fluids and circulatory support
	Alcohol: emesis, gastric lavage
	Respiratory and circulatory support
	IV glucose to prevent hypoglycemia
	If blood levels >300–350 mg/dL, consider hemodialysis, fluids
	Sedatives: ipecac emetic if recent ingestion, if sedated, use lavage and charcoal with cuffed endotracheal

continued

Table 4-18.8. *Continued*

	tube; rarely dialysis, alkalinization can speed excretion
	Benzodiazepines:
	Activated charcoal
	If respiratory depression: respiratory ventilation or flumazenil, 0.2-mg IV bolus with 0.3–0.5 mg IV up to 3–10 mg, continuous infusion, 0.1–0.2 mg/hr after response
Cholinergics	Remove clothing and wash skin; empty stomach
	Atropine, 2 mg adults and 0.01 mg/kg IV or IM in children, q15–60 min, repeat as needed if no signs of atropine toxicity
	Pralidoxime chloride (PAM): adults, 1–2 g, children, 20–40 mg/kg IV, over 15–30 min; repeat in 1h if needed
	Respiratory and circulatory support
	Do not use morphine or aminophylline
Lithium	Acute: activated charcoal (will not adsorb lithium but will bind other co-ingestants); IV fluids; urine alkalinization
	Sedation and consider hemodialysis or peritoneal dialysis
	Chronic: dose reduction and supportive care

- monitor vital signs and ECG
- establish IV access
- toxicology screen (don't forget acetaminophen and salicylate levels)
- neuroimaging, if clinically indicated

Whenever possible, it is important to try to obtain the pill bottles, count the pills, and identify any unknown pills. Have the family or someone else search the entire home for pills, pill bottles, or other evidence of overdose. Contacting the patient's physician or the pharmacy to clarify the medication regimen also can help a great deal. Collateral information from prehospital providers (EMT, firefighters, police, paramedics), family, friends, co-workers, old records, and treating specialists should be attempted. A thorough search of the patient and the belongings can help clarify things; a pill found or drug paraphernalia can be important clues. Search for track marks and unusual odors on the patient's breath, skin, or clothing (glue odor indicates toluene; fruity odor, alcohol).

If and when the patient has been assessed to be medically stable, he or she may be transferred to a psychiatric ED for the continuation of a psychiatric evaluation including a full delineation of the circumstances surrounding the event. If a suspicion of a suicide attempt is considered, the patient must be placed on an enhanced observational status while in the ED. If a patient who has overdosed must be admitted to one of the medical floors, then a psychiatric consultation will be performed, and the appropriate follow up by the psychiatry C-L team can ensue.

Lithium toxicity is a medical emergency and requires supportive medical care; this includes correction of fluid and electrolyte abnormalities, normal saline, activated charcoal, and if not effective, hemodialysis. Assessment of overdoses in particular and suicide in general must include an exhaustive interrogation of the patient and, if possible, collateral sources. The amount and types of pills taken, time of ingestion, combination of alcohol or other drugs (and amounts), as well as postgesture reactions (e.g., vomiting, drinking fluids) must be carefully explored (see Chapter 4-21). The intent and lethality of the gesture, the current thoughts regarding the failed attempt, the quality of the gesture (e.g., premeditated vs. impulsive), and family history of suicide as well as prior history of suicide are key elements in your assessment of a suicide gesture. These issues will also assist in the determination of the need for enhanced supervision on the inpatient service and/or the patient's ability to commit to safety.

DISPOSITION

Appropriate medical care and treatment are necessary. Psychiatry C-L may follow up patients once they are admitted to the medical-surgical floor if the overdose is intentional. Make certain that the necessary precautions are taken to ensure the patient's safety while on a medical-surgical service. Once medically cleared, the patient should be admitted to a locked psychiatric inpatient unit for continued management and treatment.

BIBLIOGRAPHY

Ash SR, Levy H, Akmal M, et al. Treatment of severe tricyclic antidepressant overdose with extracorporeal sorbent detoxification. *Adv Ren Replace Ther* 2002;9:31–41.

Dargan PI, Jones AL. Acetaminophen poisoning: an update for the intensivist. *Crit Care* 2002;6:108–110.

Delva NJ, Hawken ER. Preventing lithium intoxication: guide for physicians. *Can Fam Physician* 2001;47:1595–1600.

Glauser J. Tricyclic antidepressant poisoning. *Cleve Clin J Med* 2000;67:704–706.

Hopkins HS, Gelenberg AJ. Serum lithium levels and the outcome of maintenance therapy of bipolar disorder. *Bipolar Disord* 2000;2: 174–179.

Kerr GW, McGuffie AC, Wilkie S. Tricyclic antidepressant overdose: a review. *Emerg Med J* 2001;18:236–241.

Kulig K. Initial management of ingestions of toxic substances. *N Engl J Med* 1992;326:1677.

Nagappan R, Parkin WG, Holdsworth SR. Acute lithium intoxication. *Anaesth Intens Care* 2002;30:90–92.

Stoudemire A, Moran MG, Fogel BS. Psychotropic drug use in the medically ill, Part II. *Psychosomatics* 1991;32:38.

Webb AL, Solomon DA, Ryan CE. Lithium levels and toxicity among hospitalized patients. *Psychiatr Serv* 2001;52:229–231.

Chapter 4-19 Perceptual Disturbances

DEFINITION

Perceptual disturbances, such as hallucinations and illusions, are misperceived or misrepresented sensory stimuli. Hallucinations are considered false sensory perceptions, perceived stimuli with no external producing source. Illusions and distortions conversely are considered misperceived stimuli, which arise from a real external source.

PRESENTATION

Hallucinations are perceived as real phenomena by the patient and are different from illusions or distortions. Real external stimuli, if misrepresented or misperceived, can give rise to illusions. Hallucinations can arise from any of our five senses. Hallucinations are characteristic of a psychotic thought disorder. Hallucinations can, at times, be associated with delusions. It is important to distinguish the underlying cause of the hallucination. Hallucinations can cut across many different psychiatric, medical, or substance-induced disorders. An adequate and thorough assessment will permit a more precise approach to the management and treatment of the hallucination. See Table 4-19.1 for a list of medical causes and medications that can cause psychosis.

Patients with new-onset perceptual disturbances (psychosis) of less than 1 month duration may have a brief psychotic disorder, and if the duration of the symptoms is 1 month to less than 6 months in duration, they may have a schizophreniform disorder. In those patients with more than 6 months of active psychotic symptoms and functional impairment (in the absence of drug-related or causative medical conditions), schizophrenia may be the cause. Given that schizophrenia is a chronic disease, many patients have poor insight and poor adherence to antipsychotic medication, leading to recurrent episodes. Medication adherence in this population is limited; denial of illness, stigma about the illness, cultural beliefs, daily dosing schedules of medications, and unpleasant medication side effects complicate adherence.

Auditory hallucination (AH) is the most common form of perceptual disturbance in psychiatry. These are usually perceived as sounds, noises, words, or sentences, making remarks or comments about the patient. "You're no good," "Why are you doing that?" "Don't go there," etc. Voices are usually punitive in their remarks and almost never inquisitive about external events. AHs occur most frequently in schizophrenia, although many patients with schizophrenia can have multisensory hallucinations. In schizophrenia, AHs are intermittent rather than continuous, with the voices usually coming from outside the head. In the vast majority of schizophrenic patients, the voices are both male and female, with a clear message. In one third of schizophrenics, the voices are accusatory, and about one third of patients are thought to talk back to the voices. It is known that AHs diminish when people are involved in activities. The mean number of voices is

4. Acute Psychiatric Presentations **171**

Table 4-19.1. Common medical causes and medications that can cause psychosis

Cardiovascular	Anemias associated with chronic heart disease Hypoperfusion Hypoxia Pulmonary insufficiency
Infectious	Acute rheumatic fever Diphtheria HIV-related infections Legionnaire disease Malaria Pneumonia Rocky Mountain spotted fever Sepsis Syphilis Typhoid fever
Medications	Antibiotics (isoniazid, rifampin) Anticonvulsants (phenytoin, ethosuximide primidone, phenobarbital) Antidepressants (amitriptyline, doxepine protriptyline, imipramine, trimipramine) Anxiolytics (diazepam, alprazolam, clonazepam, ethchlorvynol, chlordiazepoxide) Cardiovascular agents (digitalis, disopyramide, methyldopa, captopril procainamide, reserpine, propranolol) OTC (antihistamines, antitussives, decongestants, diet or weight-reducing drugs) Other (corticosteroids, disulfiram, cimetidine, cycloserine, antineoplastic agents, cimetidine, bromides, heavy metals, L-Dopa)
Metabolic	Addison disease Cushing disease Diabetic ketoacidosis Electrolyte imbalances Hepatic dysfunctions Hyperthyroidism Hypocalcemia or hypercalcemia Hypoglycemia Hypothyroidism Pituitary dysfunctions Vitamin deficiencies Wilson disease
Neurologic	Aneurysms Angiomas Cerebral abscess Cerebral infections Chronic subdural hematoma Hypertensive encephalopathy Neoplasms Normal-pressure hydrocephalus Seizure disorder (temporal lobe and postictal states)

Table 4-19.1. *Continued*

Drugs	Alcohol
	Amphetamines
	Cocaine
	Lysergic acid diethylamide (LSD)
	Marijuana
	Mescaline
	Methamphetamine
	Phencyclidine (PCP)
	Psilocybin
Other	Collagen vascular diseases
	Depression
	Sensory deprivation
	Substance-related (abuse, dependence, intoxication, withdrawal)

HIV, human immunodeficiency virus; OTC, over the counter.

about three, although more than half of patients report hearing crowds of people mumbling or talking together. Patients complain that the most common AHs are of terms of abuse. Women usually report hearing comments about their sexual activity, denoting promiscuity or calling them a "slut," whereas men are more likely to report AHs commenting on issues of homosexuality. As the illness progresses, it is thought that the voices develop in number and complexity. Specific activities, such as working or watching TV, lying down or taking a walk, and talking to someone else can help mitigate the impact of the AH. Patients report that being alone makes the AH worse.

Visual hallucinations (VHs) are more common in organic disorders. Commonly they are of objects, animals, or normal-sized people. Small people (Lilliputian hallucinations) are reported in alcoholics, organic causes, or toxic syndromes, especially anticholinergic (atropine) toxicity. VHs are usually in color and maintain some consistency with the AHs and delusional thoughts a person may have. VHs do not change with eyes open or closed. Studies showed that people with drug-induced VHs report VHs more often with eyes closed. Shadows, flashing lights, and moving objects are commonly experienced VHs with cocaine-related hallucinatory phenomena. These types of unformed hallucinations can be seen in neurologic disorders as well. Elderly patients who report VHs should make you think about eye pathology such as cataracts.

Olfactory hallucinations (OHs) are more common in organic disorders, and especially common in temporal lobe epilepsy. OHs tend to be associated with other hallucinations and when present are usually of unpleasant odors.

Tactile (haptic) hallucinations (THs) are false perceptions from touch or surface sensation and also are usually in the context of an organic disorder, such as delirium tremens or cocaine or amphetamine intoxication. Rarely are THs reported alone.

Gustatory hallucinations (GHs) are more common in organic disorders. GHs are more often of unpleasant tastes than of pleasant tastes and are usually associated with other hallucinations; commonly seen in temporal lobe epilepsy.

Somatic or cenesthesic hallucinations are false sensations of things occurring inside the body, most often visceral in origin. Patients report a burning sensation or feeling of pressure in the brain, a pulsing sensation in the blood, or other such symptoms.

Synesthesias are a form of hallucination caused or triggered by another different sensory modality, such as hearing a smell or seeing a noise.

Hypnopompic hallucinations are a nonpathologic condition whereby a person experiences hallucinatory-like phenomena on awakening from sleep.

Hypnogogic hallucinations are a nonpathologic condition whereby a person experiences hallucinatory-like phenomena while falling asleep.

More than 600,000 ED visits annually are drug related. The drugs that are commonly responsible for these acute presentations with psychosis are alcohol, cocaine, PCP, ketamine, and MDMA. Alcoholic hallucinosis is a condition in which hallucinations occur in the context of cessation or decrease in alcohol use in an alcohol-dependent patient. These hallucinations persist throughout the withdrawal phase and, although uncommon, are more often seen in men than in women. These are characterized by vivid hallucinations, usually starting off as unpleasant noises or music and then turning into voices typically heard outside the patient's head and often commenting on the patient in third person. Insight into the hallucinations is maintained, and they last only a few days. In about 10% of the cases, the hallucinations last longer, and some even go on to become chronic. Delusions and paranoia can be seen, and the patient usually has intact orientation and no change in the level of consciousness.

In an alcohol-induced psychotic disorder, which may occur during intoxication or withdrawal, hallucinations and delusions are common. Hallucinations are commonly auditory, unstructured, and commonly of negative connotation. The hallucinations may last a week or so and although a loss of reality testing occurs, on resolution, the patient will regain insight into the hallucinatory nature of the symptom.

Close to 50% of people who use cocaine develop a cocaine-induced psychotic disorder with paranoid delusions and hallucinations. These symptoms also can be in the context of intoxication or withdrawal. It is commonly seen in IV cocaine and crack users, although it depends on the amount of cocaine used, the duration of use, and the individual's sensitivity. Auditory, visual, and even tactile hallucinations, such as bugs crawling under the skin (formication), have been described.

In patients who have used hallucinogens, it is possible to re-experience or have a flashback of hallucinogenic symptoms long after having used the drug, called hallucinogen hallucinosis. It is thought that 15% to 80% of hallucinogen users may have hallucinogen persisting perception disorder. The flashback experiences, after careful workup for medical causes (seizures or migraines), are usually triggered by stress or use of another drug such as alcohol or marijuana. The symptoms commonly described are visual distortions, geometric hallucinations, auditory hallucinations of voices or sounds, trailing phenomenon, etc. These symptoms are different from a hallucinogen-induced psychotic disorder, in which reality testing is intact and a direct temporal relation exists between the occurrence of the psychotic symptom and the use of a hallucinogen. The psychotic symptoms are time limited.

Hallucinations in the context of affective disorders (depressive, manic, or mixed episodes) are fairly common. In mania, close to half of patients will report AHs, and fewer than a third will report VHs. Hallucinations in affective disorders can be either mood congruent or incongruent. In mood-congruent hallucination, the content of the hallucination is in keeping with the affective state; in other words, a depressed person will hear negative and disparaging voices, whereas a manic patient will hear voices commenting on the patient's power. Mood-incongruent hallucinations are those with a disconnection between the content of the hallucination and the affective state. In the early stages of grief, a patient may report hearing the voice of the deceased or seeing the deceased.

Command auditory hallucinations (CAHs) are false perceptions that the voices are commanding the patient to do something, which then patient must obey or has intense difficulty resisting. The types of commands, noted in one study, were of suicide (52%), homicide (5%), injury to self/others (12%), nonviolent acts (14%), and the remainder were unspecified. Numerous studies have shown that CAHs are obeyed 10% to 80% of the time. This wide spread in percentages demonstrates that we do not have a good sense of when and why patients act on their CAHs. It is variable, but when acted on, it can be serious. As such, it is imperative to inquire carefully about the nature of the CAHs. We know that patients with CAHs are less likely to obey them if the acts to be followed are dangerous. Alternatively, it also is possible that a patient will act on the CAHs if there is a hallucination-related delusion or if it is a familiar voice. Inquire about how the patients deal with the commands. Do they ignore the voices and how? Are the commands reasonable, and do they carry them out (CAHs to go shopping or take their medications)? If the voices are not obeyed, what happens? Do the voices intensify? Become nagging? Get louder? Have they ever carried out the demands just to get the voices to stop? Remember, CAHs, whether "good" commands or "bad" commands, should be considered a high-risk factor for danger (to self or others). Discriminating the CAHs as "good versus bad" is neither helpful nor useful. Patients who have CAHs should be assessed thoroughly, and safety considerations should be taken into account before a disposition is reached.

Keep in mind that psychotic symptoms may have a significant cultural overlay that makes the assessment and diagnosis quite confusing and complex. Acute psychotic processes have a cultural component different from what may be commonly seen in this country. These presentations may be more prevalent in large ethnically and culturally diverse urban settings. These culture-bound syndromes, such as *amok, ataque de nervios, koro, falling-out, susto,* have important diagnostic and treatment implications in the ED setting. A detailed description of these important culturally bound syndromes is outside the scope of this handbook, and a general textbook should be referenced for more detailed information. Staff should be familiar with the most common ethnic and racial groups represented in their area/community and be sensitive to these cultural variables and possible variants when they appear.

Although not very common, postpartum psychosis or puerperal psychosis may be seen in the ED. The incidence is very low (0.1% of all deliveries), but the seriousness and possible negative outcomes (suicide or infanticide) can be high. These patients may have a progressive worsening clinical picture of confusion, disorientation, prominent hallucinations, and even delusions. The onset is typically 2 weeks to a month after delivery, and in many cases, the patient has a history of postpartum psychiatric illness.

MANAGEMENT

Hallucinations must be assessed carefully, with attention to the details of the hallucinations. Ask the patient:

Do you ever hear voices when no one else is around? Have you ever heard any strange sounds you can't explain? Do you understand what I mean when I ask you if you ever "hear voice"? Have you ever seen anything you can't explain? Have you ever seen colors, lights, or shapes that no one else can see? Have you ever felt any strange sensations or touches on your skin that you couldn't explain? Have you ever smelled anything, like flowers, perfume, or a bad smell, when there isn't anything around?

What is the content and clarity of the hallucination? How vivid is the hallucination? How long does it last, and how often does it occur? Are the hallucinations intermittent or continuous? How is the patient coping with the hallucination? Does he or she ignore it? Does he or she respond? What is the patient's mood during the hallucination? Are the hallucinations mood congruent or incongruent? How is the hallucination related to delusions or not? Is the patient confused about the hallucination—what is the reaction to the symptom? What makes the hallucinations better or worse?

Specific Questions to Ask about Auditory Hallucinations

Describe the AH—noises, sounds, words, phrases, etc. How many voices? Is its volume loud or soft? Is it a male or a female voice? Do they recognize the voices? Is the AH inside or outside their head? If it is a voice, what is the tone, and do they speak in first or third person? What is the patient's response in understanding and behaviors with the AH? Are the AHs accompanied by other hallucinations or delusions? Does the patient converse with the voices? What does the patient do to cope with the voices? Does the patient have any strategies to make the voices go away? Do the voices give commands? Does the patient respond and act on those commands? If not, why, and how do they stop themselves from acting on them?

Specific Questions about Visual Hallucinations

Describe the VHs—flashes, lights, objects, animals, or persons. Are they in color or black-and-white? Are the people normal sized or smaller than normal? Do the VHs change with the eyes closed or open? Are they accompanied by other hallucinations? Do they relate to a delusion?

Never challenge a patient complaining of hallucinations. Hallucinating is a distressing and painful experience. Patients may have some insight into the symptom or be totally overwhelmed by the experience and very frightened. An empathic approach with no perceived judgment on your part regarding the hallucinations is important. Try to provide a reassuring and calming environment. If the patient asks you if you hear, or see, or smell what they are experiencing, you should honestly answer that you do not, but adding that it does not mean that they are not having that experience. Perceptual disturbances can be frightening and can make a patient anxious and even agitated. Always inquire about CAHs.

Visual, tactile, olfactory, gustatory, and other types of hallucinations are more commonly seen in organic-related causes. These symptoms should lead you to determine whether there are underlying medical causes of such phenomenon. Substance intoxication and certain withdrawal syndromes can cause hallucinations. Medications like L-Dopa used in Parkinson disease and certain medical conditions, such as seizures or delirium, can cause hallucinations.

Obtain vital signs, standard laboratory values, and urine toxicology to assist in ruling out medical and/or substance-related causes. Obtain a thorough history; review any records or supporting documentation. Contact family, friends, or other collateral sources for more information. Review the medical regimen and ask carefully about current, recent, or past substance use. Inquire about amounts of drug used as well. In cases of alcohol-dependent patients, you must rule out withdrawal, which can be accompanied with hallucination from alcohol hallucinosis. It is the temporal relation with alcohol withdrawal, short duration, and intact sensorium that can assist in differentiating an alcohol-induced hallucination from schizophrenia or delirium tremens. In cases of recent hallucinogen use, symptoms start usually 1 hour after ingestion and can last up to 12 hours. "Bad trips," especially in first-time users, can be accompanied with hallucinations, especially synesthesias. Reassurance and reorientation in a quiet and calming environment are helpful during these types of presentations.

In patients with a probable psychotic disorder, the goal should be to alleviate and reduce the acute psychotic presentation and perform a thorough evaluation to assess the general medical and neurologic condition, discover any comorbid conditions, and establish a baseline for antipsychotic medication management. In addition, safety concerns, behavioral control, and symptom reduction or resolution are acute-phase management goals. In patients with chronic illness, such as schizophrenia or schizoaffective disorder, the goals remain the same, but added are the need to ascertain adequate follow-up and referral to outpatient medical and psychiatric care. Additionally, if alcohol or drugs are a confounding factor, referral to short-term or long-term substance-abuse/ dependence treatment is important.

In cases of confusing presentations, in which culture, religion, or spiritual beliefs or supernatural or mystical explanations are offered, a thorough assessment of the family, community, and its religious beliefs must be undertaken. Understanding the patient's culturally "normal" beliefs and behaviors, as well as the more common cultural manifestations of stress or symptom presentation, may help in the assessment, diagnosis, and management. Ask the family or others if the patient's symptoms are consistent with their culture and its outward manifestations of illness, or are they beyond what is normal and expected for this community. Inquire about religious or spiritual beliefs and how they may affect or influence the manifestations of symptoms. If the symptoms are outside the cultural norm, it may be important to address these findings with the patient, the family, and, if necessary, invoke the assistance of the community's elders or religious/spiritual leaders in dealing with the patient and the needed treatment recommendations. Psychoeducation will be crucial in these cases for everyone involved.

Postpartum psychosis must be assessed carefully and treated rapidly. Small doses of antipsychotics may be helpful while a thorough assessment of the child's safety, family situation, and other psychosocial variables is being addressed. A hospitalization may be required to stabilize and adequately manage this condition, with usually a favorable response to medication, good prognosis, and relatively quick resolution of symptoms.

BRIEF PSYCHIATRIC RATING SCALE

The Brief Psychiatric Rating Scale (BPRS) was developed in the 1960s as a means of assessing psychotic and other psychiatric symptoms in a rapid, valid, and reliable manner. It is divided into 18 items assessing different areas of psychiatric disorders, and each item is rated on a 7-point scale (from "not present" to "extremely severe"). The higher the score, the greater the degree of psychopathology, with a score of 35 and above being consistent with significant impairment. The BPRS is a semistructured interview, and because no individual criteria exist for each item, the interviewer must have a consistent approach, with internal anchor criteria obtained from practice and frequent use of this scale. Here are brief explanations for each item (see Appendix D).

- Somatic concern: Physical complaints or beliefs of bodily illness or malfunctioning regardless of the true organic basis; ranges from very mild concern to clear-cut somatic delusions, based on verbal report.
- Anxiety: Subjective experience of nervousness, worry, fear, apprehension, or overconcern about present or future, based on verbal report.
- Emotional withdrawal: Deficiency in relating to the interviewer as if an invisible barrier existed between you and the patient. Manifested by poor to absent eye contact, failure to orient physically to you, poor engagement, decreased verbal and nonverbal communication, based on observation.
- Conceptual disorganization: Disruption of normal thought processes; can be any formal thought disorder, based on cognitive–verbal process during the interview.
- Guilt feelings: Sense of remorse for real or imagined misdeeds, which can range from self-blame to delusions, based on verbal report.
- Tension: Overt physical manifestations of anxiety, fear, or agitation; includes fidgeting, tremors, swaying, stiffness, restlessness, frequent postural changes, pacing, hand wringing, based on observation. Do not rate signs of TD.

- Mannerisms and posturing: Unusual or unnatural or bizarre motor behaviors or postures, odd repetitive movements, awkward postures, grimaces, rocking, based on observation. TD is rated under this item but not higher than a 3.
- Grandiosity: Exaggerated self-opinion or inflated appraisal of the talents, powers, abilities, accomplishments, knowledge, importance, wealth, fame, or identity, ranging from mild boastfulness to grandiose delusions, based on the patient's current thoughts and opinions from the verbal report.
- Depressive mood: Subjective report of feeling sad, blue, down in the dumps, hopeless, helpless or discouraged, facial expressions, weeping, moaning, and other nonverbal modes of communicating mood state should be taken into account, based on subjective report.
- Hostility: Feelings of animosity, belligerence, contempt, disdain, or hatred for other people, physical manifestations score high, based primarily on verbal report. Do not rate hostility toward self or the rater here.
- Suspiciousness: Belief that others have (now or in the past) malicious or discriminatory intent toward them, from mild guardedness or distrust to persecutory delusions, based on verbal report and its influence on behavior.
- Hallucinatory behavior: Report or behavior indicating perceptions generated by an identifiable external stimuli; these can be auditory, visual, olfactory, tactile, or gustatory, based on verbal report and observation.
- Motor retardation: Reduction in energy and motor activity with slowing or lessening of movements and speech, decreased responsiveness to stimuli and reduced body tone, based on observation.
- Uncooperativeness: Resistance, hostility, unfriendliness, resentment, or lack of readiness to cooperate with the interview, based on responses of the patient.
- Unusual thought content: Beliefs that are unfounded, unrealistic, and bizarre (delusions score 4 or more), based on verbal report.
- Blunted affect: Decreased emotional responsivity, with deficits in facial expression, communicative gestures, modulation of feelings, and vocal expressions or tone; inappropriate affect rates up to 3, based on observation.
- Excitement: Heightened emotional tone with accelerated motor behavior, increased responsivity to stimuli, hypervigilance, agitation, irritability, overarousal, based on observation.
- Disorientation: Confusion or lack of proper association to person, place, and time.

Hallucinations related to drug use or as part of grief or stressor response will resolve relatively quickly. In these cases, it is best to treat with a benzodiazepine.

lorazepam (Ativan), 0.5 to 2 mg, PO or IM

In more severe cases or hallucinations with agitation, the use of neuroleptics or a combination of benzodiazepines and neuroleptics is warranted. Remember to use an anticholinergic agent in patients who are neuroleptic naive or at higher risks for developing neuroleptic-induced side effects.

lorazepam (Ativan), 0.5 to 2 mg, PO or IM
+
haloperidol (Haldol), 1 to 5 mg, PO or IM
or
Fluphenazine (Prolixin), 1 mg to 5 mg PO or IM
or
ziprasidone (Geodon), 10 to 20 mg, IM q2 to 4hr (maximum, 40 mg in 24 hours)

Also consider risperidone (oral concentrate), or olanzapine, quetiapine, ziprasidone, or aripiprazole if the patient agrees to take PO medication or is already taking one of these agents.

In alcohol- and hallucinogen-related hallucination, stay away from low-potency antipsychotics such as chlorpromazine to avoid anticholinergic side effects such as postural hypotension and exacerbation of the hallucinations.

DISPOSITION

After the careful assessment and management in the ED, disposition options are either inpatient hospitalization or discharge back to the community. This depends on the severity of perceptual disturbances and the possible underlying etiologic factors. In patients with new onset of perceptual disturbances, admission for a more thorough evaluation and medication management is indicated. Research findings and clinical experience suggest that close to 60% of patients treated with antipsychotic medication for at least 6 weeks will improve (both positive and negative symptoms) to the point of complete remission or very mild residual symptoms. The remainder will continue to have moderate to severe symptoms, whereas 8% will have no improvement or a worsening of their condition. Inquiring about the patient's prior response to medication remains a fairly reliable predictor of response to a subsequent trial. Psychoeducation and psychosocial interventions aimed at reducing the overstimulating and stressful influences on the patients are important. In patients with long-standing primary psychiatric disorders, such as schizophrenia or affective disorders, the decision to admit or discharge will depend on safety issues, level of community support, and adherence factors. Patients who have good community supports and regular aftercare plans might need observation in the ED, medication given, and aftercare plans confirmed for discharge. At times, an enhancement in the level of support might be needed. In patients with first-episode psychosis, safety concerns, poor supports, and poor adherence with aftercare plans, admission might be warranted. In alcoholic hallucinosis or other substance-induced psychosis, after immediate management, discharge to ongoing treatment, such as outpatient detoxification or rehabilitation programs, is in order. Consider referrals to 12-step programs as part of any discharge plan. Some patients might require inpatient medically supervised detoxification before they can be discharged. Hallucinogen hallucinosis usually can be dealt with in the ED, in a safe, quiet, low-stimuli setting until the symptoms abate. Talking to the patient and offering comfort and security can greatly alleviate the experience of a "bad trip" without requiring other forms of interventions.

Any patient with CAHs should be carefully assessed and managed. If CAHs persist or the patient has acted on CAHs in the past, admission might be necessary. Suicidal or homicidal thoughts and perceptual disturbances are a potentially dangerous combination, especially if CAHs are present. If so, consider admitting.

BIBLIOGRAPHY

Assad G. *Hallucinations in clinical psychiatry: a guide for mental health professionals.* Brunner/Mazel, 1990.

Assad G, Shapiro B. Hallucinations: theoretical and clinical overview. *Am J Psych* 1986;143:1088–1097.

Beck J, Harris MJ. Visual hallucinations in non-delusional elderly. *Int J Geriatr Psychiatry* 1994;9:531–536.

Cummings JL, Miller BL. Visual hallucinations: clinical occurrence and use in differential diagnosis. *Western J Med* 1987;46:46–51.

Falloon I, Talbot R. Persistent auditory hallucinations: coping mechanisms and implications for management. *Psychol Med* 1981;11: 329–339.

Forster PL, Buckley R, Phelps MA. Phenomenology and treatment of psychotic disorders in the psychiatric emergency service. *Psychiatr Clin North Am* 1999;23:735–754.

Goodwin DW, Anderson P, Rosenthal R. Clinical significance in psychiatric disorders: a study of 116 hallucinatory patients. *Arch Gen Psychiatry* 1971;24:76.

Hellerstein D, Frosch W, Koenigsberg HW. The clinical significance of command hallucinations. *Am J Psych* 1987;44:219.

Junginger J. Command hallucinations and the prediction of dangerousness. *Psychiatr Serv* 1995;46:911–914.

Leudar I, Thomas P, Mcnally D, et al. What voices can do with words: pragmatics of verbal hallucinations. *Psychol Med* 1997;27:885–898.

Lewinsohn PM. An empirical test of several popular notions about hallucinations in schizophrenic patients. In: Keup W, ed. *Origin and mechanism of hallucinations.* New York: Plenum Press, 1970: 401–403.

McNiel DE, Eisner JP, Binder RL. The relationship between command hallucinations and violence. *Psychiatr Serv* 2000;51:1288–1292.

Miller LJ. Qualitative changes in hallucinations. *Am J Psychiatry* 1996;153:2.

Mitchell J, Vierkant AD. Delusions and hallucinations of cocaine abusers and paranoid schizophrenics: a comparative study. *J Psychol* 1991;25:301–310.

Mott RH, Small IF, Andersen JM. Comparative study of hallucinations. *Arch Gen Psychiatry* 1965;12:595.

Nayani TH, David AS. The auditory hallucination: a phenomenological survey. *Psychol Med* 1996;26:177–189.

Overall JE, Gorhman DR. The brief psychiatric rating scale. *Psychol Rep* 1962;10:799.

Reischel UA, Shih RD. Evaluation and management of psychotic patients in the emergency department. *Hosp Physician* 1999;35(10): 26–38.

Resnick PJ. The detection of malingered psychosis. *Psychiatr Clin North Am* 1999;22:159–172.

Richards CF, Gurr DE. Psychosis. *Emerg Med Clin North Am* 2000;18: 253–262.

Substance Abuse and Mental Health Services Administration (SAMHSA). *Drug Abuse Warning Network (DAWN) for 2000,* http://www.samhsa.gv/OAS/Dawn.htm

Surawicz FG. Alcoholic hallucinosis: a missed diagnosis: differential diagnosis and management. *Can J Psychiatry* 1980;25:57–63.

Ziedonis D, Williams J. When psychosis and substance use coincide in the emergency service. *Psychiatr Issues Emerg Care Setting* 2002:3–13.

Chapter 4-20 Sleep Disturbances

DEFINITION

Sleep disturbances, such as insomnia or hypersomnia, are very common findings and like so many other symptoms discussed here, cut across diagnostic entities. Sleep disorders are divided, with occasional overlapping symptoms, into three major groups: dyssomnias, parasomnias, and sleep disorders that are associated with medical and psychiatric conditions. See Table 4-20.1 for a list of psychiatric, medical, and neurological conditions that can casuse sleep disorders. *Dyssomnias* are a primary sleep disorder, characterized by a disturbance in initiating and maintaining sleep or by excessive sleepiness. These include the following:

Breathing-related sleep disorder
Circadian rhythm sleep disorder
Hpersomnia
Hypersomnia related to another mental disorder
Insomnia
Insomnia related to another mental disorder
Narcolepsy.

Parasomnias are sleep disorders that have unusual or bizarre phenomena during the transition from one stage of sleep to another or during arousal or partial arousal, representing an episodic disorder in sleep. These include

Nightmare disorder
Rapid eye movement (REM) sleep behavior disorder

Table 4-20.1. List of psychiatric, medical, and neurological conditions that can casuse sleep disorders

Psychiatric conditions	Anxiety disorders
	Mood disorders
	Psychotic disorders
	Substance-related disorders (alcoholism)
Medical conditions	Chronic obstructive pulmonary disease
	Fibrositis syndrome
	Nocturnal cardiac ischemia
	Peptic ulcer disease
	Sleeping sickness
	Sleep-related asthma
	Sleep-related gastroesophageal reflux
Neurologic conditions	Cerebral degenerative disorders
	Dementia
	Fatal familial insomnia
	Parkinsonism
	Sleep-related epilepsy
	Sleep-related headaches

Sleep terror disorder
Sleepwalking disorder.

Insomnia is considered the difficulty in initiating or maintaining or insufficient sleep, whereas **hypersomnia** is excessive daytime sleepiness or an excessive amount of sleep (narcolepsy and substance-related causes are the most common type of hypersomnia). See Table 4-20.2 for common causes of insomnia and hypersomnia.

PRESENTATION
Insomnia and hypersomnia are among the most frequent types of sleep-related complaints you will encounter in an ED setting, most often as an associated finding in a primary medical or psychiatric disorder. Sleep disturbances, such as insomnia (more common) and hypersomnia (less frequently), can be common complaints.

Table 4-20.2.   Causes of insomnia and hypersomnia

Insomnia	Aging
	Anxiety disorders
	CNS lesions
	Depression
	Endocrine/metabolic disorders
	Infectious diseases
	Medication interactions
	Neoplasms
	Nocturnal myoclonus
	Pain
	Parasomnias
	Posttraumatic stress disorder
	Psychosocial stressors
	Restless leg syndrome
	Schizophrenia
	Sleep apnea
	Sleep–wake cycle disruptions
	Substance-related conditions
Hypersomnia	Depression
	Encephalitis
	Hyperthyroidism
	Hypoventilation syndrome
	Kleine-Levin syndrome
	Medication interactions
	Menstrual related
	Metabolic disorders
	Narcolepsy
	Other conditions that cause insomnia
	Poor sleep
	Sleep apneas
	Sleep deprivation
	Sleep–wake cycle disruptions
	Substance related
	Toxic conditions
	Withdrawal phenomenon

CNS, central nervous system.

More than one third of Americans have some form of a sleep disorder at some point in their lives, and more than half will have some form of intermittent sleep disturbance, commonly a poor night's sleep with some daytime sleepiness. Women, the elderly, and patients with medical, psychiatric, or substance-related disorders are at higher risk for sleep disorders.

Patients with sleep disorders infrequently seek help in the ED. Occasionally, because they have insomnia—with recent onset or of a more chronic course—or they have daytime sleepiness, and/or these symptoms are affecting their day-to-day lives, they may seek help. Patients with insomnia (which may be transient and situational, such as before an important meeting, a change of bedroom when traveling, or after the death of a loved one) seldom require an intervention. If it is more persistent and debilitating, it may drive a person to the ED with complaints of sleep problems, most often manifesting as difficulty falling asleep. Many times, anxiety plays a major role, without the patient even being aware of being anxious. These scenarios are seldom severe enough to warrant an ED visit, but at times, insomnia may be the chief complaint, and a symptom of a more serious underlying medical or psychiatric condition. Insomnia becomes a problem if functional impairment or excessive daytime sedation occurs, which can affect a person's ability to work and perform adequately, even posing a safety risk, depending on the job he or she performs.

Patients may often complain that because of stress, tension, or other psychosocial problems, they have difficulty sleeping. They may complain of frequent awakenings, anxious dreams, increased muscular tension, and feeling fatigued when they awaken. They may sleep well when away on vacation or away from home. If depressed, the patient will often complain of unsatisfying sleep, multiple awakenings, and early morning awakenings; whereas if the patient is manic, little sleep occurs, several hours at most, with or without the need for daytime naps. Patients under the influence of substances will develop severe insomnia, with increased awakenings, nightmares, and other withdrawal-related phenomena. In patients with PTSD, poor sleep may result from nightmares or bad dreams of the traumatic event. Those with sleep apnea will have a brief period of cessation in breathing with subsequent awakening and sleeplessness, whereas those patients with nocturnal myoclonus will have sleep-related periodic leg contractions followed by full or partial awakenings. Periodic limb-movement disorder and restless-leg syndrome are sleep disorders characterized by abnormal leg movements. These are both fairly prevalent in the general population and affect sleep and mental health quite dramatically. Recognition and appropriate assessment are important.

Patients with hypersomnia or excessive daytime sedation must be assessed carefully, because this symptom can affect a person's judgment, and cognitive and motor skills can be impaired. The excessive sleepiness can be either prolonged sleep episodes or daytime sleep episodes that occur almost daily and cause significant distress or impairment. A type of dyssomnia, **narcolepsy,** consists of (a) excessive daytime sedation; (b) sudden weakness or loss of muscle tone, without loss of consciousness (cataplexy); (c) hypnogogic (sleep onset) or hypnopompic (awakening) hallucinations; and (d) muscular paralysis on awakening.

MANAGEMENT

As stated earlier, normally most people will not seek help for a sleep disturbance, and if they do, a detailed and comprehensive history and examination are seldom conducted. The underlying sleep disorder is hardly ever diagnosed, and a sedative/hypnotic is the remedy of choice. Sleep disturbances can be harbingers of underlying medical or psychiatric conditions and require a full assessment, including polysomnographic testing, to reach an adequate diagnosis and treatment. Sleep, like fever or pain, should be viewed as a manifestation of a more serious underlying condition, and as such worked up thoroughly.

A careful history should include

Type? Insomnia can be subdivided into difficulty falling asleep, frequent awakening, early morning awakenings, or persistent daytime sleepiness.

Duration? Insomnia can be divided into transient insomnia (short term, a few episodes) or short-term insomnia (a few weeks), or long-term or chronic insomnia (months to years).

Severity?

Consistency?

Consequences?

Medical and psychiatric history?

Medication and other substances?

Collateral sources can help at times in corroborating the degree of daytime impairment or actual nighttime insomnia; the patient may either under- or misreport symptoms that may be important, such as snoring, restless leg movements, nocturia, or falling asleep while driving or in other circumstances.

Determining the type of sleep disorder may be hard in an ED setting, but gathering information about the nature of the sleep disturbance can assist in a better understanding of the patient's complaint and a more effective referral and even treatment selection. Patients with complaints of sleep disturbances can be provided with a copy of the Sleep Questionnaire (see Table 4-20.3), and a clinician can then review the responses, to better gauge the type of sleep disorder.

If the insomnia is secondary to medical or psychiatric causes, the goal of treatment will be to address the underlying conditions, and in those cases of situational insomnia, the treatment will be geared to relieve the precipitating factors.

DISPOSITION

Because a definitive diagnosis will be hard to make in the ED, a referral to a specialized clinic, if available, for a polysomnography is necessary to achieve an accurate diagnosis and treatment plan. Otherwise, a referral to a primary care specialist or clinic should be undertaken; provide the patient with instructions on good sleep hygiene, and also instruct him or her to keep a sleep diary until the outpatient visit; keeping track of:

Work times
Sleep times
Naps
Nocturnal awakenings

Table 4-20.3. Sleep questionnaire

Difficulty Falling Sleep	Daytime Sleepiness	Trouble During Sleeping
Do you have difficulty falling asleep?	Do you feel as if you are getting sleepy when you don't want to, such as when driving, watching TV, reading, etc.?	Do your legs jerk frequently or feel uncomfortable or restless before or during sleep?
Do you wake too early?		Have you ever had an episode of sleep-walking?
Is it difficult to get back to sleep if you awaken at night?		
Are you frequently tired in the morning?	Does daytime sleepiness interfere with your social/work responsibilities?	Do you frequently have night-mares?
Does loss of sleep affect your mood during the day, making you more irritable, tense, or depressed?	Do you sleep more than 9 hr in a 24-hr period?	Have you ever wet the bed?
	Do you snore at night?	Have you ever fallen out of bed?
Do you have variable sleep/wake times?	Have you been told you have long pauses in your breathing during sleep?	Do you grind your teeth at night?
Do you travel often?		Do you wake with jaw pain?
Do you do night-shift work?		Do you know if you have seizures in your sleep?
Is there too much light in your bedroom?	Have you ever had any accidents or near-accidents because of excessive sleepiness?	Do you thrash in your sleep?
Do you sleep in a noisy environment?	Do you fall asleep unintentionally during the day?	Do you ever awaken screaming, violent, or confused?
Does your bed partner disturb your sleep?	Are you irritable during the day?	
Do you exercise 2 hr before going to bed?	Do you take a nap?	
Do you drink any caffeinated beverages at night?	Do you have headaches on awakening?	
Do you smoke before going to bed or at night when you wake up?	Do your muscles feel very weak when you are laughing, excited, or angry?	
Do you feel that you are too stressed out to sleep?	Do you have difficulty concentrating or remembering things?	

continued

Table 4-20.3. *Continued*

Difficulty Falling Sleep	Daytime Sleepiness	Trouble During Sleeping
Have there been any recent stressors in your life?	Do you ever see or hear or feel things as you are falling asleep or awakening?	
In the last month, have you had difficulty sleeping because of: cough, difficulty breathing, frequent urination, hot flashes, pain?	Do you have night sweat?	
	Is your sleep restless?	
Are you taking medications to help you sleep?		
Are you taking any over-the-counter medications for sleep?		
Do you drink any alcoholic beverages at night?		

Hours slept
Use of sleep aids
Use of alcohol or drugs.

Improving sleep hygiene is a must, and recommendations should be made to patients with sleep problems to improve their sleep-behavior habits before attempting other treatment options. See Table 4-20.4 for a list of sleep do's and don'ts. Recommend that too much reliance on nonprescription or over-the-counter sleep remedies can be hazardous, because of risks of side effects or adverse reactions. Elderly patients should be cautioned as well about these remedies, being more sensitive, and if prescribed benzodiazepines, they should be informed that risks could include anterograde amnesia, insomnia, daytime anxiety or sedation, and even psychomotor abnormalities, including increased propensity for falls or withdrawal seizures.

A bed partner who is disruptive to a patient's ability to sleep can at times be a potential problem that is not easy to remedy. A referral for the bed partner (although not your primary patient), if he or she has a sleep disorder, may help the actual patient in the long run. A referral to couples therapy may be beneficial as well, if the source of disruption is conjugal discord, which may be played out at night in bed.

Table 4-20.4.   Sleep hygiene do's and don'ts

These do's and don'ts should be discussed with patients complaining of insomnia as part of the psychoeducation on sleep hygiene.

- Many people feel that exercising before bedtime will make them feel tired and able to fall asleep. Strenuous exercise before bedtime actually makes it harder to fall asleep. Instruct the patient to do relaxing activities before sleeping, such as reading, watching TV, listening to music, knitting, etc.
- Patients will often think that a cup of hot cocoa, tea, or a nightcap will help them sleep. Chocolate, caffeinated soft drinks, coffee, and caffeinated teas all contain caffeine, which can keep people awake. It takes several hours for caffeine to clear from one's system; thus it is important to remind patients to avoid all caffeinated drinks several hours before going to bed. Alcohol can initially make one feel drowsy, but it will likely wake them several hours later and make it difficult to get back to sleep
- Conversely, a glass of warm milk can be beneficial in helping people get to sleep; over-the-counter sleep-aid teas also can be helpful
- Remind the patient to stay away from over-the-counter tryptophan pills because of case reports of eosinophilia-myalgia syndrome
- Instruct the patient to avoid drinking too many liquids before going to sleep to avoid frequent awakening to void
- Irregular sleep schedules can disrupt a patient's body's normal sleep/wake cycle. Regular bedtime and rising times are important to keep consistent, even on weekends
- Insomnia can be caused by too much stress. Remind the patient to find time, before going to sleep, to deal with charged or emotionally intense issues. The bed should not be the place to discuss or fight with a partner
- Lying in bed, unable to get to sleep, can reinforce the inability to fall asleep. Recommend getting out of bed and doing something relaxing, such as reading or watching TV, until they become drowsy again and can go back to sleep
- Warm baths are more soothing and relaxing and are less activating than showers. A warm bath at night can help people relax
- Nicotine also can be a stimulant and affect one's ability to fall asleep. Smoking ≥1 hr before bedtime is not recommended
- Loud noises, bright lights, extremes of temperature in a person's bedroom can all negatively affect their ability to sleep
- Large meals can interfere with sleep onset
- Clocks can heighten the anxiety about sleep and hours left to sleep. Patients should try to avoid focusing on these external cues
- Remind the patient that effective treatments for sleep disorders and help are possible

In transient or short-term insomnia, a brief course of hypnotic medication might be effective. Recommend sleep-hygiene improvements, over-the-counter remedies (to be used judiciously), and teas before using a hypnotic agent. See Table 4-20.5 for a list of over-the-counter nighttime sleep aids. For patients with more chronic forms of insomnia or other forms of sleep disorder, a referral to a specialist and avoiding prescription medication until a definitive diagnosis can be reached are important.

If providing a hypnotic agent, consider these nonbenzodiazepine hypnotics:

zolpidem (Ambien), 10 mg, PO
zaleplom (Sonata), 10 mg, PO

Consider these short-acting benzodiazepines, which decrease the likelihood of daytime sedation, in cases of initial insomnia:

estazolam (ProSom), 1 mg, PO
temazepam (Restoril), 15 mg, PO
triazolam (Halcion), 0.125 mg, PO

Patients with frequent or early awakenings might need longer-acting benzodiazepines, such as

flurazepam (Dalmane), 15 mg, PO
quazepam (Doral), 7.5 mg, PO

Table 4-20.5.   Over-the-counter nighttime sleep aids

Product	Ingredient
Excedrin PM	Diphenhydramine citrate, 38 mg + acetaminophen, 500 mg
Extra Strength Bayer PM Aspirin	Diphenhydramine HCl, 25 mg + aspirin, 500 mg
Extra Strength Doan's PM	Diphenhydramine HCl, 25 mg + salicylate 500 mg
Bayer Select Nighttime Pain Relief	Diphenhydramine HCl, 25 mg + acetaminophen, 500 mg
Miles Nervine Nighttime Pain Relief	Diphenhydramine HCl, 25 mg
Nytol QuickCaps	Diphenhydramine HCl, 25 mg
Maximum Strength Nytol	Doxylamine succinate, 25 mg
Legatrin PM	Diphenhydramine HCl, 25 mg + acetaminophen, 500 mg
Sleepinal	Diphenhydramine HCl, 50 mg
Unisom Nighttime Sleep Aid	Doxylamine succinate, 25 mg
Unisom with Pain Relief Sleep Aid	Diphenhydramine HCl, 50 mg + acetaminophen, 650 mg
Maximum Strength Unisom Sleep Gels	Diphenhydramine HCl, 50 mg

Patients with depression and sleep disturbances may respond to antidepressant treatment; although several SSRIs can have a negative effect on sleep patterns and will require concomitant treatment with a hypnotic agent.

BIBLIOGRAPHY

Benca RM. Consequences of insomnia and its therapies. *J Clin Psychiatry* 2001;62(suppl 10):33–38.

Katz G, Durst R, Zislin Y, et al. Psychiatric aspects of jet lag: a review and hypothesis. *Med Hypotheses* 2001;56:20–23.

Kaufman DM. *Clinical neurology for psychiatrists.* 4th ed. Philadelphia: WB Saunders, 1995.

McCall WV. A psychiatric perspective on insomnia. *J Clin Psychiatry* 2001;62(suppl 10):27–32.

Morin CM, Daley M, Ouellet MC. Insomnia in adults. *Curr Treat Options Neurol* 2001;3:9–18.

Ohayon MM, Roth T. Prevalence of restless leg syndrome and periodic limb movement disorder in the general population. *J Psychosom Res* 2002;53:547–554.

Richardson GS, Roth T. Future directions in the management of insomnia. *J Clin Psychiatry* 2001;62(suppl 10):39–45.

Richardson GS, Roth T, Kramer JA. Management of insomnia: the role of zaleplon. *Med Gen Med* 2002;14:9.

Schneider DL. Insomnia: safe and effective therapy for sleep problems in the older patient. *Geriatrics* 2002;57:24–26, 29, 32.

Thase ME. Treatment issues related to sleep and depression. *J Clin Psychiatry* 2000;61(suppl 11):46–50.

Chapter 4-21 Suicidal Ideation/Attempts

DEFINITION

Suicide is the act of killing oneself; it is intentional self-inflicted death.

PRESENTATION

Suicidal ideation or attempts can occur in many different psychiatric disorders but are not specific to any. It can occur in patients with affective, psychotic, or personality disorders, acute intoxication or withdrawal states, and certain medical conditions. The assessment of suicidal ideation is an important aspect of any initial evaluation and an integral part of the psychiatric MSE. Suicidal ideation should always be viewed as an extreme manifestation of despair.

In an ED, suicidal ideation should be initially assessed at triage so that the necessary precautionary procedures are instituted (see Chapter 3). Primarily, the emergency physician should manage patients with overdoses (see Chapter 4-18) or with lacerations, cuts, and wounds requiring more involved medical care, with psychiatry consultation as needed. All other patients with suicidal presentations should be handle by psychiatry.

Suicide must be conceptualized on a continuum from passive ideation to a completed act. Suicide attempts manifest from superficial cuts on the wrist or forearm, to serious self-inflicted stab wounds, or the intentional ingestion of toxic agents, to the overdosing of medications and drugs. Passive suicidal ideation, for example, could be seen as a 68-year-old woman reporting, in the context of her medical and personal life stressors, that she would be "better off dead." An example of active suicidal ideation is the severely depressed 30-year-old man with schizophrenia who plans to jump off his roof to escape the "voices in his head." Suicide attempts that are half-completed tend to expose the patient's ambivalence—their struggle between the wish to live and the wish to die. Such situations afford the ED staff the greatest opportunity to intervene, to ally him- or herself with the patient's wish to live and assist the patient in seeing the opportunity for help and treatment.

Several profiles exist of patients who frequently have suicidal ideation, and I have grouped them as follows, although these do not represent the totality of patients with suicidal ideation.

Patient Profiles

Adolescent / Impulsive Type

- Commonly young adolescent girls, occasionally adolescent boys
- Recent stressors
- Respond impulsively by reporting suicidal ideation or attempting suicide
- Prior psychiatric histories and suicide attempts
- Suicide attempts are usually attention seeking, either because of familial discord, legal or school problems, or relationship conflicts
- Attempts are predominantly by overdosing or superficial self-cutting, with minimal or no intent to die; although the intent is nonlethal and more for attention or rescue, the severity and lethality can still be high
- Brought in mostly by a parent or guardian or a school or agency staff member, and rarely on their own.

Substance Abusing / Impulsive Type

- Commonly males
- Antisocial or sociopathic features
- Some have a psychiatric diagnosis besides their alcohol or substance-abuse/dependence
- Suicidal ideation occurs often in the context of acute intoxication or during withdrawal
- Associated depressive symptoms are often situational
- Frequently a history of impulsivity, violence, or self-inflicted harm
- Suicide threats or attempts are often seen as a means to an end: a meal, a token, or a hospital admission
- Most often are walk-ins or are brought in by emergency medical technicians or police after being found on the streets acting bizarrely or being disruptive

Despondent / Anxious Type

- Suicidal ideation is a predominant feature
- Often have primary psychiatric disorders, such as an affective, anxiety, or psychotic disorder

- In a primary affective disorder, depressive symptoms and hopelessness are present and overwhelming; however, usually no history of prior suicide attempts is found, and if so, a tendency to minimize its lethality
- In anxiety or psychotic disorders, the anxiety, agitation, and psychosis are the driving features and are severe enough to precipitate suicidal ideation and attempts
- Severe anxiety should be considered a risk factor–panic and anxiety, anhedonia, agitation, and ruminative thinking are signs of intense psychic turmoil
- Often state that it would be better for themselves or others if they were dead
- React with regret if they are thwarted in their suicide attempt
- Mostly referred by their family or friends and occasionally are brought in by ambulance or police

Angry/Impulsive Type
- Commonly young females
- Predominant character disorders
- Long history of recurrent suicidal ideation and many prior suicide gestures
- History of multiple treatment approaches and medication trials with significant impulse dysregulation
- Have suicide ideation in the context of real or perceived losses or separations
- Presentations are characterized by intense emotional lability, anxiety, and even dissociative symptoms
- Suicide attempts are intended as attention seeking and nonlethal, although these too can be quite serious and even deadly
- Often well known to the ED staff from frequent emergency visits and are often in established care within the hospital system
- Mostly self-referred or occasionally sent in by their primary provider or clinic.

MANAGEMENT

It is imperative that the assessment of suicidality, especially in the ED, be performed in an organized and systematic approach. Because future suicide is difficult to predict, the goal is to use sound clinical judgment within certain parameters. Studies have shown that 30% to 45% of suicide victims give no warning about their intent. For this reason, it is crucial that every clinician be aware of the known predictors and high-risk factors for suicide. It is essential to perform a thorough evaluation and diagnostic assessment to identify whether a particular patient has a psychiatric disorder that is associated with increased suicide risk, such as: schizophrenia, substance abuse, or mood, anxiety, or personality disorders. Table 4.21.1 lists the possible high-risk factors and predictors of suicide, and Table 4.21.2 lists medical conditions that can increase the suicide risk in a patient.

Paterson et al. developed the SAD PERSONS Scale for assessing the risk of suicide. The higher the number of points scored, the greater the risk (1 or 2 points scored for each factor deemed present: 0, very little risk/10, very high risk). Although the scale

Table 4-21.1.   Associated high-risk factors and predictors of suicide

General
   Males
   Older than 40 years
   Caucasians, except for certain specific groups, such as inner-city
      youths, Native-American and Alaskan Indians
   Single, widowed, or divorced
   Immigrant status
   Living alone or poor social supports
   Socially disorganized urban areas, resort towns
   Higher SES and any changes in SES
   Unoccupied, unemployed, or retired

Medical
   Incapacitating medical illness
   Dementia, confusional states, or delirium
   Organic brain syndromes

Psychiatric
   Affective disorders, schizophrenia, alcohol and substance abuse
   Prior suicide attempts
   Soon after onset of illness, at beginning of treatment, or within
      6 months after discharge from active treatment
   Depressive symptoms of persistent insomnia, dejected appearance
      and weight loss, slowed speech, loss of interest, listlessness,
      social withdrawal, hopelessness and pessimism, ideas of
      unworthiness, agitation, restlessness
   Suicidal ideation
   Irritability or angry affects
   Intense anxiety or panic symptoms
   Alcohol dependence and intoxication or withdrawal states
      Domestic and social complications of drinking
   Frequent psychiatry emergency room visits

History
   Past suicide attempts are the best indicator of future
   suicide
   Family history of affective disorders, suicide, alcoholism

Other
   Family stress or instability
   Spring/fall
   Access to weapon
   Recent loss or separation
   Preparatory acts (procuring means, putting affairs in order,
      warning statements, giving away of personal belongings,
      suicide notes)
   Unwillingness to accept help
   Precautions taken against discovery
   Violent methods and lethal drugs/poisons
   Change in resident rotation
   Reading *The Final Exit*

SES, socioeconomic status.

Table 4-21.2. Medical conditions that increase risk of suicide

CNS diseases	Seizure disorders, multiple sclerosis, traumatic brain injuries, CVAs, dementia, AIDS, Huntington disease
Endocrine diseases	Cushing, Klinefelter, porphyria
Gastrointestinal diseases	Peptic ulcer disease, cirrhosis
Genitourinary diseases	Benign prostatic hypertrophy, renal disease, hemodialysis
Other	Illness with loss of mobility, disfigurement, chronic intractable pain

CNS, central nervous system; CVA, cerebrovascular accident; AIDS, acquired immunodeficiency syndrome.

has sensitivity and specificity problems it is a good guide to make certain all pertinent risk factors for suicide are queried.

Sex	male	1
Age	<19 or >45 years old	1
Depression	endorses depressive symptoms	2
Previous attempt	yes (including prior hospitalizations)	1
Ethanol (drug) use	yes (acute or chronic)	1
Rational thinking loss	medical etiology or psychosis	2
Separated, divorced, widowed	recent or anniversary	1
Organized plan	well thought out, lethal plan	2
No social support	no friends, family, or supports	1
Stated future intent	determined or ambivalent	2

Although staff may feel uncomfortable when inquiring about current or past suicidal ideation, it is nonetheless necessary. Patients who have suicidal ideation will potentially be relieved if they are asked directly about their thoughts and will feel that the staff is interested in their condition. Specific questions that must always be asked:

• Ask about recent acute stressors or exacerbation of chronic ones
• Ask about losses or separations (this can assist in giving the clinician a better understanding of the patient's psychological framework)
• Ask about suicidal ideation, urges, and images.

Ask patients *directly* about killing themselves or dying, not just about hurting themselves; many people do not want to experience pain, and their intent to die is usually perceived as a painless way to end their suffering. Inquire about the frequency of the suicide ideation and any increase or change in its nature. Carefully assess anxiety, agitation, and fear; studies have shown that a decrease in fear and dread occurs before a completed suicide. Explore hopelessness. This is a crucial psychological factor behind suicide intent and behavior. Does the patient have negative expectations, or a sense of uselessness and disconnection from others?

ASSESSMENT PARAMETERS

Occasionally, within the context of a complicated bereavement, suicidal ideation can be a manifestation of a desire to join a deceased relative, spouse, or friend. Ask about family history of suicide, either recent or past. It is important to determine how close the patient was to the relative who committed suicide, both biologically and emotionally. Are suicidal ideation or attempts a family pattern in coping with stress? Has the young adolescent girl seen her mother make suicide threats or attempts when under stress? Special attention must be given to the actual suicide act—its intent, lethality, and meaning in the context of the particular patient. After any attempted suicide, a patient must be questioned in detail about the event, and a 24-hour "walk-through" of the preceding day should be obtained. As many specifics as possible of the patient's thoughts, emotions, activities should be explored, especially noting any change from the patient's routine. All cases of suicidal ideation or suicide attempts should be assessed with the following parameters in mind.

- What was the *action?* Was it impulsive or premeditated? Were there rehearsals of the suicide attempt? These are essential pieces of information that a clinician must gather to assess future lethality optimally. Also consider future actions, premeditation versus impulsivity, and current feelings or thoughts regarding the act. A detailed explanation of the events that led to the suicide, including all possible stressors, precipitants, variations in normal routine or functioning, and compliance with aftercare plans or medications is helpful in understanding the patient's current condition.
- What was the patient's *intent?* Inquire about his or her thoughts and feelings. How long has he or she had these thoughts? When did these thoughts start? How often do they occur? Do they have an obsessional quality? Are they passive or active? What does the patient wish to accomplish? Does the patient want to die, punish someone else, escape, or get attention? Have the patient explain his or her ideas about death and dying (an adolescent might think that death is the same as a prolonged slumber, with a very limited understanding of its finality). Does he or she want to join a departed loved one or someone who has committed suicide? How does he or she view death? Is it a positive experience? Try to assess the patient's capacity to carry out the plan—does he or she have the organizational ability and the energy to see it through? It is known that suicide potential is increased when people have more energy, such as in the early phase of recovery from a depression or because of impaired impulse control when intoxicated.
- What is the patient's *plan?* How much preparation has gone into it? Is there a specific sequence of events (method, place, or time)? How feasible is the plan, and what are the chances of rescue? People who have a plan with a greater chance of discovery may be more ambivalent than are those who have made sure no one will find them. Bizarre or psychotic plans are truly

high risk because they often have a less predictable outcome. Has the patient rehearsed the events (rigging a noose, putting a gun to head, driving near a bridge, going to rooftop)?

- What is the patient's understanding of the *lethality* (the likelihood of death) of the action? Did he or she know that taking an entire bottle of acetaminophen was potentially deadly (high lethality), or did he or she ingest four vitamin C tablets, after an argument with the spouse, knowing it could not be harmful (low lethality)? It is important to assess the seriousness of the act and the speed or severity with which the act can cause death. It is important to assess the patient's history of impulsive behaviors. Have external or internal regulatory mechanisms been effective in the past when dealing with stress, or are the coping mechanisms impaired?
- What is the planned *method*? Jumping or shooting and other violent methods are to be carefully assessed, because they are irreversible.
- What is the patient's *means* to obtain weapons, pills, knives, etc.? Remember that most people have access to lethal means at home: knives, rope, and so on; access to a weapon is not the only risk factor.
- Assess the patient's *current reaction*. Is he or she relieved that he or she did not succeed, or is he or she upset and discouraged because of failure?
- What were the *deterring factors*? What stopped him? Ask him what has prevented him from acting on his thoughts. Powerful prohibitions can exist, like religious beliefs, fear of death, dependent family/children, as well as worrisome indications of a future suicide attempt, such as access to means not yet achieved or a planned date.

The exploration of the circumstances surrounding prior attempts can at times provide a glimpse into the person's current state of mind. Inquire carefully about prior suicide attempts or other manifestations of self-destructive behavior. Remember that negative symptoms of psychosis can mask an underlying depression. The association between suicidal ideation and psychiatric illness is the strongest piece of evidence regarding prediction of suicide. It is this strong link that makes the meticulous assessment of underlying psychiatric illness so vital. The staff should let the patient know that suicidal ideation can be a common manifestation during intense stress or depression. The possibility of uncovering an undiagnosed or poorly treated psychiatric condition is fundamental in the ability to predict future risk. It provides the opportunity to implement adequate psychiatric treatment and follow-up, thus serving as a preventive intervention.

PATIENT PROFILES

- In the *despondent/anxious* patient with a mood or psychotic disorder and suicidal ideation, the lack of active psychotic symptoms does not imply lower risk. It is very important to keep in mind that a reduction in anxiety or improvement in affect can be very misleading. Such patients might have resolved their ambivalence and be prepared to act on their suicidal ideation. They may appear to be at peace with themselves and demonstrate no outward signs of concern. Much attention should be paid when patients appear emotionally removed, have very flat or constricted affect, or have made plans for their death: creating a will, giving away belongings, cleaning out their apartment, etc. Completed suicide lifetime rates among patients with schizophrenia are 9% to 13%, and lifetime suicide attempt rates are about 20% to 40%. Suicide is the leading cause of death among young patients with schizophrenia.

- In the *substance abusing/impulsive* patient, either intoxication or withdrawal can lead to acute suicidal ideation and increased risk. A significant decrease or impairment is found in a patient's judgment and release of inhibitions, which places her or him at high risk when under the influence. Although an evaluation is very difficult when a patient is intoxicated, it is important to keep the patient safe until he or she is sober, and then reassess. In this group, chronic abuse or dependence leads to prolonged risk, which can be interpreted as an element of self-destructiveness and a risk factor. Be wary of patients who relapse after a period of sobriety; they might be more inclined to have feelings of guilt, self-contempt, shame, or panic.

- The *adolescent/impulsive patient,* often brought in by family, school, or police, is usually reluctant to participate in an evaluation. Parents or guardians should be informed of the need first to evaluate the adolescent alone (to try to establish an alliance) but be reassured that they will be seen and spoken to as well. Adolescents tend to minimize or be lackadaisical about suicidal ideation. Often multiple psychosocial stressors are involved—at home, in school, with friends or family—with concomitant psychiatric symptoms. Adolescents commonly show fewer classic types of depressive symptoms ("depressive equivalents"), such as acting-out behavior, deteriorating school performance, or truancy, which can assist in clarifying a diagnosis and a treatment strategy. Coming out and sexual identity can be serious stressors for an adolescent, and suicide might be considered a way to cope. Determine whether they know someone who has attempted or committed suicide—copycat suicides can and do occur. They could feel enabled to take the next step if they had been thinking about suicide. Ask about physical, emotional, and sexual abuse at home, which also can contribute and aggravate underlying suicidal ideation.

- Both in the *angry/impulsive* and *adolescent/impulsive* patient, it is important to inquire about self-mutilatory or wrist-cutting behavior. This can point in the direction of mood, anxiety, dissociative, or personality-disorder spectrum illnesses, thus informing treatment options. A history of trauma or abuse also can be an important clue. More commonly, self-mutilatory or wrist-cutting behaviors are self-soothing acts with little or no intent to die, although these patients can eventually kill themselves. Ask the patient with self-mutilatory or wrist-cutting behavior if this helps calm them or relieve their anxiety.

Talk with and listen to relatives. In one study, it was found that 60% of patients who committed suicide had communicated their intent to their spouse within the prior year, whereas only 18% had communicated such ideation to a professional such as a psychiatrist. Corroborative information, especially regarding recent changes or periods of turmoil, followed by unexplainable calm, is crucial in better assessing suicide risk. In an ED setting, where the need for determining risk is so important, it is imperative to contact a family member or friend to increase one's database. Every effort should be made to obtain the patient's expressed verbal or written consent, but barring this, emergency situations such as these can be considered a generic exception to the rules of confidentiality. Both the American Psychiatric Association Position Statement of Confidentiality and the Principles of Medical Ethics clearly state that a psychiatrist may breach confidentiality to protect the patient from "imminent danger." Denial of current suicidal ideation is not reliable enough to dismiss the risk in the presence of other risk factors.

Suicide cuts across many different diagnostic spectrums—both medical and psychiatric. See Table 4-21.3 for a list of differential diagnoses. Treatment and management depend on the underlying diagnosis. A comprehensive psychiatric evaluation with an eye on diagnostic clarification will inform the immediate management and treatment. Any initial management will be to ascertain lethality and ultimately safety to arrive at a safe disposition. All attempts should be made to establish a rapport and an alliance with the patient. Patients who are paranoid or guarded are harder to assess, and thus it is harder to predict suicidality accurately in them.

Medical workup should be performed initially. Cuts, lacerations, or stab wounds should be thoroughly assessed and treated by the emergency physician with clear recommendations for follow-up. In cases of intentional ingestion or overdose, overdose workup protocols should be instituted. A full battery of tests should be performed, including SMA-7, LFTs, CBC, acetaminophen and salicylate serum levels, serum and urine toxicology screens, medication serum levels (e.g., valproic acid, carbamazepine, imipramine), ECG, and a phone call to Poison Control if necessary.

PATIENT PROFILES

- *Adolescent patients* should be seen first, and parents or guardians interviewed afterward. Corroborative information is fundamental because adolescents tend to be guarded. Call parents or guardians, the school, or therapist and ask to speak to their friends or significant others. The more you can piece together the history and story, the sooner you can make a decision regarding their safety.
- *Despondent/anxious* or *angry/impulsive patients* who are agitated, aggressive, or psychotic, regardless of the underlying illness, should be treated. The use of chemical or physical restraints is always an option, and the least-restrictive alternatives should always be considered first. If the agitation escalates or the patient refuses all least restrictive alternatives offered, then more serious and restrictive measures are called for, such as seclusion or restraints (see Chapters 3 and 5.2).
- *Substance-abusing/impulsive patients* who are acutely intoxicated or with withdrawal symptoms should be kept as long as needed and reassessed when more sober. Suicide and other associated psychiatric symptoms are many times transient. Keeping

Table 4-21.3. Differential DSM-IV-TR diagnosis for suicide

DSM-IV-TR category	Diagnosis
Disruptive behavior disorders	Conduct Disorder Oppositional Defiant Disorder Disruptive Behavior Disorder NOS
Delirium, dementia, amnestic and other cognitive disorders	Delirium due to . . . Substance Intoxication or Withdrawal Delirium Delirium due to multiple etiologies Delirium NOS Dementia of the Alzheimer type Vascular Dementia Dementia due to . . . Amnestic Disorder due to . . . Substance-Induced Persisting Amnestic Disorder Cognitive Disorder NOS
Mental disorders due to a general medical condition	Personality change due to . . .
Substance-related disorders	Alcohol-Related Disorders Amphetamine (or Amphetamine-like)-Related Disorders Cocaine-Related Disorders Hallucinogen-Related Disorders Opioid-Related Disorders Phencyclidine (or Phencyclidine-like)-Related Disorders Sedative-, Hypnotic-, or Anxiolytic-Related Disorders Polysubstance-Related Disorders
Schizophrenia and other psychotic disorders	Schizophrenia Schizophreniform Disorder Schizoaffective Disorder Delusional Disorder Brief Psychotic Disorder Psychotic Disorder due to . . . Substance-Induced Psychotic Disorder Psychotic Disorder NOS
Mood disorders	Depressive Disorders Bipolar Disorders Mood Disorder due to . . . Substance-Induced Mood Disorder Mood Disorder NOS
Anxiety disorders	Panic Disorder Posttraumatic Stress Disorder Anxiety Disorder due to . . . Substance-Induced Anxiety Disorder Anxiety Disorder NOS

4. Acute Psychiatric Presentations 199

Table 4-21.3. *Continued*

DSM-IV-TR category	Diagnosis
Somatoform disorders	Pain Disorder
	Somatoform Disorder NOS
Impulse-control disorders	Intermittent Explosive Disorder
	Impulse-Control Disorder NOS
Personality disorder	Antisocial Personality Disorder
	Borderline Personality Disorder
	Histrionic Personality Disorder
	Personality Disorder NOS

DSM, *Diagnostic and Statistical Manual of Mental Disorders;* NOS, not otherwise specified.

a person overnight until intoxication wears off is a viable option, unless an inpatient detoxification unit or a sobering-up station is available. Ongoing assessment of the withdrawal phenomenon should be performed, with periodic vital signs and management as indicated (see Chapter 4-14 and 4-24).

DISPOSITION

All visits to an ED must be a therapeutic intervention. Psychoeducation of patients with a high risk for suicide has been shown to be beneficial. Because suicide cuts across many diagnostic categories and can be acute as well as chronic, treatment planning in an ED setting must take into account immediate safety considerations. The plan must incorporate the clinician's impression of the patient's capacity to form an alliance, based on either past experience with the patient, the current relationship, or information from outside providers. The patient's ongoing potential for suicide, as well as available treatment options, factors into the disposition planning. These options range from outpatient follow-up through, but not limited to, a locked inpatient psychiatry unit. Less-restrictive outpatient settings, such as partial hospitalization or day-treatment programs, are effective; mobile crisis services, such as mobile crisis teams or assertive community treatment programs, also are good alternatives.

It is important to try to keep the patient and family, if present, as involved in the treatment-planning process as possible. Listen to the family and significant others; they often have a clearer sense of the situation and can provide valuable insights into the decision-making process. Incorporating and even bolstering existing treatment plans, as well as reassessing and recommending alternative medication options to the patient's outpatient providers can be quite helpful and an important intervention. It is when the patient has impaired judgment, poor insight, or lacks the capacity to make an informed decision regarding care that the physician must decide to admit involuntarily. Additionally, if a patient is unable to commit to safety outside the hospital, further evaluation and inpatient treatment must be considered, and involuntary hospitalization is required (see Chapter 7). If a patient requiring hospitalization cannot commit to safety and remains actively suicidal, safety must be ensured. Such patients require an enhanced observational status (one-on-one observation) on the inpatient floor. Inpatient staff can discontinue or modify the observational status once they are more familiar with the patient.

One of the hardest decisions to make in an ED setting is to discharge a patient after an assessment of suicidal ideation or after an attempt. Complex psychiatric, medicolegal, and ethical issues are always present when ascertaining adequately someone's level of safety. The decision to release is never easy, but not every case of suicidal ideation need be admitted. The notion of creating and holding a patient to a behavioral contract or promise to "commit to safety" is not a guarantee of future safety! Remember that safety, like suicide, can have a variable and fluctuating course. When discharging, make sure to provide an adequate and reasonable aftercare plan, and encourage the patient to resume close contact with treatment providers, family, and friends during this period.

PATIENT PROFILES

For the common types of suicidal presentations, these guidelines are not steadfast rules and can never be substituted for sound clinical judgment and experience.

- *Adolescent/Impulsive type:* These cases are the hardest. Children and adolescents, because of their age and their inability to grasp fully the severity of their actions, often pose a serious challenge. Although inpatient hospitalization is always an option, one must factor in the risks of an acute psychiatric hospitalization (preferably on an adolescent unit), with the risks of discharging back to a similar stressful environment. With minors, one must be allied with the parent when making these decisions. The parent or guardian must be involved in the admission process, whether signing in the patient voluntarily or filling out the application for involuntary admission. If the parent or guardian is not acting in the child's best interest or is the reason/precipitant for the suicide attempt or ideation, then the local child-protective agency must be brought in. Everyone should be familiar with the local and state laws regarding when to call child-protective services. Nonlethal or attention-seeking attempts usually do not require an inpatient hospitalization, and referral to outpatient services will suffice. If serious underlying psychiatric symptoms are present, an admission might be warranted to provide a full workup, assessment, and treatment (see Fig. 4-1).
- *Substance-abusing/Impulsive type:* Disposition varies according to the severity of the presentation. Most often, and when possible, the patient can remain in the ED while sobering up or "crashing" from the specific acute intoxication or withdrawal. Symptomatic management for agitation, psychosis, or anxiety can be provided, and the patient may be allowed to "sleep it off." Once symptoms abate, the patient is usually ready and willing to be discharged back to regular care, or alternatively, he or she must be provided with aftercare plans. These plans can run the gamut of services available for primary substance abuser and/or

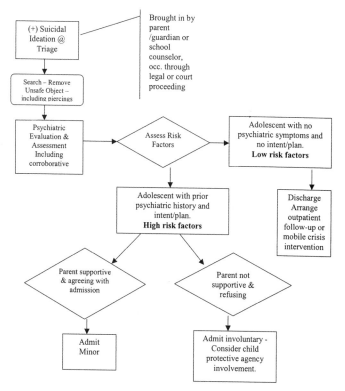

Fig. 4-1. Algorithm: Adolescents with suicidal ideation.

patients with co-occurring substance and psychiatric disorders: 12-step programs, methadone programs, inpatient or outpatient detoxification programs, inpatient or outpatient rehabilitation programs, M.I.C.A. day-treatment programs, and long-term residential programs.

- *Despondent/Anxious type:* These cases most often require an inpatient psychiatric hospitalization to provide safety, further evaluation, and stabilization. The patient is predominantly distraught and quite symptomatic, and requires a safe environment to prevent further harm to self and adequate psychiatric treatment.
- *Angry/Impulsive types:* These cases are complex; although the intent is seldom to die, lethality and risk are associated. In the context of acute or unchanging stressors, perceived loss (change in resident rotation, change in primary therapist), or poor social supports and inability to retract suicidality, these cases occasionally require an inpatient hospitalization or a slightly less-structured option, such as a partial-hospitalization program. Usually the patient is well known to the staff from prior visits,

and old medical records are available. Corroborative information and collateral sources of information inform the decision-making process. When deciding on an inpatient hospitalization, one must weigh the risk of regression and reinforcement of suicidal behavior, as well as the risk of repeated and frequent hospitalizations. If an extended observation unit is available or keeping a person overnight is possible, then a more prolonged stay, while trying to work with the patient in committing to safety, can be attempted. This type of intervention, although time-consuming and labor intensive, can be very effective if the patient and staff can work well and closely together. The goal is to try to provide a safe haven and a respite, with frequent supportive interventions over the course of the time spent in the ED. Once the patient is ready, feeling safer, and able to commit to return to the outpatient therapy, he or she should be released. Additionally, with possible recent medication nonadherence, usual medication dosages can be restarted. Attempts must be made to provide the patient with a speedy outpatient follow-up or discharge back to a structured day program.

Documentation is the key. Carefully document the decision-making process, collateral and corroborative information gathered, the patient's informed consent and capacity to make a decision regarding the care, and carefully document the aftercare plans made. If admitting, make sure the patient has capacity to understand the legal status and have the patient sign in as a voluntary patient.

BIBLIOGRAPHY

Arango V, Underwood MD, Mann JJ. Biological alteration in the brainstem of suicides. *Psychiatr Clin North Am* 1997;20:581–593.

Barraclough B, Bunch J, Nelson B, et al. A hundred cases of suicide: clinical aspects. *Br J Psychiatry* 1974;125:355–373.

Centers for Disease Control and Prevention. Vital Statistics of United States 1995, Mortality. U.S. Department of Health and Human Services, Hyattsville, Maryland, 1999.

Centers for Disease Control and Prevention. *Violence Surveillance Summary Series, No. 2.* Atlanta, GA: CDC, 1996.

Centers for Disease Control and Prevention. Surveillance for injuries and violence among older adults. *MMWR* 1999;48(SS-8):27–34.

Centers for Disease Control and Prevention. Suicide among children, adolescents, and young adults: United States, 1980–1992. *MMWR* 1995;44:289–291.

Centers for Disease Control and Prevention. Programs for the prevention of suicide among adolescents and young adults; and suicide contagion and the reporting of suicide: recommendations from a national workshop. *MMWR* 1994;43:6.

Dulcan MK, Martini DR. Special clinical circumstances. In: Dulcan MK, Martini DR, eds. *Concise guide to child and adolescent psychiatry.* 2nd ed. Washington, DC: American Psychiatric Press, 1999:191–210.

Greenhill LL, Waslick B. Management of suicidal behavior in children and adolescents. *Psychiatr Clin North Am* 1997;20:641–666.

Heila H, Heikkinen ME, Isometsa ET, et al. Life events and completed suicide in schizophrenia: a comparison of suicide victims with and without schizophrenia. *Schizophr Bull* 1999;25:519–531.

Heila H, Isometsa ET, Henriksson MM, et al. Suicide victims with schizophrenia in different treatment phases and adequacy of antipsychotic medication. *J Clin Psychiatry* 1999;60:200–208.

Hockberger RS, Rothstein RJ. Assessment of suicide potential by nonpsychiatrists using "SAD PERSONS" score. *J Emerg Med* 1988;6:99.

Ikeda RM, Kresnow MJ, Mercy JA, et al. Medical conditions and nearly lethal suicide attempts. *Suicide Life Threat Behav* 2001; 32(suppl 1):60–67.

Jacobs DG, Jamison KR, Baldessarini RJ, et al. Suicide: clinical/risk management issues for psychiatrists-grand rounds. *CNS Spectrums* 2000;5:32–53.

Jacobs DG, et al. In: Jacobs DG, ed. *Harvard Medical School guide to suicide assessment and intervention.* San Francisco, CA: Jossey-Bass, 1998:3–39.

Keith-Spiegel P, Spiegel DE. Affective states of patients immediately preceding suicide. *J Psychiatry Res* 1967;5:89–93.

Klerman GL. Clinical epidemiology of suicide. *J Clin Psychiatry* 1987;48:33–38.

Lambert MT. Seven-year outcomes of patients evaluated for suicide. *Psychiatr Serv* 2002;53:92–94.

Meltzer HY. Suicidality in schizophrenia: a review of the evidence for risk factors and treatment options. *Curr Psychiatry Rep* 2002;4: 279–283.

Meltzer HY. Treatment of suicidality in schizophrenia. *Ann N Y Acad Sci* 2001;932:44–58.

Moscicki EK. Identification of suicide risk factors using epidemiological studies. *Psychiatr Clin North Am* 1997;20:499–517.

Paris J. Chronic suicidality among patients with borderline personality disorder. *Psychiatr Serv* 2002;53:738–742.

Paterson WM, Dohn HH, Bird J, et al. Evaluation of suicidal patients: the SAD PERSONS Scale. *Psychosomatics* 1983;24:343–349.

Pfeffer C. Childhood suicidal behavior: a development perspective. *Psychiatr Clin North Am* 1997;20:551–562.

Placidi GP, Oquendo MA, Maolne KM, et al. Anxiety in major depression: relationship to suicide attempts. *Am J Psychiatry* 2000;157: 1614–1618.

Potter LB, Powell KP, Kachur SP. Suicide prevention from a public health perspective. *Suicide Life-Threat Behav* 1995;25:82–91.

Rives W. Emergency department assessment of suicidal patients. *Psychiatr Clin North Am* 1999;22:779–787.

Robins E. *The final months.* New York: Oxford University Press, 1981.

Robins E, Murphy GE, Wilkinson RH, et al. The communication of suicidal intent: a study of 134 consecutive cases of successful (completed) suicide. *Am J Psychiatry* 1959;115:724–733.

Simon RI. *Clinical psychiatry and the law.* New York: American Psychiatric Press, 1992.

Stanley B, Gameroff MJ, Michalsen V, et al. Are suicide attempters who self-mutilate a unique population? *Am J Psychiatry* 2001;158: 427–432.

U.S. Public Health Service. *The Surgeon General's call to action to prevent suicide.* Washington, DC: USPHS, 1999.

Warshaw MG, Dolan RT, Keller MD. Suicidal behavior in patients with current or past panic disorder: five years of prospective data from the Harvard/Brown Anxiety Research Program. *Am J Psychiatry* 2000;157:1876–1878.

Chapter 4-22 Treatment-emergent Syndromes

Neuroleptic malignant syndrome (NMS)
Serotonin syndrome (SS)
Lethal catatonia (LC)
Selective serotonin reuptake inhibitor (SSRI) discontinuation
  syndrome

As physicians, at times we may, in the course of a treatment intervention, induce or cause a side effect or adverse drug effect. These acute syndromes are known as treatment-emergent syndromes and can be a reason for an ED visit. These syndromes often lead to medication nonadherence; prior psychoeducation about the possibility of developing a treatment-emergent syndrome and close monitoring of the patients are hallmarks of good clinical care. See Table 4-22.1 for a comparison chart of these disorders.

NEUROLEPTIC MALIGNANT SYNDROME

Definition

NMS is an idiosyncratic drug reaction. It is a rare but life-threatening complication of antipsychotic treatment and can occur any time during the course of treatment. NMS is not dose related and can occur even after a single dose of a neuroleptic.

Presentation

Estimates of incidence vary, but in approximately 1% of patients taking neuroleptics, NMS develops. It has been reported among all ages, is twice as common in men as in women, and most commonly occurs between the ages of 20 and 50 years. It develops rapidly over a 24- to 72-hour period and is more common with high-potency antipsychotics, such as haloperidol or fluphenazine, or when neuroleptics are prescribed in high dosages and/or when dosages are titrated rapidly. It is important to keep in mind that all neuroleptics can induce NMS, including the newer atypical agents such as clozapine, risperidone, olanzapine. Certain antiemetics like prochloperazine, tricyclic antidepressants (TCAs) like amoxapine, sedatives like promethazine, properistaltic agents like metoclopramide, and other medications like phenytoin, carbamazepine, tetrabenazine, reserpine, lithium, sulpiride (presumably because of their dopamine-blocking properties) have been reported to cause NMS. See Table 4-22.2 for a list of common diagnoses in which NMS may occur.

NMS may manifest along a symptom spectrum and a severity spectrum: partial or attenuated forms of the syndrome may occur and are supported in the recent literature and in anecdotal reports of "atypical" presentations with the atypical antipsychotics.

In more than 80% of cases, mental-status changes and rigidity are the first manifestations of NMS. These early signs are not specific for NMS and do not always progress to NMS. Patients usually are first seen with:

- Muscular rigidity (95% of cases have "lead-pipe" rigidity); thoracic muscular rigidity may lead to constrictive hypoventilation requiring ventilatory support.

Table 4-22.1. Comparison chart

	NMS	Serotonin Syndrome	Lethal Catatonia	SSRI Discontinuation
History	Prolonged use of neuroleptics or recent discontinuation	Recent change of SSRI or addition of another medication	History of psychiatric disorder	Discontinuation for missed SSRI doses
Onset	Gradual (over hours or days)	Rapid	Gradual (with prodromal phase)	Rapid
Resolution	Slower (avg. 9 days)	Rapid (<24 hr)	?	Mild and fleeting to several weeks
Incidence	1% of all patients taking neuroleptics	?	?	Varies (?)
Sex ratio (related more to diagnosis and recommended treatment options)	Male > female	=	Female>male	=
Neuroleptic use	++	–	+/–	–
Recent change in meds	Yes (at times)	Yes	No	Yes
Mental status changes	+++	+++	+++	+
Muscle rigidity	+++	++	+	–
Hyperthermia	+++	++	++	–
Elevated CPK	+++	+	+	–
Dysphasia	+	–	–	–

continued

Table 4-22.1. *Continued*

	NMS	Serotonin Syndrome	Lethal Catatonia	SSRI Discontinuation
Incontinence	+	–	–	–
Sialorrhea	+	–	–	–
Myoclonus	–	+	–	–
Hyperreflexia	–	+	–	–
Ataxia	–	+	–	–
Diaphoresis	+	+	+	–
Metabolic acidosis	+	–	–	–
Elevated LFTs	+	–	–	–
Leukocytosis	++	+	–	–
Supportive medical care	Yes	Yes	Yes	No
Dantrolene	Yes	–	Yes	–
Baclofen	Yes	–	–	–
ECT	Yes	No	Yes	–
Mortality	10%–30%	?	60%	–

CPK, creatine phosphokinase; LFT, liver-function test; ECT, electroconvulsive therapy; NMS, neuroleptic malignant syndrome; SSRI, selective serotonin reuptake inhibitor.

Table 4-22.2. Diagnoses in which NMS may occur

Psychiatric diagnosis
  Schizophrenia
  Affective disorders
  Delirium
  Dementia
  Other psychosis
  Mental retardation
Nonpsychiatric diagnosis, especially patients with extrapyramidal
  disorders
  Parkinson
  Wilson
  Huntington
  Striatonigral degeneration
  Patients who have received neuroleptics or dopamine-depleting
    agents or have had dopamine agonists abruptly withdrawn

NMS, neuroleptic malignant syndrome.

- Neurologic dysfunction:
  Abnormal reflexes
  Agitation
  Aphonia
  Bradykinesia
  Chorea
  Delirium
  Dysarthria
  Dysphagia
  Dystonias
  Mutism
  Nystagmus
  Obtundation
  Seizures
  Tremor.

- Autonomic symptoms include
  Diaphoresis
  High fever (as high as 42°C)
  Hypertension
  Increased heart rate (more than 100 beats/min)

The most common progression is that the muscular rigidity develops into elevated temperature, fluctuating consciousness, and unstable vital signs. The muscular rigidity may be unresponsive to anticholinergic treatment and may be the first sign of NMS. See Table 4-22.3 for a list of associated risk factors for the development of NMS.

Management

It is important for clinicians to have a high level of suspicion for diagnosing NMS early and taking the necessary measures to minimize its progression. NMS can pose a significant challenge to

**Table 4-22.3.   Associated risk factors
for the development of NMS**

Dehydration
Poor oral intake
Elevated temperature
Prior episodes of NMS
High doses of neuroleptics, especially depot form
Rapid rate of loading
Prolonged use of restraints
Use of other medications (e.g., lithium)
Poorly controlled neuroleptic-induced EPS
Treatment-resistant EPS
Alcoholism
Organic brain syndrome or brain injury
Iron deficiency
Japanese heritage
Intense periods of psychomotor agitation or activity

NMS, neuroleptic malignant syndrome; EPS, extrapyramidal side effect.

a clinician. Careful assessment, workup, and thorough supportive care all are crucial. Differential diagnoses of NMS include CNS infections, trauma, tumors, status epilepticus, strokes, idiopathic lethal catatonia, systemic infections, heatstroke, dehydration, toxins, endocrinopathies, autoimmune disorders, and certain drugs/medications. Recommended elements of the evaluation include complete physical examination; electrolytes; renal-, thyroid-, and hepatic-function tests; serum aldolase level; CBC; serial CPKs; urinalysis and urine myoglobin; lumbar puncture; and an MRI/CT scan of the head. Other examinations to consider include blood gases, coagulation studies, blood and urine cultures, toxicology screen, lithium level, electroencephalogram, and iron deficiency tests. Patients with NMS should be medically monitored throughout the course of the syndrome. Stabilization should be a first order of priority, with withdrawal of the neuroleptic as a second-order priority. Hydration and cooling techniques are imperative.

Laboratory findings:

↑ CPK (40% to 50% of cases, extreme elevation greater than 50,000 U/L)
↑ Liver transaminases
↑ Myoglobin and myoglobinuria.
↑ Aldolase
Less common elevations in leukocytosis.

Patients with NMS are at risk for serious medical complications including acute renal failure, aspiration pneumonia, respiratory arrest, and cardiovascular collapse. Mortality estimates range from 12% to 20% and may be higher when depot neuroleptics are used, although it has been shown that specific drug and somatic therapies can reduce the mortality rate. Morbidity and mortality are commonly secondary to renal failure or respiratory failure. See Table 4-22.4 for a list of differential diagnoses.

Table 4-22.4. Differential diagnoses of NMS

Malignant hyperthermia
Lethal catatonia
Heat stroke
CNS infection
Allergic drug reaction
Anticholinergic delirium
Toxic encephalopathy
Serotonin syndrome

NMS, neuroleptic malignant syndrome; CNS, central nervous system.

Treatment is usually provided in the general adult ED or on a medical/surgical unit; for more detailed recommendations on the treatment of NMS, I would suggest you read a comprehensive emergency medicine or psychiatric textbook. These are a summary of recommended interventions:

1. Supportive and symptomatic medical treatment
   - Correcting fluid and electrolytes
   - Managing cardiovascular symptoms
   - Treating the fever (cooling techniques).
2. Discontinuation of the neuroleptic
3. Dantrolene (Dantrium), a muscle relaxant (used most often)
   - dantrolene sodium, 1 to 5 mg/kg, IV, for skeletal muscular rigidity
4. Bromocriptine (Parlodel), a dopamine agonist that can help minimize the severity
   - bromocriptine, 2.5 to 5 mg via PO/NG tube (q8h); max, 60 mg qD
   Case reports have found that the addition of dantrolene or bromocriptine significantly shortens the time to clinical response. The course of treatment is usually 5 to 10 days, unless a depot has been used.
5. Other somatic treatments tried with mixed results include
   - Amantadine (100 mg q8hr PO/NG)
   - Anticholinergics (for the initial muscular rigidity)
   - Benzodiazepines: Consider using lorazepam or alternative benzodiazepines: lorazepam (Ativan), 1 to 2 mg, IM/IV, with 1 to 2 mg, IV PRN, q8hr until relief of symptoms
   - Barbiturates
   - Verapamil
   - Pancuronium
   - Anesthesia
   - Carbidopa/levodopa
   - L-Dopa (IV)
   - Plasmapheresis
   - Electroconvulsive therapy (ECT; has good results for the syndrome and the underlying psychiatric condition).

SEROTONIN SYNDROME

Definition

SS is a disorder associated with hyperstimulation of serotonin (5-HT_{1A}) receptors in the brain and spinal cord with enhancement

of overall serotonin neurotransmission. SS is typically caused
by the combination of two or more medications with serotonin-
enhancing properties, although cases involving single agents have
been reported. Increased serotonin activity can result from

- Inhibition of serotonin metabolism [nonspecific inhibition with
  cocaine, amphetamine metabolites, or monoamine oxidase
  inhibitors (MAOIs)]
- Potentiation of serotonin activity [ecstasy (MDMA), amphetamines, cocaine, codeine, fenfluramine, dextromethorphan,
  levodopa, pentazocine, reserpine]
- Activation of serotonin receptors (LSD, buspirone, lithium,
  mescaline, sumatriptan)
- Inhibition of serotonin uptake (amphetamines, carbamazepine,
  tricyclic antidepressants, cocaine, meperidine, methadone,
  SSRIs)
- Increased substrate supply (L-tryptophan).

As mentioned earlier, SSRIs and MAOIs can cause SS, alone or
when combined with carbamazepine, dexfenfluramine, lithium,
L-tryptophan, pentazocine, phentermine, meperidine, or tricyclics.

Presentation
SS can demonstrate different gradations from mild to moderate
to severe forms. In the majority of cases, the symptoms develop
soon after the addition of a new agent, a change in the dose of one
already being taken, or the initiation of a new serotonin-enhancing
medication. This also can occur if a serotonergic agent is started
shortly after an MAOI has been discontinued. SS also has been
seen with combinations of TCAs, SSRIs, and/or MAOIs, but also
with pure MAOI overdoses.
  The classic triad seen in SS consists of

1. Altered mental status,
2. Autonomic dysfunction, and
3. Neuromuscular abnormalities.

  SS is characterized by

- Restlessness
- Nausea
- Vomiting
- Neuromuscular symptoms such as:
  Ataxia
  Myoclonus
  Nystagmus
  Hypertonicity
  Hyperreflexia
  Rigidity (especially of the lower extremities).
- Diaphoresis and generalized shivering (25%)
- Hyperthermia (greater than 39°C)
- Resting tremors
- Mental-status changes (40%) such as
  Confusion
  Agitation
  Euphoria or hypomanic-like symptoms
  Hallucinosis

Management

Most important is the careful assessment and management of these patients. First and foremost is the medical stabilization of the patient with the discontinuation of the causative agent. The presenting signs and symptoms clinically determine the required supportive measures. Laboratory findings are generally nonspecific, commonly with elevated WBC and CPK levels.

SS is usually self-limited (24 to 72 hours), with an uneventful resolution once the inciting agent has been discontinued. Partial forms (e.g., mild encephalopathy or mild autonomic instability) can persist for weeks without progression and then resolve. In its most severe presentations, it can rapidly progress to cardiac arrest, coma, seizures (14% of patients with SS have generalized tonic–clonic seizure) or multiple organ failure with disseminated intravascular coagulation and death in some cases.

The best way to make the diagnosis is to have high clinical suspicion based on a history of drug exposures that increase CNS serotonin activity, combined with signs and symptoms consistent with SS, as well as by ruling out other potential etiologies, such as CNS disorders and infections; amphetamine, ecstasy, or cocaine intoxication; thyroid storm; or sedative/opiate withdrawal. SS is hard to distinguish clinically from NMS; the precipitating medication (SSRI vs. neuroleptic) sometimes is the only difference. See Table 4-22.5 for a list of differential diagnoses of SS.

Treatment recommendations include

1. Close observation and supportive measures including
   - IV fluids
   - Cooling methods
   - Antipyretics
   - Sedative agents (lorazepam or other benzodiazepines).

Table 4-22.5. Differential diagnosis of serotonin syndrome

CNS disorders	Hyperthermia
	Infections (viral encephalitis, post-infectious encephalitis, HIV, tetanus, other bacterial, viral, or fungal agents)
	NMS
	Tumors
	Vascular or neoplastic lesions
Systemic disorders	Infections
	Heatstroke
	SLE
Drugs	Alcohol or sedative withdrawal
	Anesthetics
	Anticholinergics
	Dopamine antagonists
	Psychedelics
	Salicylates
	Stimulants
	Toxins (CO, strychnine, phenols)

CNS, central nervous system; HIV, human immunodeficiency virus; NMS, neuroleptic malignant syndrome; SLE, systemic lupus erythematosus.

2. Treatment of neurologic and cardiovascular complications
3. Serotonin-receptor antagonists such as cyproheptadine (0.25 mg/kg/day, divided in three equal doses) and propranolol (which has 5-HT_{1A}-antagonist properties), can shorten the duration of the syndrome.

LETHAL CATATONIA

Definition

Lethal catatonia (LC) is a rare syndrome that includes motor abnormalities, psychomotoric withdrawal or excitement, and bizarre repetitive behaviors. It most commonly occurs in patients receiving long-term treatment with neuroleptics. It occurs when hyperthermia or autonomic instability develops in the setting of catatonia, and it can be life threatening.

Presentation

LC is twice as common in females, with an average age at onset of 33 years, although it can occur at any age, with an estimated mortality as high as 60%. Multiple etiologies include medical, psychiatric (which account for 88% of the cases), and medication related: Dopamine antagonism or depletion is suspected in playing a major pathophysiologic role. LC also can occur in psychiatric patients NOT taking neuroleptics. Schizophrenia is the most common associated psychiatric disorder, but one third of cases have no specific psychiatric diagnosis. Some of the medical conditions that have been implicated in LC include infections such as viral encephalitis and bacterial septicemia; metabolic disorders include uremia, Addison and Cushing disease, and hyperthyroidism; and neurologic syndromes including seizure disorders, head trauma, and tumors.

The clinical course of LC frequently begins with a prodromal phase, which usually persists for an average of 2 weeks to 2 months, involving:

- Labile mood
- Anorexia
- Insomnia
- Mental-status changes
- Behavioral alterations
- Frank psychotic symptoms.

This phase then progresses to:

- Unrelenting motor agitation and excitation
- Restlessness
- Self-destructive or assaultive behavior
- Autonomic instability (fever, tachycardia).

The full syndrome is characterized by:

- Muscular rigidity
- Bizarre repetitive mannerisms and stereotypes
- Echophenomena
- Refusal of PO intake
- Intense and continued agitation and possible violence
- Motor signs including mutism, rigidity, and waxy flexibility
- Autonomic changes (high fever, rapid and weak pulse, diaphoresis, hypotension).

The last phase can last an average of 8 days, with:

- Stuporous exhaustion
- Cachexia
- Delirium
- Pronounced hyperthermia leading to coma, cardiovascular collapse, rhabdomyolysis, and even death.

Mental Status Examination Findings

- Clouding of consciousness
- Disorganized thought processes
- Pressured speech
- Hallucinations
- Delusions
- Mutism
- Negativism
- Stupor
- Impulsivity
- Combativeness
- Rarely: unprovoked physical violence and bizarre suicide attempts.

Physical Findings

Autonomic instability leads to profuse diaphoresis, tachycardia or bradycardia, labile blood pressure; hyperthermia rapidly develops and reaches up to 43°C.

Laboratory findings are nonspecific (elevated CPK level). Early diagnosis and prompt initiation of supportive measures are crucial. Acute onset, lack of prodromal phase, and lead-pipe rigidity are some of the differentiating clinical aspects between NMS and LC.

Treatment in LC of an organic origin should be directed at the underlying condition and consists of

1. Dopamine agonists (bromocriptine and amantadine)
2. Muscle relaxants (dantrolene)
3. Benzodiazepines
4. Paralyzing agents
5. ECT (effective when LC occurs with a primary psychiatric disorder but it is effective only if initiated before severe progression has occurred).

SELECTIVE SEROTONIN REUPTAKE INHIBITORS (SSRI) DISCONTINUATION SYNDROME

Definition

The SSRI-discontinuation syndrome can occur in patients who have had their SSRI medication discontinued or who have simply missed a few doses. It also has occasionally been noted in patients who have had their dosage reduced or tapered. The discontinuation syndrome occurs in patients who have been taking an SSRI for at least 1 month.

Presentations

The incidence of SSRI discontinuation syndrome varies in the literature. In postmarketing surveys, incidence rates range from 0.06% to 5.1%, whereas in other studies, incidence rates as high as 86% have been reported, depending on which SSRI has been discontinued. The syndrome has been reported across sexes, ages, doses, psychiatric disorders, and different SSRIs. The review of the recent literature has revealed that SSRIs with short half-lives, such as paroxetine (21 hours), fluvoxamine (15 hours), venlaflaxine (5 hours), compared with sertraline (26 hours) and fluoxetine (84 hours), are associated with more frequent reports of emergency discontinuation symptoms.

Symptoms characteristically appear within a week after stopping the medication but can occur as early as the second missed dose. They are typically mild and fleeting but can occasionally become severe enough to cause significant impairment in daily functioning. The symptoms are self-limited, usually subsiding within 2 weeks, and infrequently lasting up to 8 weeks. The most commonly reported symptoms of SSRI discontinuation are:

- Dizziness
- Nausea
- Lethargy
- Headache.

However, a wide range of symptoms has been reported; they can be grouped into six major categories:

1. Gastrointestinal (nausea, vomiting, diarrhea)
2. General somatic (headache, lethargy, "flu-like" symptoms); these are fairly nonspecific
3. Affective (anxiety, agitation, irritability)
4. Sleep disturbances (insomnia, vivid dreams)
5. Balance problems (dizziness, light-headedness, vertigo, gait instability)
6. Sensory abnormalities (paresthesias, "electric shock"-like sensations).

These latter symptoms stand out as unique to the SSRI-discontinuation syndrome. These CNS-like symptoms occur intermittently and can be precipitated or exacerbated by slight head movements. It is important to remember that these symptoms can appear on abrupt discontinuation of the drug as well as on reduction in dosage. The affective and sleep disturbances can mimic the original depressive or anxiety disorder, making the diagnosis much harder.

Management

It is important for the physician to diagnose SSRI-discontinuation syndrome correctly for appropriate management. Misdiagnosis may lead to unnecessary treatment and use of healthcare services. Patients who have discontinued their medications may feel as though they have a new medical illness, leading to an unnecessary workup, or their symptoms may be seen as evidence of a relapse of their original psychiatric illness, leading to unnecessary reinstatement of treatment. In addition, patients who complain of breakthrough symptoms while taking SSRIs may simply have missed doses.

The management of acute SSRI-discontinuation syndrome consists of either restarting the medication or allowing the symptoms to run their course. If clinically indicated, restarting the medications brings about a rapid cessation of the symptoms. Alternatively, allowing the symptoms to run their course leads to resolution of symptoms in from 1 to 8 weeks. Some reports state that meclizine for dizziness and/or cyclizine for nausea can be effective.

Perhaps the most important step in managing SSRI-discontinuation syndrome is patient education. Any patient started on an SSRI should have these potential discontinuation symptoms explained to them. Although the symptoms of SSRI-discontinuation syndrome are not life threatening, these symptoms can be frightening to the patient and may impair functioning and quality of life, leading to future nonadherence with antidepressant trials.

BIBLIOGRAPHY

Amdurski S, et al. Therapeutic trial of amantadine in haloperidol-induced neuroleptic malignant syndrome. *Curr Ther Res* 1983;33:225.

Bertorini T. Myoglobinuria, malignant hyperthermia, neuroleptic malignant syndrome, and serotonin syndrome. *Neurol Clin* 1997;15:649.

Black K, Shea C, Dursun S, et al. Selective serotonin reuptake inhibitor discontinuation syndrome: proposed diagnostic criteria. *J Psychiatry Neurosci* 2000;25:255–261.

Bodner RA, et al. Serotonin syndrome. *Neurology* 1995;45:219–223.

Brady WJ, Esterowitz D, Winogard SM. Life-threatening syndromes presenting with altered mentation and muscular rigidity. *Emerg Med Rep* 1999;20:51–59.

Carbone J. The neuroleptic malignant and serotonin syndromes. *Emerg Med Clin North Am* 2000;18:317–325.

Caroff SN, Mann SC, Campbell EC. Neuroleptic malignant syndrome. *Adverse Drug React Bull* 2001;209:799–802.

Coons D, Hillma F, Marshall R. Treatment of neuroleptic malignant syndrome with dantrolene: a case report. *Am J Psych* 1982;139:994.

Dhib-Jalbut S, Hesselbrock R, Brott T. Treatment of neuroleptic malignant syndrome with bromocriptine. *JAMA* 1983;250:484.

Francis A, Chandragiri S, Rizvi S, et al. Is lorazepam a treatment for neuroleptic malignant syndrome? *CNS Spectrums* 2000;5:54–57.

Gaitini L, et al. Plasmapheresis in neuroleptic malignant syndrome [Comment]. *Anesthesia* 1997;52:612.

Geduscheck J, et al. Repeated anesthesia for a patient with neuroleptic malignant syndrome. *Anesthesiology* 1988;68:134.

Haddad P. Antidepressant discontinuation reactions: discontinuation of antidepressant therapy: emerging complications and their relevance. *J Clin Psychiatry* 1998;59:541–548.

Harris M, Nora L, Tanner C. Neuroleptic malignant syndrome response to carbidopa/levodopa: support for a dopaminergic pathogenesis. *Clin Neurpharmacol* 1987;10:186.

Hasan S, Buckley P. Novel antipsychotics and the neuroleptic malignant syndrome: a review and critique. *Am J Psychiatry* 1998;155: 1113–1116.

Lejoyeux M, Ades J. Antidepressant discontinuation: a review of the literature. *J Clin Psychiatry* 1997;58(suppl 7):11–15.

Maixner SM, Greden JF. Extended antidepressant maintenance and discontinuation syndromes. *Depress Anxiety* 1998;8(suppl 1):43–53.

Mann SC, et al. Lethal catatonia. *Am J Psychiatry* 1986;143:1374–1381.

Martin TG. Serotonin syndrome. *Ann Emerg Med* 1996;28:520–525.

Mason PJ, Morris VA, Balcezak TJ. Serotonin syndrome: presentation of 2 cases and review of the literature. *Medicine (Baltimore)* 2000;79:201–209.

Michelson D, Fava M, Amsterdam J, et al. Interruption of selective serotonin re-uptake inhibitor treatment. *Br J Psychiatry* 2000;176: 363–368.

Mills KC. Serotonin syndrome: a clinical update. *Crit Care Clin* 1997;13: 763–776.

Pelonero AL, Levenson JL, Pandurangi AK. Neuroleptic malignant syndrome: a review. *Psychiatr Serv* 1998;49:1163–1172.

Price JS, Waller PC, Wood SM, et al. A comparison of the post-marketing safety of four selective serotonin re-uptake inhibitors including investigation of symptoms occurring on withdrawal. *Br J Clin Pharmacol* 1996;42:757–763.

Rosenbaum JF, Fava M, Hoog SL, et al. Selective serotonin reuptake inhibitor discontinuation syndrome: a randomized clinical trial. *Biol Psychiatry* 1998;44:77–87.

Sangel R, Dimitrejevic R. Neuroleptic malignant syndrome: successful treatment with pancuronium. *JAMA* 1989;54:2795.

Schatzberg AF, Haddad P, Kaplan EM, et al. Serotonin reuptake inhibitor discontinuation syndrome: a hypothetical definition. *J Clin Psychiatry* 1997;58(suppl 7):5–10.

Sternbach H. The serotonin syndrome. *Am J Psychiatry* 1991;148: 705–713.

Taniguchi N, et al. Classification system of complications in neuroleptic malignant syndrome. *Methods Find Exp Clin Pharmacol* 1997;19:193.

Tstsumi Y, et al. The treatment of neuroleptic malignant syndrome using dantrolene sodium. *Psychiatry Clin Neurosci* 1998;52:433.

Zajecka J, Tracy K, Mitchell S. Discontinuation symptoms after treatment with serotonin reuptake inhibitors: a literature review. *J Clin Psychiatry* 1997;58:291–297.

Chapter 4-23 Uncooperative Patient

DEFINITION

Uncooperativeness, or the unwillingness and/or inability to work with others, may be a manifestation of many psychiatric and medical conditions, or a component of a patient's ED presentation, which when severe can significantly hinder the assessment process. Conversely, the unresponsive and unconscious patient is more serious and should be considered a medical emergency requiring immediate medical evaluation and management. It is outside the scope of this handbook to expand on that topic, and I suggest you review a comprehensive emergency medicine textbook on the management of an unresponsive/unconscious patient.

PRESENTATION

One of the more frustrating scenarios in the ED usually involves an uncooperative patient. Patients may be uncooperative for a host of reasons, including being guarded, suspicious, and/or paranoid as in psychotic disorders; being withdrawn, avolitional, with slow mentation as in depression; or angry, belligerent, and oppositional as seen in children and adolescents, patients with mental retardation, and certain adults with personality disorders. Patients may be cognitively impaired, either permanently or transiently, and unable or unwilling to answer for fear of demonstrating their deficits, as in delirium, dementia, amnestic disorders, and traumatic brain injuries. At times, patients mandated to an evaluation or intoxicated may be uncooperative and hostile if they are feeling pressured or put upon by the interviewer. Uncooperativeness is not limited to a lack of participation in the interview process; it can encompass refusal to change into hospital garments, have blood tests or other diagnostic procedures, accept medications, and so on. The approach to and management of these patients, whatever their etiology, can become extremely labor intensive, time-consuming, and draining for staff.

Psychiatric causes of altered MSE and concomitant uncooperativeness can include disorders such as conversion, factitious disorder, dissociative amnesia or fugue states, malingering, and catatonic presentations. These patients will be brought in, seldom arriving on their own, and have varying degrees of unrelatedness, unresponsiveness, and changes in their MSE. These patients, despite their probable primary psychiatric condition, should be evaluated medically to determine that there is no underlying medical cause for their presentation. Patients who are unresponsive should be considered a medical emergency. Many possible differential diagnosis exist for transient loss of consciousness and coma; see Table 4-23.1. I encourage you to review a comprehensive textbook for these types of presentations.

Patients with dissociative amnesia may experience serious although reversible memory impairments, including recall of important personal information or experience, generally after an emotionally traumatic event. Patients with dissociative fugue can suddenly and unexpectedly travel away from their home location and experience impaired recall of their past; becoming confused about their former identity and assuming a new identity. Patients with factitious disorder will assume the sick role and intentionally feign or produce symptoms, which can be differentiated from malingering in that no secondary gain is possible except adopting the sick role. In malingering, a clear and defined ulterior motivation (financial, legal, or personal) must exist in the feigning or exaggeration of symptoms. In conversion disorder, patients may have symptoms that can be confused with a physical illness: for example, an illness that affects sensory (e.g., anesthesia, blindness) or voluntary motor functioning (e.g., astasia/abasia, paralysis). Usually the reported symptoms fail to conform to any known anatomic or physiological characteristics.

Patient with schizophrenia or bipolar disorder may have catatonic features, which may appear as uncooperativeness or unresponsiveness, such as

- Motoric immobility, catalepsy (including waxy flexibility), or stupor
- Extreme negativism or mutism
- Posturing, stereotyped movements, prominent mannerisms, or prominent grimacing.

Table 4-23.1. Causes of loss of consciousness and coma

Metabolic	Hypo- and hypernatremia
	Hypo- and hyperglycemia
	Hypermagnesemia
	Diabetic ketoacidosis
	Hyperosmolar states
	Hypothyroidism
	Thyrotoxicosis
	Adrenal insufficiency
	Hepatic encephalopathy
	Uremia
	Thiamine deficiency (Wernicke encephalopathy)
Vascular	Hypo- and hypertension
	Vasculitis
	CVA (thrombotic or hemorrhagic) and subarachnoid hemorrhage (aneurysm or AVM)
Neurologic	Tumors
	Hydrocephalus
	Status epilepticus
Trauma	Subdural hematoma
	Epidural hematoma
	Cerebral contusion
	Diffuse cerebral edema
Infectious	Meningitis
	Encephalitis
	Intracranial abscess
	Sepsis
Toxicologic	Carbon monoxide
	Ethanol
	Methanol
	Drug abuse and overdose
Environmental	Heatstroke
	Hypothermia
	High-altitude cerebral edema
	Near drowning
	Dysbarism
Psychiatric (usually present as transient loss of consciousness or slightly unresponsive to external stimuli)	Conversion disorder
	Dissociative amnesia
	Dissociative fugue
	Factitious disorder
	Malingering
	Catatonia

CVA, cerebrovascular accident; AVM, arteriovenous malformation.

MANAGEMENT

A thorough psychiatric evaluation may help differentiate those psychiatric disorders that demonstrate unresponsiveness and varying degrees of changes in mental status. A complete physical, medical, and serial neurologic examination is recommended. Review of pockets and belongings can assist in determining possible causes: a suicide note, a pill bottle, a medical tag, etc.

In patients who are uncooperative, the best approach is to somehow try to establish rapport, engaging the patients where they are. Forcing the interview may be counterproductive. This is not to say that you must deviate from the established procedure and protocols in the ED. If a patient is uncooperative and unwilling to, for example, change into hospital gown, attempts should be made to discuss this with the patients, work with them to change their minds, but ultimately they may need to hear and understand that they must and will be placed in hospital garments. An explanation should be offered to the patient about the ED procedures, and they must be allowed to explain their resistance or reluctance, but in the end, consistency and conforming to the rules is the best way to ensure a safe work environment. Increased staff presence or even security presence may help the patient become less uncooperative, or it may even require that the patient will have to change into a gown, or whatever the conflict may be about, by use of force.

The interview process may not happen initially, and sometimes giving the patients some time to sit and wait can help as well. Offering to assist them in their demands (for telephone, food, attention) can bring about a change in their level of cooperativeness. Again, it is imperative that the patients be told and understand that they are in the ED for an evaluation, and until you can perform that evaluation (interview), they will not be allowed to leave the ED (if that statement is appropriate). Promises of a speedy evaluation and release may help in the short term but may be unreasonable promises that will create a major split and threaten the patient–doctor relationship if they cannot be honored. Offering medication to help the patient feel more relaxed or at ease can also be beneficial in loosening up the patients and helping them become more cooperative. Stubborn and difficult patients may need repeated approaches and discussions before the interview may take place. Ultimately, in our experience, patients will come around and talk, regardless of their reliability as historians. Keeping a calm, professional, and courteous manner at all times, no matter how infuriating, demanding, or difficult a patient may be, is a decisive element in approaching an uncooperative patient. Any outward sign of frustration or anger can be seen as validation to the patient that you are either uninterested or unable to help them. Keep in mind, if a patient is making you upset by their behavior, a countertransferential feeling may be operating (these are complex unconscious feelings that a psychotherapist has toward his patient, although any clinician can have reactions to any patient), and you must make certain you do not act on that and try to explore what it may mean for you in the context of your life. If the countertransferential reactions are negative, then your ability to deliver adequate, empathic, and supportive care to the patient will most certainly be hindered. If they are positive reactions, you may unconsciously miss or minimize the patient's complaints or overextend yourself and blur boundaries, thus indirectly also affecting negatively the patient's evaluation and outcome. It is crucial that these positive or negative feelings engendered by certain types of patients be acknowledged, discussed with a supervisor or other senior staff member or in team/rounds, and processed so they are not acted on and allowed to affect patient care.

DISPOSITION

Those patients with some degree of unresponsiveness and uncooperativeness in the context of a psychiatric disorder must be evaluated and may need a psychiatric hospitalization for continued diagnostic testing, evaluation, and management.

Chapter 4-24 Withdrawal Phenomenon

DEFINITION

Withdrawal is defined as a substance-specific syndrome that follows cessation of use or reduction in intake of a psychoactive substance whose use has been heavy and prolonged, causing clinically significant impairment in social, occupational, or other area of functioning. According to DSM-IV-TR, withdrawal phenomenon is associated with the following drugs: alcohol, amphetamines, cocaine, nicotine, opioids, and sedative/hypnotics (cannabis is not known to have a clear withdrawal pattern).

PRESENTATION

When an individual persists in use of alcohol or other drugs despite problems related to its use, substance dependence may be diagnosed. Repeated use can ultimately result in tolerance to the effect of the drug, with a substance-specific withdrawal syndrome occurring when use is reduced or stopped. Withdrawal phenomenon is usually, although not always, associated with substance dependence. Many substances, such as alcohol, sedatives, hypnotics, anxiolytics; or other/unknown substances, can cause a *withdrawal delirium*. This is characterized by a rapid onset of a disturbance of consciousness, cognitive impairments, or perceptual disturbances that can fluctuate during the course of the day and is not in the context of a preexisting, established, or evolving dementia. This syndrome develops during or shortly after a substance-withdrawal episode and is quite different from typical withdrawal symptoms because of the severe cognitive impairments manifested by the patient. In one study, in almost 7% of the patients, alcohol-withdrawal delirium developed even after admission and despite benzodiazepine treatment. Several factors have been shown to assist in determining a patient's risk of developing alcohol-withdrawal delirium. These factors include current infectious disease, tachycardia, heart rate more than 120 beats/min on admission, signs of alcohol withdrawal, a history of seizures, and a history of delirium.

Patients may seek help for worsening of their withdrawal symptoms, alone, brought in by others, or by police/EMT after being disruptive or being found unresponsive. The types of symptoms these patients may have vary according to the specific drug-induced withdrawal phenomenon, the underlying medical or psychiatric conditions, and the combination of drugs and/or medications they may have ingested. Rarely will a patient have a classic "textbook" withdrawal phenomenon; often many substances are involved, with polysubstance dependence, with symptoms of either intoxication or withdrawal from different drugs and alcohol occurring concurrently.

Alcohol withdrawal is characterized by symptoms of autonomic hyperactivity (sweating, hypertension, tachycardia, coarse tremor), insomnia, anorexia, nausea or vomiting, transient visual, tactile, or auditory hallucinations or illusions, psychomotor agitation, paresthesias, hyperreflexia, malaise, fatigue, dry mouth, flushed face, muscle aches, anxiety, depressed mood, poor concentration, impaired judgment, and seizures. These symptoms generally begin 6 to 24 hours after the patient's last drink, even with high blood alcohol levels (BAL). Symptoms tend to progress from mild to severe, although this is very unpredictable, and a patient can have seizures as the first withdrawal symptom. Alcohol-withdrawal delirium, commonly known as delirium tremens (DTs), is a severe complication of alcohol withdrawal and occurs in about 5% of patients withdrawing from alcohol. Seizures or "rum fits" occur within 24 to 72 hours after the last drink, commonly precede DTs, are usually generalized tonic–clonic, and are considered a medical emergency. A patient in DTs will show distractibility, disorganized thinking, shifting levels of consciousness, marked autonomic hyperactivity (tachycardia, hypertension, tachypnea, hyperthermia, etc.), tremors, vivid hallucination (either visual or tactile; formication), delusions, or psychomotor activity changes (from lethargy to excitement). DTs occur most often within a week of decreasing or stopping alcohol consumption, usually from 24 to 72 hours after the last drink. This commonly happens in patients admitted to the hospital for medical/surgical causes, and staff neglect to ask about their alcohol (or drug) history or when they had their last drink. Risk factors for DTs include: metabolic disorders, hepatic disease, ataxia, and polyneuropathy. Untreated mortality can be as high as 20%, and treated mortality is still not too good, at 5% to 10%, usually from hyperthermia, volume depletion, infection, or cardiovascular collapse.

Wernicke-Korsakoff is seen in about 5% of alcoholics and is related to thiamine deficiency. Wernicke-Korsakoff syndrome can appear in the ED with neurologic signs (sixth nerve palsy, oculomotor paralysis, ataxia, dysarthria) and changes in MSE. These changes include amnesia, confabulation, and psychosis (a poor prognostic indicator).

Amphetamine withdrawal, after the heavy use of amphetamines or amphetamine-like substances, is characterized by intense lack of energy, apathy, tremors, hunger, muscle aches, chills, depressed mood, anxiety, irritability or agitation, and drug cravings. Patients also can experience insomnia or hypersomnia with vivid or unpleasant dreams. These symptoms commonly occur 3 or 4 days after decrease or cessation of heavy amphetamine use; depression can linger for months, and suicidality can be an associated symptom.

Cocaine does not have a specific physiological withdrawal phenomenon but does have behavioral manifestations that can prompt an ED visit. Stimulants (cocaine, crack, amphetamines, methamphetamines) are commonly used in either intermittent binges or in chronic high-dose use with similar withdrawal symptoms. Normally intense craving for the drug occurs, with symptoms that vary in intensity depending on the amount used, route, and the last use. Additionally, muscle aches and cramps, fatigue, irritability, hunger, restlessness, depressed mood, insomnia or hypersomnia with vivid or unpleasant dreams, and paranoia, suicidality, or hallucinations can occur in some cases. When patients appear in the ED, they are usually quite symptomatic, and the degree of irritability and potential suicidality/volatility is high. Often these patients also are abusing other drugs and may be reacting to specific withdrawal phenomena from one or more of these agents. Many of these patients will be uncooperative and hostile, preferring to "sleep it off" and "crash" in the ED. Many of those who are homeless or in some type of trouble with the law may seek refuge in the ED and heighten the level of symptomatic complaints and reports of suicidal ideation and attempts.

Opioid withdrawal can occur from either cessation or reduction in opioid use that has been heavy and prolonged (several weeks or longer) or because of the administration of an opioid antagonist after a period of opioid use. The withdrawal symptoms may be divided into three categories depending on the level of severity.

- *Major:* Vomiting, diarrhea, increased bowel sounds, hypotension, seizures (rare)
- *Moderate:* Restlessness, insomnia, hypertension, tachycardia, tachypnea, diaphoresis; pulse, 10 beats/min over baseline or more than 90 beats/min if baseline is unknown; systolic blood pressure more than 10 mm Hg over baseline or more than 160/95 mm Hg, in the absence of known hypertension
- *Minor:* Dilated pupils, sweating, goose-bumps, rhinorrhea, lacrimation, yawning, myalgias, cramping, anorexia, or perspiration.

Withdrawal symptoms always indicate opioid dependence and are more severe for short-acting opiates, like heroin or meperidine. Although not life-threatening, they are uncomfortable and distressing symptoms, and patients may be agitated and demanding. Withdrawal phenomenon for heroin or morphine begins on average 8 to 12 hours after the last dose and can last up to 5 to 7 days. Methadone conversely can begin 12 hours after the last dose and peak on the third day or later, with symptoms gradually subsiding, although at times continuing for 3 weeks or longer. *Levo*-α-acetylmethadol (LAAM), which was approved by the FDA in 1993 as a maintenance medication, can have withdrawal symptoms similar to those of methadone.

Sedative, hypnotic, or anxiolytic withdrawal is quite similar to alcohol withdrawal. Patients are generally very uncomfortable and can become quite agitated, with increased anxiety levels. It is characterized by autonomic hyperactivity; tremor; insomnia; nausea or vomiting; transient visual, tactile, or auditory hallucinations or illusions; drug craving; and anxiety. Serious complications include grand mal seizures, delirium, and even death. These agents used at therapeutic dose or higher when stopped will produce a withdrawal syndrome—the dosage amount used (low dose vs. high dose) will produce a qualitatively different withdrawal syndrome. Short-acting agents (see Table 4-24.1 for common benzodiazepine agents) will have onset of withdrawal symptoms beginning 12 to 24 hours after the last dose, peaking between 24 and 72 hours. In patients taking longer-acting agents, the withdrawal symptoms may peak 5 to 8 days after the last dose. The withdrawal syndromes can develop more slowly in patients with liver disease or in the elderly. In patients taking therapeutic doses of benzodiazepines for protracted periods, the withdrawal can be accompanied by a 1- to 2-week transient increase in symptoms or symptom rebound, which tends to be a rebound worsening of the patient's original symptoms. Other patients, after termination or discontinuation of the benzodiazepine, may have a protracted withdrawal syndrome, including irritability, anxiety, insomnia, and mood instability.

Nicotine withdrawal is not a common ED presentation. Many patients, if asked (and motivated), may inquire about nicotine-withdrawal techniques as part of their visit, but hardly ever will this be a primary ED concern. Occasionally a patient may complain of recent cessation of heavy nicotine use and report depressed mood, insomnia, irritability, frustration, anger, anxiety, difficulty concentrating, restlessness, and increased appetite or weight gain.

Marijuana does not have an acute withdrawal syndrome, although some patients may complain of irritability and insomnia several days after their last use. Rarely do these patients come to the ED for these symptoms.

MANAGEMENT

In cases of substance-withdrawal phenomenon, you must make certain medical supportive care is provided if clinically indicated. Vital signs, IV access (if necessary), and medical assessment are crucial at first. You must try to determine the type of substance used, the amount, and the last use. Obtain basic laboratory examinations, urine toxicology screen, relevant blood levels if warranted, and a Breathalyzer test. Determine comorbid medical or surgical problems, especially important because of the serious comorbid conditions that exist in this population and the limited access to health care. Assess any behavioral manifestations, acting-out behavior, agitation, aggressivity or impulsivity, or threats, and institute safety measures immediately. In mild cases, nonnarcotic analgesics, antidiarrheas, or antacids can offer symptomatic relief.

It is important to keep in mind that many patients in the ED with withdrawal symptoms may be abusing or dependent on more than one drug; once you have ascertained the drugs being used, you should follow these treatment recommendations:

Alcohol and stimulants: treat the alcohol abuse
Alcohol and benzodiazepines: treat with phenobarbital
Cocaine and benzodiazepines: treat the benzodiazepine withdrawal
Cocaine and opiates: treat the opiate dependence
Cocaine and amphetamines: symptomatic management.

Table 4-24.1. Common benzodiazepine agents

Generic	Brand	Dosage	Onset (After Oral Dose)	Dose Equivalents
Alprazolam	Xanax	0.25-, 0.5-, 1-, 2-mg tablets	Intermediate	0.5
Chlordiazepoxide	Librium	5-, 10-, 25-mg tablets/capsules	Intermediate	10
Clonazepam	Klonopin	0.5-, 1-, 2-mg tablets	Intermediate	0.25
Clorazepate	Tranxene	3.75-, 7.5-mg tablets/capsules 15-mg tablets	Rapid	7.5
Diazepam	Valium	2-, 5-, 10-mg tablets	Rapid	5
Estazolam	ProSom	1-, 2-mg tablets	Intermediate	0.33
Flurazepam	Dalmane	15-, 30-mg capsules	Rapid, intermediate	30
Lorazepam	Ativan	0.5-, 1-, 2-mg tablets 2 mg/ml and 4 mg/ml parenteral	Intermediate	1
Midazolam	Versed	1 mg/ml, 5 mg/ml parenteral	Intermediate	1.25–1.7
Oxazepam	Serax	10-, 15-, 30-mg capsules 15-mg tablets	Intermediate, slow	15
Quazepam	Doral	7.5-, 15-mg tablets	Rapid, intermediate	15
Temazepam	Restoril	7.5-, 15-, 30-mg capsules	Intermediate	5
Triazolam	Halcion	0.125-, 0.25-mg tablets	Intermediate	0.1

With opiate use, several clues or indications can help make the diagnosis of opiate abuse or dependence:

- Exaggerated pain complaints in relation to physical findings
- Drug-seeking behavior
- Multiple recent visits with similar pain complaints and narcotic requests
- Allergic to every analgesic except the one the patient specifically requests
- Withdrawal signs: hyperthermia, hypertension, tachycardia, diaphoresis, nausea
- Needle marks
- Positive urine toxicology screen
- A demanding, unruly, or agitated patient
- Threats to leave AMA.

It is crucial that when interviewing a patient with potential substance abuse or dependence that you speak to them in a manner they will understand, but if they use street or drug-culture lingo that you do not understand, you should ask. See Table 4-24.2 for a list of some common street drug names and terms.

Treatment also will vary according to the underlying substance used. Specific detoxification procedures exist, as well as general principles of treatment. These general principles are listed in Table 4-24.3.

Alcohol withdrawal is best treated with benzodiazepines; close monitoring of vital signs and medicating progression of symptoms while offering supportive care can help prevent a major withdrawal from occurring. Consider

lorazepam (Ativan), 1 to 2 mg PO/IM, q6hr (and PRN if needed), and start taper, preferable because of predictable elimination half-life; or if needing an IM route chlordiazepoxide (Librium), 25 to 100 mg, PO, q6hr (and PRN if needed); smoother detoxification due to its longer half-life; poor IM absorption

Seizure and DTs are medical emergencies and must be handled in the adult ED, requiring IV benzodiazepines and inpatient management. DTs accompanied by perceptual disturbances (such as auditory, visual, or tactile hallucinations) respond to antipsychotic medications.

haloperidol (Haldol), 0.5 to 2 mg, PO, q4hr (patients who are vomiting or unable to take medications by mouth can be given haloperidol IM). Low-potency atypical antipsychotics, such as chlorpromazine, should be avoided because of the increased risk of seizures.

Other mediations that have been used to treat alcohol-withdrawal symptoms include carbamazepine (Tegretol); reports exist of its effectiveness, although no double-blind placebo-controlled studies have been carried out comparing it with benzodiazepines. Certain β-blockers, such as atenolol (Tenormin) or propranolol (Inderal), can be used to treat the autonomic symptoms, such as tachycardia, hypertension, sweating, and tremors. These medications do not prevent hallucinations, seizures, or other withdrawal symptoms and may even increase the risk of delirium and hallucinations during the withdrawal.

Table 4-24.2. Common street terms and drug names

Explanation	Street Term
1,4 BD	Pine needle oil, Serenity, Revitalize Plus, Enliven, GHRE, SomatoPro, NRGE, Thunder Nector, Weight Belt Cleaner, Cherry fx Bombs, Lemon fx Drops, Orange fx Rush
Addict	Junkie
Amobarbital (Amytal)	Blue heavens, blue devils, blue birds
Amobarbital + secobarbital (Tuinal)	Double trouble, rainbows
Amphetamines	Bennies, black beauties, crosse, hearts, LA turnaround, speed, uppers
Annabolic Steroids	Roids, juice
Benzadiazepines (other than Flunitrazepam)	candy, downers, sleeping pills, tranks
Cocaine	Blow, crack, flake, gold dust, green gold, rock, snow, Cadillac of drugs, Dama Blanca, Pimp's drug, toot, Charlie
Cocaine + alcohol	Liquid lady
Cocaine measure	Dose, hit, line, spoon, snort
Codeine	Loads, doors and fours, pancake and syrup, captain cody, cody, school
Cyanide, strychnine, battery acid	Death hit
Dime	$10 bag of drugs
Drawing blood in/out of syringe	Booting
Fentanyl	China white, apache, china girl, dance fever, fiend, goodfella, jackpot, TNT, tango and cash
Flunitrazepam (Rohypnol)	Date-rape drug, rophies, roofies, roach, rope, Mexican valium, R2, Rivotril (in Mexico)
GBL (γ-butyrolactone)	Revivarant, RenewTrient, Firewater, Blue Nitro Vitality
GHB (γ-hydroxybutyrate)	Grievous bodily harm, Georgia home boy, liquid ecstasy, liquid X, liquid E, soap, easy lay, scoop, salty water, g-riffick, cherry meth, somatomax, organic quaalude
Hashish	Boom, chronic, gangster, hash, hash oil, hemp
Heroin	Dope, skag, horse, H, white stuff, Lady Jane, shill, brown sugar, smack

Table 4-24.2. *Continued*

Explanation	Street Term
Heroin + cocaine	Speedball
Inhalants	laughing gas, poppers, snappers, whippets
Inhalation of pyrolysate	Chinese blowing
Injection of transiently suspended insoluble particles	Cold shake
Internal jugular injection	Pocket shot
Intradermal injection	Skin popping
Intranasal use	Snorting
Intrarterial injection	Pinkie
IV injection	Mainlining
Ketamine	Special K, vitamin K, K, super K, Ketaset, jet, Super acid, green, purple, mauve, Special LA coke, cat valiums
LSD (lysergic acid diethylamide)	Acid, blotters, boomers, abes, micro-dot, yellow sunshines
Marijuana	Blunt, dope, ganga, herb, joint, Mary Jane, pot, reefer, skunk
MDA	Love drug
MDMA	Ecstasy, XTC, Adam, E, hug drug, M&M, lover's speed, STP, X
Mescaline	Buttons, cactus, mesc, peyote
Methamphetamine	Speed, meth, chalk, ice, crank, crystal, glass, fire, go fast
Methaqualone	Quaalude, sopor, parest, ludes, mandrex, quad, quay
Methylphenidate	Jif, MPH, B-ball, Skippy, the smart drug, vitamin e
Morphine	M, miss emma, monkey, white stuff
Needing a dose because addicted	Strung out
Nickel	$5 bag of drugs
Occasional opiate use	Chipping
Onset of high	Rush
Opium	Big O, black stuff, block, gum, hop
Overdose	OD, nod out, or fall out
Paregoric and tripelennamine	Blue velvet
PCP (phencyclidine)	Angel dust, crystal, crystal joints, dust, goon, hog, horse, PCP, rocket fuel, super grass, super weed, animal tranquilize, ele-

continued

Table 4-24.2. *Continued*

Explanation	Street Term
	phant tranquilizer, KJ (kristal joint), mintweed, PeaCe Pil, surfer, tic, tac, wow
Pentazocine (Talwin)	Ts and blues
Pentobarbital (Nembutal)	Yellows, yellow jackets, nemmies, nebbies, nimbies
Phenobarbital (Luminal)	Phennies, purple hearts, goofballs
Postinjection fever	Cotton fever
Psilocybin	magic mushroom, purple passion, shrooms
Scars	Tracks
Secobarbital (Seconal)	Reds, red devils, red birds, marshmallow reds, Mexican reds
Site to buy and inject drugs	Shooting gallery
Somnolence	Nod or nodding
Syringe	Works, tab, spike, fix, cooker
Withdrawal	Jones

All patients with alcohol dependence and in withdrawal should receive

Thiamine, 100 mg, PO/IM STAT, and then t.i.d.
Folate, 1 mg, PO STAT, and then qd
Multivitamin, PO STAT, and then b.i.d.

Table 4-24.3.   Principles of detoxification

- Alcohol and other drug dependencies require more than detoxification alone for adequate treatment.
- Only medication regimens or detoxification protocols with established safety and efficacy should be used.
- Patients should be informed about the safety of all procedures, especially those that may not have been established as safe and effective.
- During detoxification, the clinical staff should closely monitor access to medications.
- Detoxification procedures and management of withdrawal symptoms should be individualized.
- Clinicians should try to substitute a long-acting medication for a short-acting drug of addiction.
- The intensity of the withdrawal is difficult to predict, and every case should be individualized and monitored closely.
- Every effort should be made to treat the patient's signs and symptoms of withdrawal. Patients should start participating in follow-up supportive therapeutic interventions such as peer groups, family therapy, individual counseling or therapy, 12-step groups, and other educational programs.

In patients with Wernicke-Korsakoff syndrome, IV thiamine is indicated immediately—avoid dextrose solutions before thiamine replacement because of symptomatic worsening.

Amphetamine-, cocaine-, or other stimulant-withdrawal symptoms should be monitored symptomatically, and the medical or psychiatric symptoms treated as they manifest, because no specific treatment exists for stimulant withdrawal. Usually symptoms are self-limited, subside over 2 to 4 days, and can be dealt with in a calm, accommodating environment with basic supportive care. Anxiety may respond to anxiolytics, and psychotic symptoms may need a low dose of a high-potency neuroleptic or low-dose atypical antipsychotic agent.

Sedatives, hypnotics, and/or anxiolytics, all having cross-tolerance, must be dealt with as you would with alcohol. The options include gradual reduction of the agent, substitution with phenobarbital, or substitution with a longer-acting benzodiazepine. In the latter option, you would substitute a short half-life benzodiazepine with a longer-acting benzodiazepine, such as clonazepam (Klonopin) or chlordiazepoxide (Librium). This will provide a smoother and less complicated detoxification. In cases of barbiturate or other mixed sedative/hypnotics, a phenobarbital taper can be used. This will allow a safer detoxification, because phenobarbital produces few changes in blood levels between doses, has clearly observable signs of toxicity (nystagmus, slurred speech, ataxia), and phenobarbital intoxication does not produce a high, so patients do not view it as a drug of abuse. You can calculate the dose of phenobarbital by using a phenobarbital equivalency chart (see Table 4-24.4). Once you have converted the patient's daily sedative/hypnotic dose to a phenobarbital equivalent, you should divide it into three or four daily doses. In acute withdrawal, you can administer the first dose of phenobarbital intramuscularly. Unless signs of phenobarbital toxicity develop, you can then decrease the dose by 30 mg/day, while monitoring carefully for signs of toxicity or withdrawal. Another way to calculate the phenobarbital equivalent dose is with a pentobarbital challenge test: give the patient 200 mg of pentobarbital and observe the level of intoxication after an hour. If no signs of intoxication appear, then give another 100 mg, q2hr until signs and symptoms of intoxication develop (sedation, slurred speech, nystagmus) up to a maximum of 500 mg. Add the amount needed to produce mild intoxication, and then substitute for phenobarbital (using the chart). Newer anticonvulsants are being slowly used in withdrawal from benzodiazepines, sedatives, and even alcohol.

Opiate withdrawal must be determined by objective signs, such as piloerection, hypertension, and lacrimation, rather than solely on the patient's reports. Patients will occasionally inflate the amount of drug used, to get a larger dose of methadone for detoxification. If they are enrolled in a methadone maintenance program, verify the dose and the last dose given. Supportive care and reassurance are usually needed, as well as medications recommended for symptomatic relief of opiate withdrawal (see Table 4-24.5).

Clonidine (Catapres) helps reduce the nausea, vomiting, and diarrhea. It can be administered as a test dose of 0.1 mg (0.2 mg in patients weighing more than 200 pounds), with careful moni-

Table 4-24.4.   Phenobarbital equivalency chart

Drug Class	Generic Name	Brand Name	Dose Equivalent (mg) of 30 mg of Phenobarbital
Barbiturates	Amobarbital	Amtytal	100
	Butobarbital	Butisol	100
	Butalbital	Fiorinal, Sedapap	100
	Pentobarbital	Nembutal	100
	Secobarbital	Seconal	100
Other sedative– hypnotics	Chloral hydrate	Noctec, Somnos	500
	Ethchlorvynol	Placidyl	500
	Glutethimide	Doriden	250
	Meprobamate	Milltown, Equanil	1,200
	Methyprylon	Noludar	200
Benzodiazepines	Alprazolam	Xanax	1
	Chlordiazepoxide	Librium	25
	Clonazepam	Klonopin	2
	Clorazepate	Tranxene	7.5
	Diazepam	Valium	10
	Estazolam	ProSom	1
	Flurazepam	Dalmane	15
	Lorazepam	Ativan	2
	Oxazepam	Serax	10
	Temazepam	Restoril	15
	Triazolam	Halcion	0.25

toring of vital signs, especially signs of orthostatic hypotension. The sublingual route may be used if the withdrawal symptoms are acute. This is followed by 0.1 to 0.3 mg, PO, t.i.d. A transdermal clonidine patch (Catapres-TTS) can be used, more often in recovery-oriented treatment programs, with some advantages over the oral clonidine: minimizing drug cravings, avoiding disruptions from oral administration of medications, avoiding missed doses, and preventing the build-up of withdrawal symptoms during the night, as well as patient preference.

Methadone can be given initially at 5 to 10 mg, PO, q4 to 6hr; seldom is more than 40 mg required in the first 24 hours. Patients should be monitored for the first couple of hours after their dose. If the patient is sleepy, the next dose can be reduced by 5 mg, or if the patient has objective signs of opiate withdrawal, the next dose should be increased to 15 mg. Once an established daily dose is determined, the methadone should be tapered by 5 mg every day; alternatively for mild to moderate withdrawal symptoms, methadone, 20 mg, PO, b.i.d., and 5 mg PRN q6hr can be used with a similar taper regimen.

Buprenorphine is an FDA-approved medication for pain and is available in an injection form as Buprenex. Some evidence sup-

Table 4-24.5. Recommended oral medications for symptomatic relief of opiate withdrawal

Abdominal cramps	Dicyclomine (Bentil), 10mg q6hr
Anxiety or insomnia	Hydroxyzine (Vistaril), 25 to 50 mg q8hr Zolpidem (Ambien), 10 mg PO qhs Zaleplon (Sonata), 10 mg PO qhs
Constipation	Milk of Magnesia, 30 mL every other day
Headache	Acetaminophen (Tylenol), 650 mg q4hr
Indigestion	Antacid (Mylanta) 30 mL between meals and qhs
Loose stools	Bismuth-subcarbonate (Pepto-Bismol), 30 mL after each loose stool up to 8 doses total, no more than 2 days total
Bone, joint, or muscle pain	Ibuprofen (Motrin, Advil), 600–800 mg q6–8hr

ports its use in the treatment for heroin dependence, and it even can assist in methadone discontinuation.

Cocaine withdrawal can last up to 2 weeks, which is why so many patients will "medicate" the withdrawal or prevent withdrawal from occurring by continuing to use cocaine. Relapse rates are high, and patients are intensely dysphoric and irritable. Safety assessment because of suicidality is important; a safe, calming environment can assist in decreasing the agitation. Avoid confrontational approaches with these patients; try to accommodate as much as possible, obtaining the needed information and workup while allowing the patient some quiet time, food, and even sleep, if possible.

Remember that many of these patients have either limited access to health care or do not regularly use health care, preferring the ED as a source of primary care. Performing a thorough evaluation may uncover undiagnosed or untreated medical/surgical issues that should be addressed, either as an inpatient or as an outpatient.

The options for nicotine-dependence treatment include nicotine gum, patches, nasal sprays, nicotine vapor inhaler, sublingual nicotine tablets, as well as individual or group therapy, bupropion (Zyban), and less-traditional methods like hypnosis or acupuncture.

DISPOSITION

Often patients who are in withdrawal may require inpatient hospitalization. Alcohol, sedatives/hypnotics, and anxiolytics can all have quite serious consequences and must be treated in a safe environment. Inpatient medically supervised units (when available) or general medical services should be considered. Several outpatient nonmedical detoxification or intensive outpatient detoxification programs can potentially manage these syndromes on an outpatient basis. If co-occurring psychiatric symptoms are seen or suicidality is serious, an inpatient psychiatric admission should be considered. If a specialized dual-diagnosis unit can attend to both disease states, in an integrated fashion, that would be preferable.

The lack of adequate integrated care for those patients who are severely mentally ill and substance abusing or dependent leads to an increase in the likelihood of their becoming homeless, hospitalized frequently, or incarcerated. If you discharge the patient, you must gauge the level of commitment to seek help and provide psychoeducation about harm reduction and abstinence. Medical follow-up should include referrals to specialty clinics as needed. Referral to 12-step or other self-help groups in the local community, as well as different program options, like outpatient detoxification, rehabilitation, long-term residential rehabilitation (harder to arrange from an ED setting), and dual-diagnosis clinics are all viable discharge plans.

BIBLIOGRAPHY

Amato L, Davoli M, Ferri M, et al. Methadone at tapered doses for the management of opioid withdrawal. *Cochrane Database Syst Rev* 2002;2:CD003409.

Bialer PA. Designer drugs in the general hospital. *Psychiatr Clin North Am* 2002;25:231–243.

Covington EC. Anticonvulsants for neuropathic pain and detoxification. *Cleve Clin J Med* 1998;65(suppl 1):SI21–SI29.

Dyer JE, Roth B, Hyma BA. Gamma-hydroxybutyrate withdrawal syndrome. *Ann Emerg Med* 2001;37:147–153.

Foley KM. The treatment of cancer pain. *N Engl J Med* 1985;313:85.

Gelenberg AJ, Bassuk EL, Schoonover SC, eds. *The practitioner's guide to psychoactive drugs.* 4th ed. New York: Plenum, 1997.

Goldsmith RJ. Overview of psychiatric comorbidity. *Psychiatr Clin North Am* 1999;22:331–349.

Gonzalez G, Oliveto A, Kosten TR. Treatment of heroin (diamorphine) addiction: current approaches and future prospects. *Drugs* 2002;62:1331–1343.

Hurt RD. New medications for nicotine dependence treatment. *Nicotine Tob Res* 1999;1(suppl 2):S175–S177.

Johnson ME, Brems C, Burke S. Recognizing comorbidity among drug users in treatment. *Am J Drug Alcohol Abuse* 2002;28:243–261.

Olmedo R, Hoffman RS. Withdrawal syndromes. *Emerg Med Clin North Am* 2000;18:273–288.

Palmistierna T. A model for predicting alcohol withdrawal delirium. *Psychiatr Serv* 2001;52:820–823.

Siqueland L, Crits-Christoph P. Current developments in psychosocial treatments of alcohol and substance abuse. *Curr Psychiatry Rep* 1999;1:179–184.

Smith NT. A review of published literature into cannabis withdrawal symptoms in human users. *Addiction* 2002;97:621–632.

Wesson DR. *Detoxification from alcohol and other drugs: treatment improvement protocols no. 19.* Rockville, MD: U.S. Department of Health and Human Services, Substance Abuse and Mental Health Services Administration, Center for Substance Abuse Treatment, 2001.

Zealberg JJ, Brady KT. Substance abuse and emergency psychiatry. *Psych Clin North Am* 1999;23:803–817.

Zweben JE. Severely and persistently mentally ill substance abusers: clinical and policy issues. *J Psychoactive Drugs* 2000;32:383–389.

5

Special Topics

Chapter 5-1 Specific Policies and Procedures

COBRA/EMTALA REGULATIONS

All staff with primary or supervisory responsibility for patients should be familiar with the various regulations that apply to patient care and the transfer of patients to and from the Emergency Department (ED). The Congressional Omnibus Budget Reconciliation Act (COBRA) was enacted by Congress to prevent hospitals from refusing to treat individuals requiring emergency care or inappropriately transferring or discharging individuals with nonstabilized emergency conditions, better known as anti-dumping legislation. Violations of these provisions are commonly called "dumping."

An emergency condition, as defined by COBRA, is a condition manifesting itself by acute symptoms of sufficient severity, including severe pain, such that the absence of immediate medical attention could reasonably be expected to result in placing the health of the individual or unborn child in serious jeopardy; serious impairment to any bodily function; or serious dysfunction of any bodily organ or part. A psychiatric emergency is defined under the "emergency medical condition" as "a behavioral condition placing the health of such person and others in serious jeopardy." It also takes into account that if a participating hospital has specialized capabilities or facilities, they cannot refuse to accept an "appropriate" transfer of an individual who requires such specialized capabilities or facilities if the hospital has the capacity to treat the individual. This act also requires that peer-review organizations assess whether a participating hospital has committed violations and provide reports on its findings to the Office of the Inspector General, which could impose a civil monetary penalty.

Subsequently, a federal law against patient dumping was enacted, known as the EMTALA, Emergency Medical Treatment and Active Labor Act (42 USC 1867). A participating hospital must comply with the requirements as listed; adopt and enforce policies and procedures to ensure compliance; maintain medical and other records related to individuals transferred to or from the hospital for 5 years from the date of transfer; maintain a list of physicians who are on call to provide treatment necessary to stabilize an individual with an emergency condition; and post in the ED a conspicuous sign(s) informing individuals of their rights to examination and treatment, and appropriate transfer, as necessary, for emergency medical conditions and women in labor, regardless of ability to pay.

Six requirements are placed on hospitals that have emergency departments:

Medical Screening Requirement: If any individual comes to the hospital requesting examination or treatment of a medical condition by qualified medical personnel, the hospital must provide a medical screening examination within the ED's capabilities including all ancillary services available and appropriate to the individual's medical complaint, regardless of insurance status or ability to pay, sufficient to determine whether an emergency condition exists. The individual has to be on hospital property, which includes ambulances owned and operated by the hospital (even if the ambulance is not on hospital property), ambulances (not owned by the hospital) on hospital property, all areas within 250 yards of the main hospital campus, and all areas owned by the hospital (parking lots, sidewalks, driveways, etc.) to be protected by this law.

Necessary Stabilizing Treatment for Emergency Medical Conditions and Labor: If any individual, regardless of insurance status or ability to pay, comes to the hospital, and the hospital determines that the individual has an emergency condition, the hospital must provide medical examination and treatment to stabilize the condition, or transfer to another facility. If the hospital offers the individual further medical examination and treatment, or offers to transfer the individual to another medical facility and informs the individual of the risks and benefits of such examination and treatment or transfer, but the individual refuses to consent, the hospital is deemed to have met this requirement. The hospital should, however, take all reasonable steps to secure the individual's written, informed consent to refuse the examination and treatment or transfer.

Restricting Transfer Until an Individual Is Stabilized: If the individual has an emergency medical condition that has not stabilized, the hospital may NOT transfer that individual. That same individual (or legally responsible person acting on the individual's behalf) may request, in writing, transfer to another facility after being informed of the hospital's obligations under this act and of the risks and benefits of transfer. The hospital must assure that a physician sign a certification based on information available at the time of transfer that the medical benefits expected from the provision of appropriate medical treatment at another facility outweigh the increased risks to the individual or unborn child from effecting the transfer. A transfer to another facility will be considered "appropriate" only in those cases in which the transferring hospital has provided medical treatment within its capacity to minimize the risks, documents the receiving facility's capacity to treat, and documents that the receiving facility has agreed to accept the transfer and to provide appropriate medical treatment. It also must send all medical records related to the emergency condition, observation of signs or symptoms, preliminary diagnosis, treatment provided, tests results, informed written consent or certification, and the name of the receiving physician. The transferring hospital must assure that the transfer is effected through qualified personnel and transportation equipment.

Nondiscrimination: A hospital with specialized capabilities or facilities must accept the appropriate transfer of an individual requiring those specialized capabilities and facilities.

No Delay in Examination or Treatment: The hospital must not delay examination or treatment to inquire about the individual's method of payment or insurance status.

"Whistle Blower" Protections: Participating hospitals may not penalize a physician because he or she refused to authorize a transfer of an individual with an emergency condition that has not been stabilized or against hospital employees because they report a violation of any of these requirements.

An individual whose emergency medical condition has been "stabilized," as defined by the law, does not require an "appropriate" or protected transfer. Conversely, if an individual does require specialized equipment, personnel, or arrangements and communication with the receiving hospital during the transfer, he or she is not "stabilized," according to the law. For emergency conditions, the individual is "stabilized" if a transfer or discharge would not be accompanied by reasonable medical probability of deterioration of the individual's condition. Where there is such a risk, the law does permit an "appropriate" or protected transfer if it is requested by the patient, or medically required and so certified by a physician. All psychiatric conditions may be considered emergencies if they meet the general requirements of an emergency as defined by the law.

The requirements for an "appropriate" transfer include the following.

Transferring physician must contact the receiving physician before the transfer

Transferring physician must accurately relate the patient's medical status to the receiving physician

Patient or guardian must consent to transfer

If the patient or guardian refuses, the transferring physician must document that benefits outweigh risks in transferring

Transferring physician must document that no further harm will occur to patient during transfer

Receiving physician must accept transfer

Transferring hospital must provide transportation and send all medical records and diagnostic tests.

If a hospital fails to meet the requirements as described in the law, federal agencies may impose large financial penalties and potential exclusion from Medicare and Medicaid programs.

BELL COMMISSION

In 1989, the recommendations of the Bell Commission became law, as part of the New York State Health Code (Title 10, paragraph 405.4). The Resident Physician Section of the American Medical Association (AMA) recently passed a resolution substantially similar to New York's Code 405, and other states are sure to follow. Sections relating to work hours read as follows:

"On call" duty in the hospital during the night-shift hours by trainees in surgery shall not be included in the 24-hour limit contained in clause (b) and the 80-hour limit contained in clause (a) of this paragraph if:

1. The hospital can document that during such night shifts, trainees are generally resting and that interruptions for patient care are infrequent and limited to patients for whom that postgraduate trainee has continuing responsibility;
2. Such duty is scheduled for each trainee no more often than every third night;

3. A continuous assignment that includes night-shift "on call" duty is followed by a nonworking period of no less than 16 hours; and
4. Policies and procedures are developed and implemented to relieve a postgraduate trainee from a continuing assignment immediately when fatigue due to an unusually active "on call" period is observed.

In determining limits on working hours of postgraduate trainees, the medical staff shall require that scheduled on-duty assignments be separated by not less than 8 nonworking hours. Postgraduate trainees shall have at least one 24-hour period of scheduled nonworking time per week.

The elements of the Bell Commission directly applicable to the ED is with regard to consecutive hours worked and states, ". . . postgraduate trainees and attending physicians shall be limited to no more than 12 consecutive hours per on-duty assignments in the emergency service . . ." or ". . . schedule limit of up to 15 hours for attending physicians in a hospital emergency service on determination that . . . volume of patients examined and treated during the extended period is substantially less than that for other hours of the day; and adequate rest time is provided between assignments and during each week to prevent fatigue. . . ."

VISITOR POLICY

In ED settings in which space, comfort, and volume are hardly ever optimal, visitors can pose an added challenge. Many EDs try to limit the number of visitors and times when they are allowed, and many specialized psychiatric EDs have no-visitor policies, except at a clinician's discretion, and then for very brief periods. Often patients being evaluated will be permitted to have one visitor at a time, unless the ED is full, and the visitor cannot be accommodated. With the exception of adolescents, patients on enhanced observational status should not be allowed to have visitors unless prior approval is obtained from the clinical staff for each and every visit/visitor. Everyone must be alert to the possible transfer of contraband material or other personal items to a patient on an enhanced observational status by visitors, and they must be educated to what is and is not allowed to be shared with the patient (e.g., glass bottles, cans, plastic knives, cigarettes, or matches).

For reasons of safety and protection, children should not be permitted in an ED, except for possibly brief periods at the absolute discretion of the clinical staff and if clinically acceptable. If no one is available to care for the young child of a patient in the ED, commonly the hospital or ED social worker will determine the necessary arrangements needed. In that event, someone whom the patient knows and trusts should be contacted as soon as possible to take over the care of the child, or other options will have to be discussed, including child-protection agency placement.

BIBLIOGRAPHY

American College of Emergency Physicians. Policy statements on appropriate interhospital patient transfer, 1997.

The Emergency Medical Treatment and Active Labor Act, as established under the Consolidated Omnibus Budget Reconciliation Act (COBRA) of 1985 (42 USC 1395 dd), Section 9121, as amended by the Omnibus Budget Reconciliation Acts (OBRA) of 1987, 1989, and 1990. Rules and regulations published Federal Register June 22, 1994;59:32086-32127.

Frew S. EMTALA Online. Health Law Resource Center. www.med-law.com, 2002.

New York State Health Code (Title 10, paragraph 405.4)

Quinn DK, Geppert CMA, Maggiore WA. The Emergency Medical Treatment and Labor Act of 1985 and the practice of psychiatry. *Psychiatr Serv* 2002;53:1301–1307.

Chapter 5-2 Restraints and Seclusion

Restraints and seclusion should used as a final response to emergency and imminently dangerous behavior. Restraints and seclusion are solely to protect the patient from harm to self or from harming others because of the psychiatric condition. Restraints and seclusion are never to be used:

- As a means of punishment or retribution for an agitated, demanding, or disruptive patient
- For the convenience of staff
- As a substitute for a treatment program.

Restraints are considered "the direct application of physical force to a patient, with or without the patient's permission, to restrict their freedom of movement. This physical force may be human, mechanical devices, or a combination thereof." This does not apply to any brief interactions with a patient to redirect or assist in their activities of daily living, such as hygiene or feeding, nor the "use of psychotropic medication that is not a usual and customary part of medical diagnostic or treatment procedure, and that is used to restrict a patient's freedom of movement," which is called a chemical restraint. Seclusion means "involuntary confinement of a person in a locked room."

It is crucial during implementation of restraints or seclusion to preserve the patient's rights and dignity at all times. This can be achieved by

- Ensuring the patient's privacy as much as possible
- Ensuring that restraints are as individualized as possible
- Ensuring that restraints are conducted professionally
- Allowing participation in care decisions by the patient or the patient's significant others
- Ensuring that restraints are the least-restrictive measure necessary for the protection of the patient and others
- Providing ongoing assessment and monitoring
- Providing physical care and comfort during the time in restraints and seclusion.

Once the decision has been made to proceed with restraints or seclusion, a team leader must be identified who has experience in the implementation of restraints or seclusion. Sufficient trained personnel must be available so that the procedure can be carried out safely and effectively, especially if physical force becomes warranted. At all times, the staff must convey confidence and calmness, and proceed with implementation as if it were a standard and familiar procedure.

The list highlights the indications used for seclusion and restraints as per the guidelines of the American Psychiatric Association.

American Psychiatric Association indications for seclusion and restraint:

To prevent imminent harm to the patient or other persons when other means of control are not effective or appropriate

To prevent serious disruption of the treatment program or significant damage to the physical environment

For treatment as part of an ongoing plan of behavior therapy

To decrease stimulation a patient receives

For use at the request of a patient.

Once it is determined that a need exists to cross the line of mandatory physical control, the overriding principles are that it be done swiftly and humanely, and that the patient be reassured that this is believed to be in the patient's best interest. This intervention has an inherent physical and psychological impact on the patient as well as on staff. Many institutions have policies that include staff (sometimes with the patient and family included) debriefing after a patient is placed in restraint or seclusion. This helps to identify the event and possible ways to have handled it differently, to determine whether all the important aspects of implementation were conducted adequately, and to reassess or modify the patient's treatment plan.

Restraints and seclusion are often used as quality performance indicators and monitored closely, both internally and externally, by many regulatory agencies, including Joint Commission on Accreditation of Healthcare Organizations (JCAHO).

Restraints

Restraints, whether chemical or physical, should be reserved for use in only the most extreme cases of behavioral dyscontrol, that which is clinically considered most likely to result in harm to the patient's self or to others. In a study of teaching hospital EDs, it was noted that 25.2% restrained at least one patient per day, whereas another study had averaged 4.5 patients per day or 3.7% of all patients requiring seclusion or restraints. The discrepancy and the differences between these findings vary greatly depending on

- The characteristics of the ED
- The size
- The staff
- The patient population
- The training of the professional staff, which includes the ED physicians, nurses, support staff, and security personnel who are most frequently involved in the management of the violent patient.

Several studies have shown that the vast majority of patients requiring restraints in the ED have medical or surgical diagnoses, and nearly half require medical or surgical admission. The most common diagnoses include dementia, delirium, seizure disorders, mental retardation, and substance intoxication and/or substance-induced psychiatric disorders. It is important to underscore and highlight, especially for all ED physicians, a study that found that more than half of the patients who ended in restraints or seclusion had arrived through the emergency medical services (EMS) system. This is important because many of the patients brought in by EMS have little information, arrive with no family, and have unclear medical and psychiatric status.

The proper use of restraints must be applied by those who are specifically trained and competent in the assessment, implementation, care, and evaluation of patients requiring restraints, because it can be a very hazardous procedure in which the improper application of restraints can lead to injury of staff or patient. The mere presence of staff may assist in reassuring and calming the patient, thus eliminating the need for restraints. The list stipulates the Emergency Medicine Practice Committee: Use of Restraints Standards.

- *American College of Emergency Physicians* **supports the careful and appropriate use of patient restraints after careful assessment when a patient is a danger to self or others by virtue of the medical or psychiatric condition.**
- **Restraints should be individualized and should afford as much dignity to the patient**
- **Restraints should be humanely and professionally administered**
- **Protocols to ensure patient safety, such as observation, treatment, and periodic assessment, should be developed.**
- **Careful documentation should include the reason, means, and periodic assessment of restraints. Conformity with applicable laws, rules, regulations, and accreditation standards should be assured.**
- **Least-restrictive method necessary should be used for the protection of the patient and others.**

Once the decision to place a patient in restraints has been made, it should be carried out calmly, swiftly, and without vacillation. Remember to offer chemical agents before restraints. Be prepared to have many staff present: the more staff present, the easier it will be to carry on with the procedure, and the presence of staff might even assist in the patient calming down without requiring restraints. A minimum of five staff members is recommended, one for each limb, and if staff is unavailable, then the use of trained hospital security or even local police can be considered. A team "leader" must be selected or designated, and the leader will instruct the others on what to do. The patient or significant other should be informed of the reasons for restraints and be told in a calm and reassuring manner what the procedure will entail. An ongoing explanation regarding the need for restraints should be provided. The patient should be positioned on a bed or stretcher, with legs spread apart and arms securely positioned by the sides. Restraints—preferably soft-leather, which have been shown to be the most effective—should be applied securely to the bed frame and leave at least one finger space between the skin surface and the restraint. The wrist restraints should be secure enough to prevent biting or impairment of circulation. The wrist restraints should be placed in a way that intravenous (IV) fluids or blood accessioning can occur if needed. The patient's head should be slightly elevated to minimize the risks of aspiration. All four limbs should be secured to minimize injury. When in restraints, the patient should again be offered medications, and if still refusing and still agitated, involuntary medication can be considered until the patient is calm. Hospital policies will dictate the frequency and parameters of patient monitoring during restraint (i.e., skin integrity, vital signs, range of motion, toileting, pulses). The patient should be seen and evaluated periodically by a physician, preferably at least once every 30 minutes or at more-frequent intervals to reevaluate the need for continued restraints. Once the patient has calmed down, an adequate search for weapons and contraband must be conducted if not done already.

Each hospital will have its own policies on restraints, most requiring a licensed practitioner who is credentialed by the medical board of the hospital to write orders, and these must be time-limited and renewed periodically. Orders, whether written or oral, are time-limited:

- 4 hours for patients older than 18 years
- 2 hours for children and adolescents aged 9 to 17 years
- 1 hour for children younger than 9 years.

A standing or as-needed (PRN) order for restraints or seclusion must never be made. At the time the order expires, the licensed practitioner must conduct a reevaluation in person to determine the need for continuation or discontinuation, although if clinically appropriate, the restraints or seclusion can be discontinued before the elapsed time.

Documentation is very important, and a description of the reasons for restraints, the reason that less restrictive methods were not effective or used, family and patient involvement, medications (if given), course of treatment, and the patient's response while in restraints should be included. It is imperative that every use of restraints be fully documented and that all required forms be correctly filled out. The reason for this meticulous attention is the extreme circumstances under which restraints are used, and the fact that many ED's quality-assurance or performance-improvement projects are based on their use of restraints, as well as outside agency monitoring.

Nursing monitoring of a patient in restraints or seclusion will often be documented on a special form. These usually include

- Monitoring vital signs
- Addressing nutritional/hydration status
- Checking circulation and range of motion of the extremities
- Addressing physical and psychological status of the patients
- Helping the patient meet behavioral control to discontinue restraints or seclusion, recognizing the readiness for discontinuation of restraint or seclusion
- Recognizing incorrectly placed restraints.

Once the patient is in control, the staff must decide to remove the restraints, which should be done one at a time while monitoring the patient carefully for behavioral control. It is customary to inform the family or guardian that the patient was placed in restraints, if the patient has/had consented to keep the family informed. Restraints or seclusion should be ended and removed at the earliest possible clinically feasible time.

Seclusion

Seclusion denotes a place of involuntary confinement where the patient is prevented from leaving the room, with or without a locked door. A seclusion room, if available in the ED, must have all the required design specifications to ensure optimal safety for patients while in seclusion. The seclusion room must be thoroughly tamper-proof and without any objects that could be used to injure the patient. Certain regulations govern the use of seclusion in certain types of patients (e.g., pregnancy or mental retardation), which must be taken into account. Medical conditions that are unstable and require close physical interactions or monitoring preclude the use of seclusion. Seclusion can be useful for agitated patients by decreasing the external stimuli and permitting the patient a "break" to regain behavioral control. "Time-out" is different from seclusion, in that this is considered a behavioral intervention used to assist a patient in regaining control by restricting him or her to a quiet area or unlocked room for 30 minutes or less.

Once the decision to use seclusion has been made, the patient must be made aware of the plan, and enough staff members must be present to enforce seclusion. At first the door can remain open and unlocked, but if agitation continues, the door must be locked for safety. The patient is made aware that the door will remain locked for a set amount of time, and throughout the management, the patient must be aware of the consequences of his or her behavior. Medications can be offered to prevent or dissuade further restrictive measures of containment. Before seclusion, the patient is searched, and potentially dangerous items are removed. While in seclusion, the patient should be checked no less than every 15 minutes and preferably monitored with closed-circuit television. The patient must be given periodic opportunities to comply with staff's defined parameters of behavioral control to be released from seclusion. If agitation and violence persist, the patient must be placed in four-point restraints to prevent further injury. As with restraints, staff must clearly document and justify the need for seclusion, intervening steps, and medications given.

BIBLIOGRAPHY

American College of Emergency Physicians. Emergency physicians' patient care responsibilities outside of the emergency department [policy statement]: approved September 1999. *Ann Emerg Med* 2000;35:209.
American Psychiatric Association. *Resource guide on seclusion and restraint.* May 1999.
Bell CC, Palmer JM. Survey of the demographic characteristics of patients requiring restraints in a psychiatric emergency service. *J Natl Med Assoc* 1983;75(10):981–987.
Comprehensive accreditation manual for hospitals: The official handbook. Oakbrook Terrace, Illinois: Joint Commission on Accreditation of Healthcare Operations, 2001.

Lavoi FW. Consent, involuntary treatment, and the use of force in an urban emergency department. *Ann Emerg Med* 1992;21:1.

Lavoi FW, Carter GL, Danzl DF, et al. Emergency department violence in United States teaching hospitals. *Ann Emerg Med* 1988;17:1227–1233.

New York State Department of Health Regulations (405.7) 1995.

White CD, Paris PM. Field management of combative patients. *Ann Emerg Med* 1988;17:751(abst).

Chapter 5-3 Social Issues

CHILD ABUSE

Child abuse and neglect can occur in children of both sexes, of any ethnic or racial makeup, and of all socioeconomic classes. Child abuse and neglect are associated with many emotional and psychiatric symptoms.

The identification and reporting of child abuse is a mandated responsibility for all physicians in all states. Some states have elder-abuse reporting as a requirement, whereas others do not. It is important that, as in all issues that involve medicolegal aspects, you become familiar with your local, state, and federal laws. Federal legislation, the Child Abuse Prevention and Treatment Act (CAPTA; amended and reauthorized in October 1996) defines and identifies a minimum set of acts or behaviors that characterize neglect, physical abuse, or sexual abuse of a child.

CAPTA defines abuse or neglect as any act or failure to act by a parent or guardian (including employees of a residential facility or a staff person providing out-of-home care) that results in imminent risk of serious harm, death, serious physical or emotional harm, or sexual abuse or exploitation of a child (anyone younger than 18 years). CAPTA also defines sexual abuse as the use, inducement, persuasion, enticement, or coercion of any child to engage in, or assist any other person to engage in, any sexually explicit conduct or any visual depiction of such conduct. Additionally, it goes on to include rape and in cases of caretaker or interfamily relationships, statutory rape, molestation, prostitution, or incest with children.

Each state is responsible for providing definitions of child abuse and neglect within its civil and criminal codes/statutes. You must be familiar with these in your state. These statutes mandate the obligatory reporting of known or suspected cases of abuse. Each state designates individuals, typically by professional group, who are mandated by law to report child maltreatment. Any person, however, may report incidents of abuse or neglect.

Individuals typically designated as mandatory reporters have frequent contact with children. These include

- Healthcare workers
- School personnel
- Day-care providers
- Social workers
- Law-enforcement officers
- Mental health professionals.

In 2000, three million referrals concerning the welfare of approximately five million children were made to child-protection agencies throughout the United States. Almost one third of investigations or assessments (32%) resulted in a finding that the child was maltreated or at risk of abuse. Approximately 879,000 children were found to be victims of some type of child abuse, 63% suffered neglect (including medical neglect), 19% were physically abused, 10% were sexually abused, and 8% were psychologically maltreated.

Child fatalities are the most tragic consequence of child abuse. In 2000, approximately 1,200 children died of abuse or neglect, a rate of 1.71 per 100,000 children in the population. Fatalities from neglect account for 30% to 40% of deaths caused by child maltreatment. Young children are the most vulnerable; children younger than 1 year accounted for 44% of child fatalities, and 85% of child fatalities were in children younger than 6 years.

Presentations

These are some common physical findings:

- Unexplained skin lesions or bruises on different parts of the child's body
- Evidence of old fractures or unexplained fractures
- Head injuries, missing patches of hair
- Lesions with distinctive patterns
- Unexplained burns, including those made by a cigarette or by immersion into hot water (glove- and sock-like distribution).

These are some common emotional/behavioral findings:

- Child with fear of going home or extremely wary of adults
- Extreme behavioral manifestations out of character for a child
- Child frightened by parents or caretakers
- Delinquency or inappropriate antisocial behavior
- Running away
- Overly fearful behavior or development delays.

Physical findings of sexual abuse:

- Sexually transmitted disease
- Pain or irritation in the genital areas
- Bruising or perineal bleeding
- Difficulty sitting or walking
- Pregnancy.

Childhood failure to thrive, when no medical cause can be found, or an apparent lack of supervision or medical care also can be indicative of neglect. During an evaluation, children must be listened to, because many will report injury, lack of supervision at home, or sexual behaviors or assault by caretakers.

Management

If abuse is suspected, child and family members must be interviewed separately. Interviewing the child with each caretaker separately also can be helpful to determine the relationships, fears, anxieties, and attachments, although it is hard to draw conclusions from one interview about family dynamics. A thorough physical examination is important, including a genital examination, looking for scars and bruises and other telltale signs of abuse. Radiographs can help shed light on fractures, current or in varying stages of repair. Many times outward signs of sexual abuse are not readily seen, and therefore a careful and thorough interview is fundamental. The use of anatomically correct dolls can help children explain their abuse. Physicians must make certain never to lead a child in any direction regarding abuse; frightened or impressionable children are easily swayed and will report what they think the interviewer wants to hear. Children with development delays or mental retardation (see Chapter 6-1 and 6-4) have higher rates of abuse and concomitant difficulty in expressing it.

When child abuse or neglect is suspected, the physician and staff must call in a report to the local child-protection agency. The child-protection agency will determine, after an evaluation of the case and child, what placement will be indicated. Many times, the child must be admitted to the hospital or placed in an out-of-home setting, pending this evaluation, if the suspicion of abuse or neglect is serious enough not to allow the child to return home with the parent or caretaker. Several known risk factors increase a child's risk of abuse:

- Parents with histories of abuse
- Lack of support systems
- Parents with increased stressors, debts, illness, unemployment, and substance abuse
- Marital conflicts or custody disputes between parents
- Single-parent home.

Most hospitals have policies and procedures on how to assess, document, and report suspected child abuse or neglect. Familiarize yourself with these procedures. Victims of abuse, whether they be children, elderly, disabled individuals, or victims of domestic violence, must be assessed carefully and identified. Studies suggest that children are seriously affected by victimization and witnessed violence in their homes and neighborhoods. It is considered a predictor of childhood aggression, depression, anxiety, and anger. Neglecting to identify adequately such a person can place the child at continued risk. Remember, if you do not suspect abuse, you will not find abuse. Keep it present so you are more attuned to suspect abuse and ask about it.

ELDER ABUSE

Elder abuse goes often unrecognized but is a very serious public health problem, with estimates ranging at half a million elders suffering from abuse a year. To tackle this problem, in 1987, the Federal government defined elder abuse in the Amendments to the Older Americans Act. These were set as guidelines for identifying the problems but not for enforcement purposes; each state defines it, so significant variation is found from one jurisdiction to another in terms of what constitutes abuse, neglect, or exploitation of the elderly. The three basic categories of elder abuse are (a) domestic elder abuse, (b) institutional elder abuse, and (c) self-neglect or self-abuse.

Elder abuse can include neglect, physical, sexual, or emotional abuse, financial or material exploitation, abandonment, and even self-neglect. More than two thirds of elder-abuse perpetrators are family members of the victims, typically serving in a care-giving role. Spouses make up a large percentage of those, as do adult children who live with the elder, often being dependent on them for financial assistance, housing, and other forms of support. Other reasons or factors may be care-giver stress, personal characteristics of the elder (such as dementia, disruptive behaviors, problematic personality traits, and significant needs for assistance), which may all increase an elder's risk of being abused. Often the elder abuse is part of a complex cycle of family violence that may include child abuse or domestic violence. Similar factors responsible for elder abuse, poverty, inadequate housing, mental illness, substance abuse, care-giver burnout, etc.

In the ED, it is a physician's responsibility—and in some states, it is mandated—that elder abuse be assessed, managed, and reported, just as in child abuse. Be familiar with your local and hospital statutes on this issue; some jurisdictions leave the decision to report up to the practitioner if the patient is competent. Elderly patients in the ED, either brought in through EMS or with family, may have a variety of physical signs and symptoms. The patients will rarely talk about the abuse, either for fear of reprisals or because of embarrassment. Your level of suspicion should be high if any of the signs or symptoms listed in Table 5-3.1 are present. Assess for dementia and delirium, as well as for exacerbation of underlying psychiatric and medical conditions. Thorough medical and neurologic examinations are needed, with laboratory tests and neuroimaging as clinically indicated.

Try to interview the patient alone; collateral information can be obtained after the interview. Try to engage, in a supportive and reassuring manner—never confront the patient—and inquire about the findings and what the patient's thoughts are about the injuries. Many times patients will have vague and inconsistent stories or will change their stories often when confronted with the inconsistencies. Explain to the patient your suspicion, and in cases of mandated reporting, include social service staff to help in the discussion with the patient about the need to report your suspicions of abuse. If not mandated, discuss with the patient the option of reporting and then the alternatives for referral, usually victims' services, criminal justice systems, or other community-based agencies that deal with elder abuse. Keep in mind that if the patient is competent, it is his or her ultimate decision to make, and you must respect these wishes. Family members present may become suspicious and increasingly more hostile if they suspect that staff has concerns about the patient, and this situation is potentially violent and must be addressed quickly and expeditiously before escalation. Plan ahead and make certain that a volatile situation will not ensue in the ED with hostile family members; security presence may be required.

Adult Protective Services (APSs), which exist in some form in most jurisdictions, are designated as the agency to receive and investigate allegations of elder abuse and neglect. As with child abuse, if abuse or neglect is found, arrangements for services to help protect the victim will be made. Additional resources include State Elder Abuse Hotlines, usually a 24-hour toll-free number for receiving confidential reports of abuse. Many local police or sheriff's offices may investigate elder abuse, especially if there is assault or sexual abuse; mandating reporting will require that when elder abuse is suspected, you call your local area law enforcement office. If your suspicion is about institutional elder abuse, since passage of the 1975 Older Americans Act, every state has had a long-term care ombudsman program to investigate and resolve

Table 5-3.1.   Elder abuse

Abuse	Findings
Neglect 　Refusal or failure to provide an elderly person with such life necessities as food, water, clothing, shelter, personal hygiene, medicine, comfort, personal safety, and other essentials included in an implied or agreed-on responsibility to an elder	Malnourishment Dehydration Unclean skin or hair Untreated illness or injuries Unsafe or unhealthy living environment (e.g., improper wiring, no heat, or no running water, dirt, fleas, lice on person, soiled bedding, fecal/urine smell, inadequate clothing) Untreated bed sores, and poor personal hygiene Report of being mistreated
Emotional abuse 　Verbal assaults, insults, threats, intimidation, humiliation, and harassment 　Treating an older person like an infant; isolating an elderly person from his/her family, friends, or regular activities 　Giving an older person the "silent treatment"	Enforced social isolation Emotionally upset or agitated Being extremely withdrawn and noncommunicative or nonresponsive Unusual behavior usually attributed to dementia (e.g., sucking, biting, rocking) Report of being verbally or emotionally mistreated Confusion Excessive fears Insomnia Unusual weight loss or gain Depression
Physical abuse 　Hitting, beating, pushing, shoving, shaking, slapping, kicking, pinching, and burning 　Inappropriate use of drugs and physical restraints, force-feeding, and other forms of physical punishment	Bruises, black eyes, welts, lacerations, or rope marks Bone fractures, broken bones, and skull fractures Open wounds, cuts, punctures, untreated injuries in various stages of healing Sprains, dislocations, and internal injuries/bleeding Broken eyeglasses/frames, physical signs of being subjected to punishment, and signs of being restrained Laboratory findings of medication overdose or underutilization of prescribed drugs Report of being hit, slapped, kicked, or mistreated Sudden change in behavior Caregiver's refusal to allow visitors to see an elder alone Missing teeth Missing patches of hair

Table 5-3.1. *Continued*

Abuse	Findings
Sexual abuse Unwanted touching, all types of sexual assault or battery, such as rape, sodomy, coerced nudity, and sexually explicit photographing	Bruises around the breasts or genital area Unexplained venereal disease or genital infections when patient not sexually active Unexplained vaginal or anal bleeding Torn, stained, or bloody underclothing Report of being sexually assaulted or raped Difficulty sitting or walking

Financial abuse
  Illegal or improper use of an elder's funds, property, or assets, on cashing an elderly person's checks without authorization/permission
  Forging an older person's signature; misusing or stealing an older person's money or possessions
  Coercing or deceiving an older person into signing any document (e.g., contracts or will)
  Improper use of conservatorship, guardianship, or power of attorney
	Inaccurate or confused knowledge of their finances
	Sudden inability to pay for their basics (food, bills, rent)
	Depression
	Family member expresses interest in their assets
	Sudden changes in bank account or banking practice, including an unexplained withdrawal of large sums of money by a person accompanying the elder
	Inclusion of additional names on an elder's bank signature card
	Unauthorized withdrawal of the elder's funds using the elder's ATM card
	Abrupt changes in a will or other financial documents
	Unexplained disappearance of funds or valuable possessions
	Discovery of an elder's signature being forged for financial transactions or for the titles to his/her possessions
	Sudden appearance of previously uninvolved relatives claiming their rights to an elder's affairs and possessions
	Unexplained sudden transfer of assets to a family member or someone outside the family
	Report of financial exploitation

Abandonment Desertion of an elderly person by an individual who has assumed responsibility for providing care for an elder, or by a person with physical custody of an elder	Desertion of an elder at a hospital, a nursing facility, or other similar institution Desertion of an elder at a shopping center or other public location Report of being abandoned

continued

Table 5-3.1. *Continued*

Abuse	Findings
Self-neglect Behavior that threatens their health or safety such as refusal or failure to provide themselves with adequate food, water, clothing, shelter, personal hygiene, medication (when indicated), and safety precautions	Dehydration, malnutrition, untreated or improperly attended medical conditions, and poor personal hygiene Hazardous or unsafe living conditions/arrangements (e.g., improper wiring, no indoor plumbing, no heat, no running water) Unsanitary or unclean living quarters (e.g., animal/insect infestation, no functioning toilet, fecal/urine smell) Inappropriate and/or inadequate clothing, lack of the necessary medical aids (e.g., eyeglasses, hearing aids, dentures) Grossly inadequate housing or homelessness

nursing home complaints. Ask your social service department or State Unit on Aging or Area Agency on Aging to see whether the long-term care ombudsman program in your area can help in any given situation. Every State Attorney General's office is required by Federal law to have a Medicaid Fraud Control Unit (MFCUs) to investigate and prosecute Medicaid provider fraud and patient abuse or neglect in healthcare programs that participate in Medicaid, including home healthcare services. Most local area agencies that deal with elder abuse have an information and referral (I & R) line that can refer people to a wide range of services for people aged 60 years and older; this can be particularly helpful in locating services that can help prevent abuse and neglect.

Admission to a medical or psychiatric unit, depending on the presenting symptoms, may be needed while an investigation is taking place, alternative placement is being sought, or for the management and care of the medical/psychiatric conditions and injuries.

DISABLED PERSONS ABUSE
Individuals with hearing, visual, or physical impairments and those with developmental disabilities will have a harder time describing or relating their abuse or assault, given their differing levels of disability. Changes in behavior, personality, or aggressiveness can signal that an underlying problem may be present. Often they have vague complaints of injury without physical evidence of trauma or have multiple injury sites, attributed to their disability. Caretakers, if present, might try to conceal these findings and explain them as part of the individual's illness or self-inflicted. Many times, signs of depression, fatigue, or anxiety, along with bruises, abrasions, lacerations, headaches, or abdominal or unexplained pain can be harbingers of abuse at home or in a res-

idence. Worsening of the underlying medical condition and frequently missed follow-up appointments also can be indicative.

PHYSICAL AND SEXUAL ABUSE

Victims of physical and sexual abuse can be women or men, adults or children, and have very singular medical, psychological, and legal needs when they are seen in the ED. Access to emergency care should be prompt and as dignified and supportive as possible, and extraordinary care in collecting evidence should be undertaken in all cases. Most hospitals, in coordination with local and state laws, should have a detailed policy on how to deal with sexually abuse victims; some may even have a separate program in the hospital, which responds to the ED when needed. Specially trained personnel with the appropriate understanding of the policies and needed equipment for evidentiary collection are fundamental in the management of a sexually assaulted victim. Counseling and pregnancy testing as well as testing and treatment for sexually transmitted diseases and human immunodeficiency virus (HIV) all are recommended. Careful attention to policies and protocols, as well as concise and clear documentation, is fundamental in these cases.

Findings can range from typical outward manifestations, such as bruises, scratches, bite marks, eye injuries, missing teeth or patches of hair, broken or fractured bones, to multiple injury sites with even evidence of rape or sexual assault. This can occur in women as well as men; especially in men, it must be considered and the subject addressed, because most often men will be embarrassed or too ashamed to report that they were physically or sexually assaulted. Levels of suspicion should be increased in patients with these physical findings and other nonspecific findings such as depressed mood, anxiety, fears, suicidal ideation, changes in behavior, withdrawal, resignation, etc. At times the explanation of the injuries does not match what would be expected, or the injuries are in various levels of healing, suggesting that the infliction of the abuse was over time.

DOMESTIC VIOLENCE

Presentations to the ED of battered individuals seldom are clear and simple. We do know that women make up 85% of the adult domestic violence cases reported, these being perpetrated predominantly by the current or former partner. Women experience 5 to 8 times as many incidents of violence by an intimate than do men, and half of these are by a spouse or ex-spouse—20% of these were with a weapon. Estimates range from 960,000 incidents of domestic violence to 3.9 million a year—regardless, the numbers are enormous, and many more certainly are unreported.

Domestic violence is a complex phenomenon whose understanding and manifestations are disconcerting. Domestic violence cuts across all variables; it can affect women and men of all races, ethnic groups, socioeconomic status, and educational backgrounds. Domestic violence and abuse occurs in close to half of women who have children in the home, and 50% of men who abuse their spouses also abuse their children. Statistics show that close to 75% of the victims of murder by an intimate partner were women, which places battered women in a high-risk homicide category. Additionally, in these contexts, elder abuse, sexual assaults, rapes, or stalking can be common.

Women or men who are battered may appear in the ED with multiple injuries or other manifestations but hardly ever will admit the true reason until they are ready to make a change. Domestic violence can be many different things, and an ED clinician must be aware of the possibilities and be able to have a high level of suspicion in certain cases. Battered women can often be severely injured, and many of these women will visit the ED for their injuries related to ongoing domestic violence, but it is thought that one in four women who attempt suicide or have a psychiatric complaint or seek prenatal care may be victims of domestic violence. Depending on the survey, 17% to 46% of lesbians and gays report abuse by their partner or current partner. A consequence of domestic violence, besides the physical injuries and even death in certain cases, is the psychological sequelae; posttraumatic stress disorder (PTSD) and depression are found in much higher rates among battered women.

Domestic violence (partner abuse, spouse abuse, or battering) is the establishment through violence, intimidation, threats, or psychological abuse of control and fear in a relationship. Through these direct and indirect techniques, a batterer is able to coerce and control the other person; the actual violence is a hidden but ever-present terrorizing factor in the battered individual's life. Some of the most common violence women experience from their partners does not leave bruises. Emotional or psychological abuse may precede or accompany physical violence as a means of controlling through fear.

Physical abuse can be grabbing, punching, pinching, shoving, slapping, biting, or hair pulling. Other forms of abuse are subtler but no less painful or potentially damaging, such as withholding access to resources necessary for proper maintenance of health (such as medical care, sleep, food) or forced use of alcohol or drugs. Emotional abuse is considered the attempt to undermine a person's sense of self-worth through repeated criticism, belittling, name calling, put-downs, and manipulation of the other person's feelings or emotions. Spiritual abuse can mean not allowing the person to have or maintain his or her own spiritual belief system, or being forbidden to attend church or religious gatherings. Another subtle form of abuse is psychological abuse, wherein the perpetrator attempts to instill fear through intimidation, threats, menacing, blackmail, harassment, or by the isolation from friends, family, school, or work. Sexual abuse is considered the coercion or attempt to coerce sexual contact(s) without consent (e.g., rape, forced sex after a beating, attacks on the sexual parts of the body, forced prostitution, and pornography) as well as the attempt to undermine a person's sexuality by accusations of infidelity or withholding sex.

As an ED physician and patient advocate, you must be aware of the magnitude of this issue, try to identify it, and with the assistance of social services, provide psychoeducation, support, resources, and optimally, a viable solution to break the cycle of domestic violence. Because no specific clinical presentation, demographic characteristics, or predictive indicators of domestic violence are known, it is a priority to inquire about it in women seen in the ED. Certain medical findings should make you be more suspicious and inquire directly about domestic violence:

- Multiple types of injures (abrasions, contusions, lacerations, ecchymoses, etc.) over different sites
- Delays between the time of injury and seeking treatment, and injuries that are inconsistent with the patient's explanation
- Injuries during pregnancy
- Injuries that suggest a defensive posture or central or bathing-suit pattern injuries: bruises over chest, breasts, abdomen, and pelvis—areas that are not visible to others
- Repeated patterns of ED visits or an ED visit because of a sexual assault or rape
- Evidence of alcohol or drug use or a suicide gesture.

Interpersonal relationship patterns observed in the ED can be very telling. Verbal or physical hostile interactions between the patient and the spouse can trigger some concerns. A guarded, defensive, evasive, or apathetic patient with an overly solicitous and accommodating spouse answering all the questions also may cause concern. An angry, obstructionistic, and aggressive spouse who interferes with the care of his partner in the ED should not only be of concern as far as domestic violence is concerned but also should heighten the need for a safe environment. These individuals may be agitated and even violent, especially if intoxicated or feeling as if they are being confronted, and can become violent with staff or with the patient while in the ED.

Medical and psychiatric evaluations should be conducted as per routine; laboratory test, radiographs, or neuroimaging may be indicated to rule out fractures or head injuries. Many victims may come in for nonspecific complaints, such as headaches, pain, gastrointestinal (GI) distress, or depression, anxiety, or insomnia. Admission is determined by clinical status. Referral to a battered women's shelter may be an option if the woman is ready to make that decision.

Remember that assault, battering, and domestic violence are crimes.

Research has shown that men, if questioned, will admit to being batterers or perpetrating violence on their domestic partner. This raises the possibility and the dilemma of making this part of the ED screening and, if positive, then intervening.

You must be familiar with your hospital and local jurisdiction's policies on mandatory reporting of domestic violence. Certain states require mandatory arrests of batters, and some will even pursue a batterer despite the partner's refusal to press charges. Mandatory reporting against a patient's will is a very complex issue with increased risk of injury or death for the patient. You cannot force or coerce someone into leaving the abusive relationship. Many patients will not be ready to leave the relationship, and providing emotional support and reassurance as well as psychoeducation about domestic violence and options may be the only thing you can do in the ED. See Table 5-3.2 for some of the commonly reported reasons that women do not leave abusive spouses. Sometimes, even if it is not discussed in the ED visit, but you are suspicious, providing the victim with a handout of resources can be helpful.

Table 5-3.2.   Top 10 reasons cited
by women victims of domestic violence

1. Fear of harm to self, children, family, partner, or fear of increased violence
2. Lack of resources (often these women have at least one dependent child, are not employed outside of the home, have no property, lack access to cash or bank accounts, fear being charged with desertion, and losing children and joint assets)
3. Lack of job skills and/or education or face a decline in living standards for herself and her children
4. Lack of information or safe accessible resources, especially undocumented women, disabled women, lesbians, women of color, Orthodox Jewish women
5. Lack of support or isolation. Many women become isolated from friends and families, either by the jealous and possessive abuser, or to hide signs of the abuse from the outside world. The isolation contributes to a sense that there is nowhere to turn
6. Love for the partner and hopes that things will change. The abuser rarely beats the woman all the time. During the non-violent phases, he may fulfill the woman's dream of romantic love. She believes that he is basically a "good man." If she believes that she should hold onto a "good man," this reinforces her decision to stay. She also may rationalize that her abuser is basically good until something bad happens to him, and he has to "let off steam"
7. Religious values and beliefs or family pressures. Clergy and secular counselors are often trained to "save" the marriage at all costs. Many women are taught that their identity and worth are contingent on their marital status; do not believe divorce is a viable alternative; believe that a single-parent family is unacceptable, and that even a violent father is better than no father at all; believe that they are responsible for making their marriage work—failure to maintain the marriage equals failure as a woman
8. Many women rationalize their abuser's behavior by blaming stress, alcohol, and problems at work, unemployment, or other factors
9. Police officers often do not provide support to women. They treat violence as a domestic "dispute," instead of a crime where one person is physically attacking another person, and even try to dissuade women from filing charges
10. Prosecutors are often reluctant to prosecute cases, and judges rarely levy the maximum sentence on convicted abusers. Probation or a fine is much more common

HOMELESSNESS

Homelessness is not only a major public health problem, but also a serious social and moral dilemma that our country must ultimately face and resolve. Homelessness affects the ED directly, with more frequent visits, misuse of services, draining of resources, and lack of coordinated care across clinical services. Homeless patients frequently have more physical health problems, such as tuberculosis, asthma, bronchitis, HIV, and higher rates of mental disorders and substance abuse; rates of morbidity and mortality are higher as well.

Homeless patients are a heterogeneous group, with a wide variety of sociodemographic factors; risk factors; medical, psychiatric and substance-related diagnostic considerations; and functional performance and employment or residential histories. Homelessness, for many a temporary situation, is difficult to define and measure. Many more people are thought to be homeless, with a large turnover rate, and many, although not on the streets, live in crowded apartments, shuffling between friends and families, or in places where researchers traditionally do not look. Examples of these would be living in vehicles, boxcars, tents, boxes, caves, or campgrounds. Although complex and certainly multifactorial, important social and economic factors contribute to becoming homeless, such as sudden loss of employment or prolonged unemployment, domestic violence, mental illness, substance abuse, and lack of affordable housing. Women and children have now become a major segment of the homeless population with less access to health insurance and regular health care. Homeless women were found to be at higher risk for mental illnesses, substance abuse, injection-drug use, trading drugs for sex (especially in crack cocaine–dependent women), and consequently higher risk for HIV transmission. Homeless women were found to have increased rates of physical and sexual abuse, with a relationship to psychopathology as well. The United States Senate Judiciary Committee on Violence Against Women–Victims of the System (1991) found that close to 50% of homeless women and children in the United States are on the streets because of violence in the home.

To achieve a more appropriate measure of the number of homeless people, many consider the number of people who are homeless over time, not the number of "homeless people." Most studies, though, conduct a time-specific count of people who are in shelters, accessing soup kitchens, or on the streets as a measure of homelessness, yielding lower numbers than actually exist. Several national estimates have been made, depending on the methods used, of the number of homeless people in the United States. These range from 500,000 to 600,000 homeless people found in shelters, eating at soup kitchens, or congregating on the street during 1 week in 1988 to an estimate of more than 700,000 people homeless on any given night, and up to 2 million people who experience homelessness during 1 year (using a 5% yearly increase in numbers). Another study conducted in 1995 demonstrated that close to 7 million people had been literally homeless at some point in their lives; further refinements to this study revealed that the number was closer to 12 million. A study from 1994 demonstrated a consistent 3% rate of homelessness in many regions across the United States. Indirectly another measure of the growth of homelessness is the parallel increase—two- to threefold—in the number of shelter beds over the years. The reality is that the capacity of the emergency shelter system is overloaded, and many people apply without receiving shelter when requested. Almost every city in the United States has greater official homeless counts than shelter beds and transitional housing slots.

Deinstitutionalization with the consequent lack of adequate and appropriate projected community-based resources has been blamed for creating a large homeless problem. Current growth in the mentally ill homeless population also results from other factors, some of which can be attributed to poor discharge planning, managed-care cost containment, and loss of low-income housing units in major urban centers with the economically prosperous 1990s. These may have contributed to large numbers of mentally ill patients becoming homeless or in the criminal justice system. It is estimated that approximately 25% of homeless persons have a serious mental illness, and of those, on average 10% are thought to have schizophrenia. These patients, who struggle with the double burden of homelessness and mental illness, are largely the most disenfranchised, marginalized, and the most vulnerable segment of the homeless population. Factors related to poverty and mental illnesses are intricately related to lack of education, poor employment histories, substance abuse, family dysfunction (instability and violence), crime, and abuse histories, among others. Co-occurring substance-related disorders only compound an already complex paradigm. Being homeless places individuals among the poorest of the poor in the United States, and it can become a barrier to employment, which in many is further complicated by mental, physical, and substance-abuse problems. Although many homeless people will work or attempt to work, these physical and mental health barriers and substance-abuse disorders impede their ability to maintain employment for long. Accessibility to disability and other entitlements also is fraught with a myriad of confusing and difficult-to-navigate processes, and the outcome is that homeless persons have less access to health care but higher rates of illness and disability. These patients will use much more acute hospital-based care, such as EDs, for their healthcare services. Countless studies, research projects, and innovative programs (outreach, case management, housing placement, assertive community treatment) have been created to meet this increasing demand, with very mixed results. Employment and permanent residential placement often are not the only solution to this challenge.

Because the prevalence of homelessness varies greatly, it is especially the large urban emergency centers that share the brunt of primary care for these patients. Findings have shown that homeless patients have higher rates of ED use. These higher rates were correlated with the following factors: less stable housing, victimization, involvement with the criminal justice system, physical and mental illnesses, social isolation, and substance abuse. These patients have significantly worse outcomes when compared with other populations and have more chronic medical conditions such as hepatitis B and C and HIV, as well as coinfection.

In the ED, the standard of care for these patients remains the same. Chief complaints, whether medical or psychiatric, must be identified, assessed, diagnosed, and treated accordingly. Social services intervention from the outset can assist greatly at the time of creating a disposition plan. The clinical management must transcend the patient's actual homeless status, despite the frustration and impotence felt by staff with frequent ED users who are homeless and return periodically. After many visits, the staff's patience and empathy with these patients wear thin, and potential suboptimal care may be delivered, placing the patient, the staff, and the institution at higher risk. Staff meetings or reports should include a frank discussion about their feelings with these patients and optimally assist them in working through the frustration and negative transference that these patients can often engender. Treatment plans are usually clinically dictated, with admission to medicine, surgery, or psychiatry, if warranted, or discharge. Remember that homeless persons have higher rates of schizophrenia and other primary psychiatric disorders, substance abuse (primarily alcohol), and chronic and acute medical conditions that can be alone or comorbid. Engaging the person in the ED and trying to make a referral to alternative available services/programs might be the only contact that person has had or will have if he or she returns to living on the streets. These are important opportunities to make a difference and to make an effort at engaging the patients in follow-up care and optimally into a system that will allow them to achieve permanent housing and greater personal satisfaction.

Discharge poses a challenge; certain jurisdictions have well-established emergency shelter systems or drop-in units, but others may not. Knowing the resources in your community and how the shelter system works will be quite helpful when confronted with the need to discharge a homeless person from your emergency service. Policies on feeding, bathing, and sleeping overnight in the ED are institution specific and must be understood by each clinician at the ED. Car fare, tokens, or other forms of transportation for discharged homeless patients are another institution- and even local/state-specific issue that is addressed in hospital policies or procedures.

Nonprofit agencies offer the vast majority (85%) of homeless assistance programs in the United States: secular nonprofits offer 51% of all programs, whereas religious nonprofits offer 34%. Government agencies operate 14% of all programs, and for-profit firms account for a mere 1%. These programs include:

Outreach and engagement teams
Emergency shelters
Transitional housing
Mobile crisis teams
Assertive community teams
Permanent housing for formerly homeless clients
Voucher distribution for housing
Food pantries
Soup kitchens/meal-distribution programs
Mobile food programs
Physical health programs
Mental health programs
Alcohol and/or drug programs
HIV/AIDS programs
Outreach programs
Drop-in centers.

Discuss with the patient and the social service team what the most appropriate disposition plan would be for that patient. Determine the patient's wants and needs at that moment, and remember to address issues of entitlements, substance-abuse treatment (inpatient or outpatient), and aftercare medical and psychiatric plans.

BIBLIOGRAPHY

Child and Elder Abuse

American College Emergency Physicians Policy Statement on Child Abuse, Policy # 400279, 2000.

American Psychiatric Association. *Opinions of the ethics committee on the principles of medical ethics with annotations especially applicable to psychiatry.* 2001.

Berkowitz CD. Fatal child neglect. *Adv Pediatr* 2001;48:331–361.

Child Abuse Prevention and Treatment Act (CAPTA) of 1974 (P.L. 93-247) & Child Abuse Prevention and Treatment Act Amendments of 1996 (P.L. 104–235.)

Johnson RM, Kotch JB, Catellier DJ, et al. Adverse behavioral and emotional outcomes from child abuse and witnessed violence. *Child Maltreat* 2002;7:179–186.

Domestic Violence

American College Emergency Physicians. *Policy statement on domestic violence*, Policy # 400286, 1999.

American College Emergency Physicians. *Policy statement on support for violence victims*, Policy # 400266, 1998.

American College of Emergency Physicians. Mandatory reporting of domestic violence to law enforcement and criminal justice agencies. *Ann Emerg Med* 1997;30:561.

Bureau of Justice Statistics. Criminal victimization in the United States, 1995. *NCJ* 2000;171129.

Bureau of Justice Statistics. Female victims of violent crimes, *NCJ* 1996;162602.

Bureau of Justice Statistics. Intimate partner violence in the United States, May 2000. *NCJ* 178247.

Butterfield MI, Panzer PG, Forneris CA. Victimization of women and its impact on assessment and treatment in the psychiatric emergency setting. *Psychiatr Clin North Am* 1999;23:875–896.

Cheung RC, Hanson AK, Maganti K, et al. Viral hepatitis and other infectious diseases in a homeless population. *J Clin Gastroenterol* 2002;34:476–480.

Cohen B, Cohen M, Cohen B. *America's homeless: numbers, characteristics, and programs that serve them.* Washington, DC: The Urban Institute, 1989.

Cohen B, Cohen M. *Practical methods for counting homeless people: a manual for states and local jurisdictions.* 2nd ed. Washington, DC: The Urban Institute, Publications Sales Office, 1996.

Cohen JH, Friedman DI. Health care use by perpetrators of domestic violence. *J Emerg Med* 2002;22:313–317.

Culhane D, et al. Public shelter admission rates in Philadelphia and New York City: implications of turnover for sheltered population counts. *Housing Policy Debate* 1994;2:107–140.

D'Amore J, Hung O, Chiang W, et al. The epidemiology of the homeless population and its impact on an urban emergency department. *Acad Emerg Med* 2001;8:1051–1055.

Dickey B. Review of programs for persons who are homeless and mentally ill. *Harv Rev Psychiatry* 2000;8:242–250.

Draine J, Salzer MS, Culhane DP, et al. Role of social disadvantage in crime, joblessness, and homelessness among persons with serious mental illness. *Psychiatr Serv* 2002;53:565–573.

Echert LO, Sugar N, Fine D. Characteristics of sexual assaults in women with a major psychiatric diagnosis. *Am J Obstet Gynecol* 2002;186:1284–1288.

Elliot L, Nerney M, Jones T, et al. Barriers to screening for domestic violence. *J Gen Intern Med* 2002;17:112–116.

Elliot P. Shattering illusions: same-sex domestic violence. In: Renzetti CM, Miley CH, eds. *Violence in gay and lesbian domestic partnerships.* Binghamton, NY: Haworth Press, 1996:1–8.

Folsom D, Jeste DV. Schizophrenia in homeless persons: a systematic review of the literature. *Acta Psychiatr Scand* 2002;105:404–413.

Gleason W. Mental disorders in battered women: an empirical study. *Violence Vict* 1993:8:53–68.

Gonzalez G, Rosenheck RA. Outcomes and service use among homeless persons with serious mental illness and substance abuse. *Psychiatr Serv* 2002;53:437–446.

Hatton DC. Homeless women's access to health services: a study of social networks and managed care in the US. *Women Health* 2001; 33:149–162.

Heinzer MM, Krimm JR. Barriers to screening for domestic violence in an emergency department. *Holist Nurs Pract* 2002;16:24–33.

Housing and Homelessness, National Alliance to End Homeless, 1987. Homelessness: Programs and the People They Serve. Findings of the National Survey of Homeless Assistance Providers and Clients. Highlights. Interagency Council on the Homeless, December, 1999.

Inciardi JA, Surratt HL. Drug use, street crime, and sex-trading among cocaine-dependent women: implications for public health and criminal justice policy. *J Psychoactive Drugs* 2001;33:379–389.

Jainchill N, Hawke J, Yagelka J. Gender, psychopathology, and patterns of homelessness among clients in shelter-based TCs. *Am J Drug Alcohol Abuse* 2000;26:553–567.

Kilbourne AM, Herndon B, Andersen RM, et al. Psychiatric symptoms, health services, and HIV risk factors among homeless women. *J Health Care Poor Underserved* 2002;13:49–65.

Koegel P, et al. The causes of homelessness. In: *Homelessness in America.* Washington, DC: Oryx Press, 1996.

Kramer A. Domestic violence: how to ask and how to listen. *Nurs Clin North Am* 2002;37:189–210.

Kushel MB, Perry S, Bangsberg D, et al. Emergency department use among the homeless and marginally housed: results from a community-based study. *Am J Public Health* 2002;92:778–784.

Kushel MB, Vittinghoff E, Haas JS. Factors associated with the health care utilization of homeless persons. *JAMA* 2001;285:200–206.

Lamb HR, Bachrach LL. Some perspectives on deinstitutionalization. *Psychiatr Serv* 2001;52:1039–1045.

Lee D, Ross MW, Mizwa M, et al. HIV risks in a homeless population. *Int J STD AIDS* 2000;11:509–515.

Lim YW, Andersen R, Leake B, et al. How accessible is medical care for homeless women? *Med Care* 2002;40:510–520.

Link B, et al. Life-time and five-year prevalence of homelessness in the United States. *Am J Public Health* 1994;84:1907–1912.

Link B, et al. Life-time and five-year prevalence of homelessness in the United States: new evidence on an old debate. *Am J Orthopsychiatry* 1995;3:347–354.

Metraux S, Culhane D, Raphael S, et al. Assessing homeless population size through the use of emergency and transitional shelter services in 1998: results from the analysis of administrative data from nine U.S. jurisdictions. *Public Health Rep* 2001;116:344–352.

National Aging Information Center (naic@aoa.gov). *The National Elder Abuse Incidence Study; Final Report.* Washington, DC: National Aging Information Center, 1988.

National Center on Elder Abuse. *Fact sheet.* Washington, DC: National Center on Elder Abuse, http://www.elderabusecenter.org.

National Child Abuse and Neglect Data System (NCANDS). *Summary of key findings from calendar year 2000.* April 2002 [http://www.calib.com/nccanch/pubs/factsheets]

National Law Center on Homelessness and Poverty. *Out of sight, out of mind? A report on anti-homeless laws, litigation, and alternatives in 50 United States cities.* Washington, DC: National Law Center on Homelessness and Poverty, 1999.

Odell SM, Commander MJ. Risk factors for homelessness among people with psychotic disorders. *Soc Psychiatry Psychiatr Epidemiol* 2000;35:396–401.

Strauss MA, Gelles RJ. How violent are American families? In: Strauss MA, Gelles RJ, eds. *Physical violence in American families: risk factors and adaptations to violence in 8,145 families.* New Brunswick, New Jersey: Transaction Publishers, 1990:95–112.

Sullivan G, Burnam A, Koegel P. Pathways to homelessness among the mentally ill. *Soc Psychiatry Psychiatr Epidemiol* 2000;35:444–450.

The Commonwealth Fund. *First Comprehensive National Health Survey of American Women, July, 1993;* http://www.cmwf.org.

U.S. Department of Justice, Office of Justice Programs, Bureau of Justice Statistics. *NCJ* 1998;167237.

U.S. Department of Justice, Bureau of Justice Statistics: Violence by intimates. 1998 *NCJ* 167237.

Zachary MJ, Mulvihill MN, Burton WB, et al. Domestic abuse in the emergency department: can a risk profile be defined? *Acad Emerg Med* 2001;8:796–803.

Zuvekas SH, Hill SC. Income and employment among homeless people: the role of mental health, health and substance abuse. *J Ment Health Policy Econ* 2000;3:153–163.

Chapter 5-4 Consultation-Liaison Psychiatry Issues

Consultation-Liaison (C-L) psychiatry has become an increasingly important component of the work performed by psychiatrists. It is an established part of residency training education and has a strong recommendation from the American Psychiatric Association that it be recognized as a subspecialty. A C-L psychiatrist must have an in-depth knowledge of psychiatry and medical illnesses and their comorbidities, the impact of psychosocial stressors on medical and psychiatric illnesses, drug–drug interactions and the newest drug therapies in medical illnesses, the ability to work well with a medical multidisciplinary team, and the skills needed to communicate clearly and precisely their findings to the medical team. These last items are what make "liaison" such an important part of C-L psychiatry; including the teaching of psychiatry and psychosocial variables that impinge on the care of medically ill patients to nonpsychiatric staff.

Some key elements must be taken into account when performing a psychiatric consultation:

- Talk with staff from the requesting service about the consultation, clarifying the reasons and concerns, and assisting the staff to formulate a clear reason if the consult is confusing or unclear.
- Review chart thoroughly, including nursing notes, and, if possible, family or other collateral sources of information, before consultation.
- Perform a thorough psychiatric evaluation including a detailed mental status exam.
- Document findings in a clear, legible, and concise manner; detailing only the relevant and important data that the medical team will require. Document a working diagnosis and a differential diagnosis.
- Make recommendations about diagnostic testing, management on the service, medications (with special considerations for drug–drug interactions or adverse events listed), and clear plan to follow.
- Be available for crisis situations or emergencies, and help provide support and guidance in patients who are behaviorally dyscontrolled.
- Assist in and facilitate the transfer process to psychiatry once the patient has been medically cleared, especially around legal admission issues.
- Provide patient and family with psychoeducation and relevant information pertaining to your understanding of the current situation, diagnostic impression, and recommended treatment plans, including possible risks and benefits. Convey the same information to the medical team.
- Follow up the patient while hospitalized as often as clinically needed, and help elaborate a discharge plan with specific recommendations for aftercare plans.

SUICIDE ASSESSMENT ON A MEDICAL/SURGICAL UNIT

If called to assess suicidality in an admitted medical/surgical patient, several parameters should be followed:

Determine whether medical causes are present (delirium, severe pain, or alcohol withdrawal)

Ask patients about suicidal thoughts: Are they upset about their medical condition? Have they been tearful? What types of thoughts go through their minds when they are discouraged and tearful? Have they ever thought that life would not be worth living under these circumstances? Have they come to a point where they seriously think about ways of ending their life? If so, what types of thoughts have they had? What things could mitigate their suicidality?

Obtain collateral sources of information from staff, family, caretakers, etc.

Recommend treating the underlying causes: anxiety, depression, psychosis, delirium, or optimization of pain management

Make the environment as safe as possible, remove lethal or dangerous objects, consider need for enhanced observational status (one-on-one observation) or transfer to psychiatry if medically feasible

Continue to follow up on the medical/surgical unit until a psychiatry bed is available or medically/psychiatrically stable for discharge with concrete psychiatric aftercare plans.

COMPETENCY/DECISION-MAKING CAPACITY

The determination of competency or medical decision-making capacity is a task that a C-L psychiatrist will be called on to perform very often. The two types of competency are legal or *de jure* and clinical or *de facto*. Everyone is legally competent except minors or those declared incompetent by a judicial determination. Competency in the medical field is referred to as clinical capacity (decision-making capacity), and the lack thereof is considered incapacity. To have the capacity to make a healthcare decision requires that the patient have

- Some basic cognitive and mental abilities to understand the treatment being proposed
- The ability to make a decision based on that understanding
- The ability to communicate that decision to the staff.

In patients who are clinically determined to lack decision-making capacity, all efforts must be made to obtain other legally valid methods of authorization for treatment. When confronted with the task of assessing someone for a capacity to refuse treatment or to leave the hospital (common requests for capacity assessment), make sure you approach the patient unencumbered by the actual notion that he or she may lack capacity. Many times the questioning will lead to an understanding that there are potential interpersonal difficulties with staff, depression, delirium, lack of adequate information about the procedure, uncomfortable surroundings and certain needs not being met, lack of visitation from family, fears and concerns not expressed or verbalized to staff, or simply denial of severity of illness. Often sitting with the patient and discussing some of these issues and addressing others can resolve the capacity issue. Certain other elements must be present as well to determine competency/capacity, those being the absence of interfering negative motivational pressures or negative relationships that may be influencing the patient's decisions. An example would be a patient who has a court appearance and is refusing treatment or asking to be released AMA to avoid missing the appointment. Another may be an overbearing and demanding spouse who cannot care for him- or herself without the presence of the patient and is unduly influencing the patient to leave or refuse treatment to satisfy the spouse's own internal struggles. Additionally, it is important to gauge the patient's awareness of what a reasonable person or society would determine in similar circumstances and why they are deviating from that standard.

Questions to ask:

What is your understanding of your illness?
What treatments have the doctors recommended?
What have the doctors told you would happen if you do not receive the treatment?
What is your understanding of the risks if you do not receive this treatment?
What other options did the doctors discuss with you?

The cases that fall in the middle or are unclear may require further assistance from legal counsel or a court determination, although in certain emergency cases, no time may exist to arrange these contingencies, and a decision must be made, with erring on the side of community-standard treatment as the only viable option. When faced with the decision to treat a patient involuntarily or detain a patient at risk whose capacity is questionable, staff must be prepared to prevent these patients from leaving the medical/surgical unit. Legal precedents have held staff and the hospital liable for injuries incurred by escaped or incapacitated patients not fully evaluated or whose capacity was unclear or questionable.

Occasionally a C-L psychiatrist will be called to assist in the determination of a patient requesting to sign out AMA with a potential active tuberculosis (TB) illness. Because a potential public safety issue is at stake, it is important to handle this situation carefully. Most hospitals have some internal policy and procedure for dealing with these situations, usually involving the infection-control nurse, a nursing administrator, or staff from the ID Department. Many jurisdictions may even have a TB-Hotline run by the local Department of Health, which can assist in answering questions or concerns regarding involuntary retention. The Department of Health has regulations that determine when a suspected TB patient can be detained. This is usually the case with persons who are potentially infectious, as evidenced by a cavitary lesion on chest radiograph (CXR) or a (+) smear for acid-fast bacillus (AFB).

BIBLIOGRAPHY

Mahler J, Perry S. Assessing competency in the physically ill: guidelines for psychiatric consultants. *Hosp Community Psychiatry* 1988; 39:856–861.

6

Special Populations

Chapter 6-1 Children and Adolescents

The age cutoff for psychiatric emergency departments (EDs) is quite variable, compared with the definitive age cutoff between a pediatric and an adult general ED. This age cutoff depends on many variables and specifically on the existence of specialized on-site child/adolescents services and staffing availability. Many general hospitals do not have a specialized child/adolescent psychiatry department or even consultants available after hours and on weekends or holidays to respond to children and adolescents. It is outside the scope of this handbook to provide a comprehensive approach to this topic, but certain clinically relevant themes, especially focused on adolescents, are highlighted.

Because most presentations to an ED are in response to crises, prompted often by concerned parents, guardians, schools, pediatricians, therapists, or other legal or social agencies, they involve multiple informants and a reluctant, frightened, anxious, oppositional, or guarded child or adolescent. The approach to a child or adolescent is relatively more complex and time-consuming, because you must invariably deal with the child/adolescent and these other key players. The assessment must include all of the aspects we elaborated for adults but also include developmental functioning, both normal and abnormal, in the context of the child/adolescent's age, gender, and sociocultural background. Developmental history should include milestones for pregnancy, birth and neonate period, infancy, toddler stage, preschool- and school-age, and adolescence temperament, as well as a detailed school and family history. Other important variables to determine are current habits, hobbies, activities and interests, relationships with family members, risk-taking behaviors, sexual development and behavior, traumatic events, academic performance, and relationships with peers. A child or adolescent must always be viewed in light of the family and its culture, ethnicity, and value system. It is important to remember that certain behaviors and actions may be appropriate at one age but not at another. Sometimes asking a child, or even an adolescent, to describe "three wishes" can provide information on the fantasy life and projective and future-oriented thinking. Another important assessment point, when inquiring about sexual behaviors, a difficult and embarrassing topic for many adolescents, is to remain neutral in your inquiries about their love interests. Presuming that a boy has girlfriends or a girl has boyfriends may alienate the adolescent if he or she is struggling with sexuality or is gay or lesbian. Never presume, and keep these types of questions free of personal bias or prejudices; the more open and supportive you can be with them, the more they will open up and talk about their issues, even those that are hardest.

Many major Axis I disorders can begin in childhood or adolescence, as well as many "disorders usually first diagnosed in infancy, childhood, or adolescence" that are frequent reasons for an

ED visit. *Diagnostic and Statistical Manual of Mental Disorders* (DSM-IV-TR) also lists other conditions that can prompt an ED visit, these being the "V" codes, or other conditions that are a focus of clinical attention:

- Academic problems
- Bereavement
- Borderline intellectual functioning (IQ of 71 to 84, coded on Axis II)
- Child or adolescent antisocial behavior
- Identity problems
- Neglect of a child
- Noncompliance with treatment
- Parent–child relational problem
- Physical abuse
- Relational problems related to a mental disorder or general medical condition
- Sexual abuse
- Sibling relational problem
- Issues and problems related to foster placement.

One of the major difficulties in assessing children or adolescents in the ED is that many times they are brought unwillingly, or worse yet, under false pretenses; in other words, they are "tricked" into coming. This sets the stage for a rather contentious and tenuous patient–doctor relationship to be established. Engaging a child or adolescent is a hard task, although explaining the purpose of the interview and soliciting their help can assist in breaking the ice. Adolescents should always be seen before the parents to make them feel that they will be heard first and valued in what they have to say. It helps minimize the anxiety and make the adolescent feel that the parents and staff are not in collusion or will gang up on them. The downside is that it also reinforces the notion that the adolescent is the designated problem or troublemaker, when the reality often lies in a more complex family dynamic, as well as the false impression that there is truly nothing wrong because adolescents tend to minimize their symptoms and dangerousness. Interviewing the parents alone also is helpful in finding the reasons for referral and gathering data on developmental history. Occasionally it may be useful to interview the adolescent and the parents together, and with a lot of structure, it can yield valuable evidence about how the family works and interacts.

Because the ED focus of an assessment is to establish safety and determine the best course of action for the child or adolescent, many times these goals are at odds with the parent's wishes, motives, or needs. The main goal is the children/adolescents and their safety; whether it is because of suicidal/homicidal thoughts, or physical or sexual abuse, this can engender intense reactions in parents. The degree of parental anxiety, hostility, denial, guilt, and avoidance can make the interview and assessment quite laborious.

Confidentially must be preserved and respected with an adolescent, as it would be with an adult. Sexual history, drug use, and other sensitive information that is divulged during the evaluation must be kept confidential. Parent and patient should be made aware of this from the outset. However, as with adults, information about potential risk to self or others is the exception.

Certain jurisdictions may have local or state mandates for the reporting of certain information to a parent, such as pregnancy status, and you should be familiar with these rules to spell out clearly at the beginning of the interview what you are obliged to keep confidential and what you are not.

The interview and assessment must be conducted at the child's or adolescent's level of development and never above or below that, with the ultimate purpose to establish a diagnostic impression and a treatment plan. In a recent survey of EDs, carried out by the American Association of Emergency Psychiatry, the most common types of emergency presentation to an ED were suicide threats or gestures and violent or threatening behaviors.

Medical workup in the ED must follow the same protocols as established for adults and/or clinically indicated. Urine toxicology and urine pregnancy tests may be warranted in adolescents. Serum blood levels of common therapeutic agents should be determined to verify compliance. The management of an acute overdose as a suicidal gesture must be handled primarily in a pediatric ED with pediatricians, with a psychiatry consultation as needed, or more definitive involvement once the patient is stable.

Human immunodeficiency virus (HIV) risk behaviors and seroprevalence are particularly high among street youth with very low rates of use of healthcare services. In addition, these homeless youths are prone to higher rates of severe partner violence. Gay, lesbian, bisexual, and transgender youths have even higher rates of victimization, drug use, mental disorders (depression, substance-related disorders, dysthymia) and more frequent HIV risk-taking sexual behaviors and sexually transmitted diseases (STDs). Suicide risk and rates, in this population, also are higher; for boys, these factors include being gay, emotional distress, drug use, and friends with suicidality, whereas for girls, the factors were lower age, low self-esteem, emotional distress, assaults, and friends with suicidality. Such patients in the ED should be thoroughly assessed medically and psychiatrically and engaged in treatment and services as often as possible.

Recent traumatic events, like the terrorist attacks on September 11, 2001, and subsequent events, have raised the level of concern about the welfare of children and adolescents. Children exposed to trauma (or violence) are known to have psychiatric consequences from these; level of exposure, psychiatric history, and level of social supports all play a major role in psychopathology. It is important, based on the current understanding, that children exposed to traumatic events be assessed carefully and monitored closely, especially if they are in a high-risk-factor group. Responses to disaster and traumatic events will manifest themselves quite differently in children and adolescents compared with adults. Among children and adolescents, the differences in reactions will be dictated by developmental level and age. In a preschool child, reactions may involve bed-wetting, fear of darkness, clinginess, speech difficulties, and fear of being left alone. In a school-age child, these reactions will be more in keeping with regressive behaviors, thumb sucking, whining, clinginess, irritability or aggressiveness at home or school, school avoidance, fears, and withdrawal; a preadolescent conversely may have sleep and/or appetite disturbances, rebelliousness, refusal to do chores or homework, and loss of interest in school or peers. Adolescents will have symptoms of headaches or other physical complaints, depression, poor concentration and school performance, risk-taking behaviors, aggressiveness or irritability, indifference, and changes in personality and relationships at home or at school.

After assessing the child or adolescent, the disposition plans must be carried out with, ideally, full cooperation of the family or in conjunction with the external agencies that are involved in the care of the patient. Treatment generally will involve the active participation of the parents or guardian as well as the teachers, counselors, and other agencies. As with adults, the treatment options run the gamut from different types of therapies through medication management but also include emergency placement by child-protective services, foster care, residential treatment facilities, and even mobile crisis teams.

SUICIDE IN CHILDREN, ADOLESCENTS, AND YOUNG ADULTS

For people aged 15 to 24 years, suicide is the third leading cause of death, after accidents and homicide. Approximately 4,500 adolescent-completed suicides occur per year. In 1998, more deaths by suicide were found among this age group than those from cancer, heart disease, acquired immunodeficiency syndrome (AIDS), birth defects, stroke, pneumonia and influenza, and chronic lung disease combined. From 1980 to 1997, the rate of suicide among whites aged 15 to 19 years increased by 11% (13.6 per 100,000 for males and 3.6 per 100,000 for females), and among persons aged 10 to 14 years, by 109%. Interestingly, during the same period, the suicide rate for African-American males aged 15 to 19 years increased dramatically by 105%. Such increases may be due to greater rates of substance abuse, the increase in family instability, and greater prevalence of depressive disorders in this age group. More than 40% of overdoses are associated with anti-depressant medications, indirectly indicating the rate of these disorders in this age group.

More than 60% of the increase in the overall rate of suicide for children, adolescents, and young adults was related to the use of firearms. In 1997, nationwide, 21% of high-school students had considered attempting suicide within the past year, and 8% had attempted suicide within the past year. Although females are more likely than males to attempt suicide, males are more likely to die in their first attempt than are females: the male-to-female ratio of completed suicide is 3:1. Males will use more lethal methods, such as firearms and hanging, whereas females will resort to ingestion of toxics, jumping, and carbon monoxide poisoning.

Suicide in children and adolescents is more often related to depressive disorders.

Completed suicides are rare in those younger than 12 years, although the significant increase in the rate among children aged 10 to 14 years illustrates the need for careful assessment and public education. Several specific risk factors for this population:

- Being male
- Substance abuse
- Access to a lethal weapon
- Poor impulse control

- Recent loss
- Severe stressors
- Prior suicide attempt
- Friend or family member who has committed suicide
- Exposure to recent news story or movie about suicide
- Poor social support
- Victim of physical or sexual abuse
- Pathological family dynamics (uninvolved or uninterested parents, problems not taken seriously, overly angry or punitive parents, parents unwilling or unable to provide help or support)
- Being pregnant
- Running away.

Establishing rapport and engaging the patient after a suicide gesture is crucial. Obtaining collateral information, even (if granted permission) from friends or significant others, can help clarify the surrounding contextual framework of the gesture. A 24-hour walkthrough also can help to clarify the patient's thinking and experiences surrounding this event. The decisions to admit must to be made depending on many variables. Medical complications from an overdose or other more lethal attempt will require a pediatric-medical admission. A gesture in the context of severe psychiatric symptoms such as depression, mania, psychosis, or substance abuse, although medically clear, may require a psychiatric admission. Admission to a locked psychiatric unit is preferable when a specialized child or adolescent unit is available. Mixing adolescent with adults can at times be of concern, but ultimately must be decided depending on the services available in the community and the severity of the presentation. Minors usually are signed in by a parent if voluntarily being admitted, or involuntarily admitted by the ED physician. Customarily, voluntary admission is preferable, denoting a willingness and active participation of the parents in their child's need for admission and treatment and in anticipation of a better alliance with the future treatment team. See Algorithm 4-21.1, for admission of adolescents with suicidality.

VIOLENCE OR PHYSICALLY ASSAULTIVE BEHAVIORS

Adolescents who are brought in because of violence (about one fourth of adolescent emergency psychiatric evaluations) or become physically assaultive and combative while in the ED pose a special concern. As explained, safety becomes the number one priority for the patient and the staff. The causes for out-of-control behavior are many, both psychiatric and medical. Psychotic disorders, especially with paranoia; affective disorders with irritability; impulse-control disorders and disruptive behavioral disorders, such as oppositional-defiant disorder (ODD) or conduct disorder (CD); mental retardation; and states of intoxication or withdrawal from illicit drugs can all demonstrate out-of-control behavior. Head trauma, seizures, delirium, adverse medication reaction, metabolic or endocrine abnormalities, and toxic ingestion are additional medical causes for behavioral dyscontrol. See Table 6.1 for a list of risk factors associated with juvenile delinquent behavior. These can help in the assessment—and hopeful intervention—of an out-of-control adolescent who may be at risk for committing juvenile crimes.

Table 6-1.1. Risk factors associated with delinquent behavior

Individual	Admiration of antisocial behavior
	Early onset of delinquency
	Low intelligence, cognitive, learning, and language problems
	Poor impulse control
	Poor social skills
	Working more than 20 hours/week
Family	Conflict and hostility at home
	Criminal history
	Ineffective discipline
	Low education levels
	Physical/sexual abuse
	Poverty
	Psychiatric disorders
	Substance abuse
Peers	Association with delinquency
	Association with alcohol/drug use
	Membership in gangs
School	Falling behind same-age peers
	Poor attendance
	Poor grades/achievements
	Sense of isolation or prejudice
Community	Availability of drugs/weapons
	Frequent family moves
	Isolation from neighbors
	Living in dangerous neighborhoods
	Poor support network

Depending on their size and the degree of agitation manifested, the management—chemical or physical restraints—will be different. A large and strong adolescent may require management like that for an adult, whereas a smaller adolescent or child may require a different approach and even smaller doses of medication. Restraint or seclusion is a viable option, and psychopharmacologic management, dependent on the presumed underlying cause of the agitation, is another. Time-out in a room can be helpful to de-escalate the situation, and sometimes just approaching the patients in a calm and reassuring manner with the promise to hear their side of the story can have a calming effect. Asking the patients if they may need anything to help them calm down or feel better also can help. A quick assessment, to thwart the progression of out-of-control behavior from turning into a violent act, is truly important. At all times, keep the patient and family aware of the steps that will be taken, especially when giving medication and using restraints or seclusion.

Psychopharmacologic management in children and adolescents has not been studied as assiduously as that for adults, and many of the agents are not Food and Drug Administration (FDA) approved for use in children or adolescents. Agitation that does not respond to less restrictive measures can be treated with neuroleptics or, in some cases, with benzodiazepines. Monitor carefully for hypotension or acute dystonic reactions when using neuroleptics or oversedation with benzodiazepines.

In children aged 12 years or older:

haloperidol (Haldol), 0.5 to 2 mg, PO/IM
chlorpromazine (Thorazine), either 25 to 50 mg, PO (or 25 mg IM)
fluphenazine (Prolixin), 0.5 to 2 mg, PO/IM
lorazepam (Ativan), 0.5 to 1 mg PO/IM.

SUBSTANCE-RELATED DISORDERS

This is a serious public health issue, in that a continued increase is found in the use of substances among adolescents, a decrease in the age at first diagnosis of substance-related disorders, and the causal relation—with increased morbidity and mortality—between substances and adverse outcomes, such as motor-vehicle accidents, suicide, violence, etc. No current distinction in diagnostic criteria for substance-related disorders is made for adults and adolescents. The distinction between experimental use, casual use, and the transition to abuse is difficult. Applying DSM-IV-TR criteria to adolescents may not be clinically accurate—dependence is harder to diagnose—however, the psychiatric and social ramifications of the increase in substance use among adolescents are quite evident. High-risk factors for adolescents with substance-related disorders include:

- Aggression or impulsivity
- Alienation from parents
- Criminal justice involvement
- Experimentation before age 15 years
- Family violence
- Homelessness and runaways
- Low self-esteem
- Physical and sexual abuse
- Poor social integration
- Posttraumatic stress disorder
- Rebelliousness
- Relationship with peers who have substance-use problems
- School-performance difficulties.

A very large percentage of those adolescents with substance-abuse disorders also have a concurrent psychiatric disorder, ranging from conduct disorders and attention deficit–hyperactivity disorder to anxiety, mood, and psychotic disorders. Complete psychiatric and medical evaluations are indicated in these cases, and a high level of suspicion must be maintained (in general) with any adolescent who arrives or is brought into the ED with acute emotional, psychiatric, behavioral, or cognitive changes. Approach the adolescent with a nonjudgmental manner, making sure to ask about all types of drugs, including cigarettes, alcohol, and club drugs. Determine amount, frequency, context of use (alone or with friends), impairments, peers and their use, use at school, and outcomes of use, such as truancy; declining school performance; worsening family conflicts; loss of friends; lack of interest in hobbies, sports, or activities; risky behaviors (driving while intoxicated, unprotected and promiscuous sex). Collateral information gathering is important; adolescents tend to minimize or underreport the impact of use or even the amount of use. Certain adolescent-specific screening tools can be used, and urine toxicology and/or Breathalyzers also can be used in the assessment.

Although prevention is an important intervention strategy, in the ED, the focus is a thorough assessment and determination of an adequate disposition plan. Unless the adolescent has serious and acute psychiatric symptoms that require hospitalization, most will require specialized outpatient treatment programs. Understanding the social context of the adolescent (family) as well as the resources that are available will be crucial to developing a good disposition plan. Many communities lack adequate specialized services for adolescents with substance abuse and even fewer for those with dual diagnosis. EDs should have a resource list of programs readily available and if possible even linkage agreements with some of them to facilitate appointments or admissions. Group therapy, 12-step programs, individual therapy, psychopharmacologic management, family therapy, inpatient dual-diagnosis units, and residential treatment programs are all options that must be considered individually in each case.

BIBLIOGRAPHY

Auerswald CL, Eyre SL. Youth homelessness in San Francisco: a life cycle approach. *Soc Sci Med* 2002;54:1497–1512.

Boris NW, Heller SS, Sheperd T, et al. Partner violence among homeless young adults: measurement issues and associations. *J Adolesc Health* 2002;30:355–363.

Centers for Disease Control and Prevention. Suicide among children, adolescents, and young adults: United States, 1980–1992. *MMWR* 1995;44:289–291.

Centers for Disease Control and Prevention. Surveillance for injuries and violence among older adults. *MMWR* 1999;48(SS-8):27–34.

Centers for Disease Control and Prevention. Unpublished mortality data from the National Center for Health Statistics (NCHS) Mortality Data Tapes.

Cochran BN, Stewart AJ, Ginzler JA, et al. Challenges faced by homeless sexual minorities: comparison of gay, lesbian, bisexual, and transgender homeless adolescents with their heterosexual counterparts. *Am J Public Health* 2002;92:773–777.

De Hert M, McKenzie K, Peuskens J. Risk factors for suicide in young people suffering from schizophrenia: a long term follow-up study. *Schizophr Res* 2001;47:127–134.

Dulcan MK, Martini DR. *Concise guide to child and adolescent psychiatry.* 2nd ed. Washington, DC: American Psychiatric Press, 1999.

Dyegrov A, Mitchell JT. Work with traumatized children: psychological effects and coping strategies. *J Trauma Stress* 1992;1:5–18.

Greenhill LL, Waslick B. Management of suicidal behavior in children and adolescents. *Psychiatr Clin North Am* 1997;20:641–666.

Halamandaris PV, Anderson TR. Children and adolescents in the psychiatric emergency setting. *Psychiatr Clin North Am* 1999;22:865–874.

Kaminer Y. Addictive disorders in adolescents. *Psychiatr Clin North Am* 1999;22:275–288.

Klein JD, Woods AH, Wilson KM, et al. Homeless and runaway youths' access to health care. *J Adolesc Health* 2000;27:331–339.

Klerman GL. Clinical epidemiology of suicide. *J Clin Psych* 1987;48: 33–38.

Leon SC, Lyons JS, Uziel-Miller ND. Variations in the clinical presentations of children and adolescents at eight psychiatric hospitals. *Psychiatr Serv* 2000;51:786–790.

Leslie MB, Stein JA, Rotheram-Borus MJ. Sex-specific predictors of suicidality among runaway youth. *J Clin Child Adolesc Psychol* 2002;31:27–40.

Milner K, Katz DM. The state of child and adolescent emergency psychiatric services. *Emerg Psychiatry* 2002;8:5–9.

Moscicki EK. Identification of suicide risk factors using epidemiological studies. *Psychiatr Clin North Am* 1997;20:499–517.

Noell JW, Ochs LM. Relationship of sexual orientation to substance use, suicidal ideation, suicide attempts, and other factors in a population of homeless adolescents. *J Adolesc Health* 2001;29:31–36.

Parmlee DX. Child and adolescent psychiatry. In: Parmlee DX, ed. *Mosby's neurology psychiatry access series.* St. Louis, MO: Mosby, 1996.

Pfeffer C. Childhood suicidal behavior: a development perspective. *Psychiatr Clin North Am* 1997;20:551–562.

Pine DS, Cohen JA. Trauma in children and adolescents: risk and treatment of psychiatric sequelae. *Biol Psychiatry* 2002;51:519–531.

Quinlan PE, Berney J, Milner K. An algorithm for the reduction and management of aggression in pediatric patients in the emergency room. *Emerg Psychiatry* 2002;8:17–20.

Rohde P, Noell J, Ochs L, et al. Depression, suicidal ideation and STD-related risk in homeless older adolescents. *J Adolesc* 2001;24: 447–460.

Schetsky DH, Benedek EP, eds. *Principles and practice of child and adolescent forensic psychiatry.* Washington, DC: American Psychiatric Publishing, 2002.

Tomb D. Child psychiatry emergencies. In: Lewis M, ed. *Child and adolescent psychiatry: a comprehensive textbook.* 2nd ed. Baltimore: Williams & Wilkins, 1996:929–934.

U.S. Public Health Service. *The Surgeon General's call to action to prevent suicide.* Washington, DC: U.S. Public Health Service, 1999.

Weddle M, Kokotailo P. Adolescent substance abuse: confidentiality and consent. *Pediatr Clin North Am* 2002;49:301–315.

Wiener JM, ed. *Textbook of child and adolescent psychiatry.* 2nd ed. Washington, DC: American Academy of Child and Adolescent Psychiatry, 1997.

Chapter 6-2 Human Immunodeficiency Virus/Acquired Immunodeficiency Syndrome

As of June 2001, the cumulative number of AIDS cases reported to the Centers for Disease Control and Prevention (CDC) was 793,026; adults and adolescents make up a total of 784,032, and 8,994 AIDS cases in children younger than 13 years. Of those, 649,186 cases were in male and 134,845 cases were in female patients. Given that the overall prevalence of HIV/AIDS has increased because of a decline in AIDS deaths, patients with HIV/AIDS will continue to be seen quite often in the ED, because of either an associated medical complication, a comorbid psychiatric disorder, or HIV/AIDS-related neuropsychiatric manifestation. Many HIV/AIDS patients prefer the ED to a clinic; ethnic minorities, the poor, and those with psychiatric symptoms are known to have higher rates of ED use. These patients, especially those with chronic mental illnesses, are in a special category, in that their assessment, management, and treatment, generally similar in all respects to those of any other patients, require a bit more thought and planning.

Psychiatric disorders can often be the first manifestation of HIV infection, and many patients with HIV have psychiatric and/or drug-dependence disorders, these patients now being labeled "triply diagnosed patients." Psychiatric symptoms like anxiety or depression often can be a reaction to the realization and acceptance of an HIV diagnosis and its associated societal connotations. Psychiatric disorders also can increase the risk of acquiring HIV and also increase the morbidity of HIV-related illness because of poor adherence to treatment and high-risk behaviors. Because a neuropathologic involvement of the brain is found in 75% to 90% of autopsied brains of AIDS patients, close to 50% of patients with HIV have a diagnosed neuropsychiatric complication, and in approximately 10% of patients, these are the first indications of illness, a careful assessment and approach are important. It is essential to recognize and differentiate patients with preexisting psychiatric conditions and HIV infection from those patients with no prior psychiatric disorders and HIV infection with new-onset psychiatric symptoms. Because the prevalence of HIV illnesses has continued to grow, it is safe to assume that the co-occurrence of these illnesses also will increase steadily. The ED evaluation of any patient with new-onset symptoms is a challenge and can be a mystery that must be carefully assessed and managed. Patients with HIV/AIDS and psychiatric/substance-related disorders are still confronted with stigma and for many reasons have less access to health care.

It has been reported that 4% to 40% of HIV-infected patients meet criteria for depressive disorders; the variation in reported prevalence rates might be related to the diagnostic criteria used as well as the overlap of symptoms, which can be attributed to HIV infection *per se*. More often that not, when someone is triaged with an acute psychiatric complaint, such as suicidality, depression, auditory hallucinations, or paranoid delusions, the patient is sent to the psychiatry ED or a psychiatric consultation is called for. Regardless of their ultimate location in the ED, these patients with new-onset psychiatric symptoms must have a thorough medical evaluation.

In obtaining a history, it is important to determine the patient's HIV risk, sexual history, and HIV status. The clinician must be familiar with all of the high-risk behaviors asked about and the terminologies used, and then must use these with a nonjudgmental attitude. Asking about sexual orientation, sexual practices, drug use, and other personal information can at times be hard, but if the clinician can feel comfortable asking and conveying that to the patients, they will likely be more open to discussing these topics openly and with great relief. Inquiring about recent HIV testing is important; many patients are reluctant to be tested for HIV because of their fears, anxieties, and the stigma that is still attached to HIV/AIDS. Ask about depression, suicidality, dangerous behaviors, or even anger—common findings in patients with HIV/AIDS. A large number of women are being dually diagnosed with HIV and substance-use disorders, with HIV infection predominantly through injection-drug use, whereas many more are using drugs but not injecting. This has serious implication in terms of quality of life, health and illness status, and treatment recommendations and outcomes.

The challenge for the ED physician is to reconceptualize the order of thinking about psychiatric symptoms and place what is usually a secondary or tertiary differential diagnosis on the top. Patients with abrupt onset of psychiatric symptoms can potentially have an underlying medical condition or a medication/substance causing or exacerbating their current condition. This is especially true in patients with HIV illness and new onset of symptoms. The ability to think of medical causes as a potentially implicating factor in an acute presentation will allow the physician to provide the patient with the optimal management, care, and treatment.

Remember that, as with all other patient healthcare information, the ED is bound to ensure the confidentiality of patients with HIV; special forms are to be used for requiring a release of medical information. Universal precautions are to be followed when handling blood and bodily fluids from the patient with HIV infection, as is the case with ALL patients. Attempts should be made to obtain collateral information; contacting the patient's family, friends, significant other, physician, or social worker to increase the database and clarify medications and adherence to medications, psychiatric or medical.

Psychiatric symptoms in HIV-infected individuals are thought to have several possible underlying etiologies. Psychotic symptoms may be attributed to either a direct effect of the HIV infection on the brain or an effect of infection of the brain by other viruses or agents. Also postulated are theories of coinfection of the brain by two or more viruses, coincidental association of psychiatric symptoms with HIV infection, or the overload of major life stressors that would cause psychotic symptoms in people without HIV as well.

Abrupt-onset psychiatric symptoms can be an early symptom of an encephalopathy, and delirium should be the first diagnosis to rule out because it is common in HIV infection. Common causes include psychoactive substance–induced toxicity, neoplasms, metabolic alterations, infections, some antiretrovirals or other medications, or street drugs. Regardless of the underlying etiology, it is important to recognize and institute treatment quickly, given the associated morbidity and mortality. Causes for cognitive impairments can be HIV-associated dementia, HIV-associated minor cognitive motor disorder, or HIV-associated progressive encephalopathy. These have progressive cognitive decline, behavioral changes, and differing levels of neurologic involvement.

Complete medical workup is crucial to rule out all treatable and reversible causes of psychiatric presentations. CD4 and viral load counts can be done in the ED, although a correlation is not always found between these changes in mental status and CD4/viral load count. Complete neurologic examination, neuroimaging, lumbar punctures, Mini Mental Status Exam, and toxicology screens are all useful laboratory tests to perform in the ED.

Acute psychotic symptoms in HIV-infected or AIDS patients call for, as part of the differential diagnosis, a range of Axis I psychiatric disorders including primary psychotic disorders such as schizophrenia, mood disorders, delirium due to causes other than HIV, dementia, and substance-related disorders. The frequency or rates available in the literature on new-onset HIV-associated psychosis vary from 0.02% to 15% depending on the author, population, and methods used.

One must always keep in mind the psychological factors that affect this illness including people's adaptation/processing of their diagnosis. As with many chronic illnesses and their potential to cause, exacerbate, or affect a patient's possible psychiatric condition, HIV in particular, requires a close and collegial cooperation between ED services and the primary clinicians/workers. Programs aimed at providing on-site psychiatric evaluations and treatments or the use of in-service training of staff in the early detection and referral process to a psychiatric service, including the ED, are the best possible patient care. If the patient has not been tested, psychoeducation about the need for testing must be carried out—pretest HIV counseling, which in many hospitals is usually conducted by a specialized service or team when and where available. Disposition plans should be geared to the patient's clinical needs, whether a medical or psychiatric admission or a discharge.

General psychopharmacologic management in such patients must be done with caution, as with the geriatric and child populations. Titrate slowly and with care. Use simple dosing schedules and avoid combining medications that have similar side effects or that share metabolic pathways.

Remember: go slow and start low!

In general, benzodiazepines and/or neuroleptics must be used carefully especially when a patient is taking antiretroviral medication because there can be changes in blood levels.

Atypical neuroleptics and at lower doses are often the treatments of choice, given that the risk for neuroleptic-induced extrapyramidal side effects can be higher in patients with HIV. Benzodiazepines can worsen cognitive functioning and cause oversedation. Remember that many of the psychiatric medications used in clinical practice can have potential drug–drug interactions with a patient's antiretroviral medications.

Because significant comorbidities occur, it is crucial to coordinate the aftercare with mental health and medical providers. Providing or sharing clinical information is fundamental to keep all of the patient's providers abreast of the patient's condition. Psychoeducation will be an important part of the ED intervention, discussing the importance of addressing substance abuse or dependence, medication and/or aftercare nonadherence, high-risk sexual practices, psychiatric disorders and treatments, disclosure to family and/or partners, etc.

BIBLIOGRAPHY

New research adds support for ED at-risk testing. *Aids Alert* 2002;17(1): 7.2(abst).

Angelino AF, Treisman GJ. Management of psychiatric disorders in patients infected with human immunodeficiency virus. *Clin Infect Dis* 2001;15;33(6):847–856.

Babcock IC, Wyer PC, Gerson LW. Preventive care in the emergency department, Part II: Clinical preventive services: an emergency medicine evidence-based review; Society for Academic Emergency Medicine Public Health and Education Task Force Preventive Services Work Group. *Acad Emerg Med* 2000;7(9):1042–1054.

Bing EG, Burnam MA, Longshore D, et al. Psychiatric disorders and drug use among human immunodeficiency virus-infected adults in the United States. *Arch Gen Psychiatry* 2001;58:721–728.

Centers for Disease Control and Prevention. *Semiannual HIV/AIDS surveillance report.* Atlanta, GA: CDC, 2001.

Cohen MAA. Biopsychosocial aspects of the HIV epidemic. In: Wormser GD, ed. *AIDS and other manifestations of HIV infection.* 2nd ed. New York: Raven Press, 1992:349–371.

Cohen MAA. Psychiatric care for patients with AIDS in the long-term care setting. *Dir Psychiatry* 2001;18:365–383.

Derse AR. HIV and AIDS: legal and ethical issues in the emergency department. *Emerg Med Clin North Am* 1995;13:213–223.

Doyle ME, Labbate LA. Incidence of HIV infection among patients with new-onset psychosis. *Psychiatr Serv* 1997;48:237–238.

Gifford AL, Collins R, Timberlake D, et al. Propensity of HIV patients to seek urgent and emergent care: HIV Cost and Services Utilization Study Consortium. *J Gen Intern Med* 2000;15:8330.

McDermott BE, Sautter FJ Jr, Winstead DK. Diagnosis, health beliefs, and risk of HIV infection in psychiatric patients. *Hosp Community Psychiatry* 1994;45:580–585.

McKinnon K, Cournos F, Herman R. HIV among people with chronic mental illness. *Psychiatry Q* 2002;73:17–31.

Moser KM, Sowell RL, Phillips KD. Issues of women dually diagnosed with HIV infection and substance use problems in the Carolinas. *Issues Ment Health Nurs* 2001;22:23–49.

Otto-Salaj LL, Stevenson LY. Influence of psychiatric diagnoses and symptoms on HIV risk behavior in adults with serious mental illness. *AIDS Read* 2001;11:197–204.

Robinson MJ, Qaqish RB. Practical psychopharmacology in HIV-1 and acquired immunodeficiency syndrome. *Psychiatr Clin North Am* 2002;25:149–175.

Sewell DD. Schizophrenia and HIV. *Schizophr Bull* 1996;22:465–473.

Chapter 6-3 The Elderly

As the life expectancy in the United States continues to increase and the largest growth in the population remains among the elderly, EDs will be confronted with elderly patients with acute psychiatric presentations ever more frequently. The most commonly occurring psychiatric disorders in the elderly are depressive disorders, phobias, cognitive disorders, alcohol-related disorders, disorders secondary to medical conditions, and drug-induced disorders. Studies have shown that 15% to 20% of the elderly have depression, 20% to 40% of patients with stroke have depression, 10% to 20% of elderly have anxiety disorders, and the risks for dementias increase with age. Elderly individuals have a high risk for suicide. Several known risk factors predispose the elderly to have psychiatric disorders, including:

• Co-occurring medical conditions
• Decline in cognitive abilities
• Decline in social interactions
• Decreased autonomy
• Financial burdens
• Loss of friends and family
• Occupational loss.

In addition to all of these, many acute presentations, if adequately assessed, diagnosed, and treated, can be alleviated or even reversed. As with children and adolescents, concerned family, friends, or caretakers will bring an elderly patient to the ED. Changes in behavior, cognition, or emotional status, although normally occurring gradually in the elderly, can manifest quite abruptly and are frequent reasons for an ED visit. Abrupt onset of hallucinations, delusional thinking or paranoia, incoherent or disorganized thinking, suicidal ideation or gestures, lack of motivation, or severe social withdrawal can all be reasons for concern. These are more dramatic and frightening presentations, but more subtle changes, when monitored closely by the patient's caregiver, may prompt an ED visit. See Table 6-3.1 for a list of some

**Table 6-3.1. Common causes
for an emergency department visit**

Anhedonia
Avoidant behavior
Bouts of increased energy
Changes in appetite
Changes in sleep pattern
Confusion and disorientation
Decrease in physical activities
Deterioration in activities of daily living (ADLs)
Impulsivity
Labile moods
Medication or treatment noncompliance
Memory disturbances
Outbursts or tantrums
Personality changes
Preoccupation with death and related themes
Sexually inappropriate behavior
Social withdrawal or preferring to stay alone
Unexplained fears
Worsening of bladder/bowel incontinence

of these causes. Dementia and its behavioral manifestations, sleep disturbance, psychosis, or agitation are common presentations. Medical or medication-related disorders, causing delirium, are another common finding in these patients.

In the elderly, anxiety and depressive symptoms must be assessed carefully. In many cases, anxiety can be a recurrence or worsening of a preexisting anxiety disorder. Anxiety also is comorbid with other psychiatric and medical conditions, and all efforts should be made to evaluate and treat any underlying conditions. Cognitive–behavioral therapy and relaxation techniques as well as selective serotonin reuptake inhibitors (SSRIs) are the preferred treatment options. Depression and minor depression in the elderly carry significant risk and increased mortality because of suicide, increased disability, associated medical illnesses, and poorer quality of life. Many possible contributing factors in the elderly are found in the development of depressive symptoms, not reaching major depression proportions—more consistent with a minor depression—such as loss, bereavement, loss of independence, poorer health status, retirement, nursing home placement, diminishing social supports, and cognitive impairment. These minor depressive symptoms (fewer and less severe depressive symptoms that last 2 weeks or more) may be attributed to the coexisting psychosocial stressors, making the diagnosis easy to miss and treatment unavailable.

Geriatric patients are generally triaged in the adult ED to determine the level of medical stability before being sent to a psychiatric ED, if the primary complaint is clearly psychiatric. As we have seen, many of the acute psychiatric complaints can be caused by medical and medication-induced causes. If the patient is deemed medically unstable, he or she should remain in the general ED for evaluation, with a consult from the psychiatry team. Once medically cleared and stabilized, the patient can be admitted to a psychiatric unit if clinically indicated or be sent to the psychiatry ED for continued evaluation and management. If the patient during the course of the ED workup requires a medical admission, the psychiatrist or psychiatry team should write a consultation note with a formulation, diagnosis. and plan including plans for psychiatry follow-up during the hospital admission.

The assessment, depending on level of orientation and cognitive abilities, remains the same as that with adults. Often external sources of information are the most important to determine baseline functioning and behaviors, as compared with current presentation. Family or caregivers, primary care physicians or gerontologists, therapist, visiting nurse services, and old ED records (if available) are all important sources of collateral information for an elderly patient in the ED. The thoroughness of the medical workup in geriatric patients cannot be underestimated. The possibility of ameliorating and reversing certain causative medical conditions if they are properly diagnosed is fundamental. Crucial components are detailed current and past psychiatric, surgical, and medical histories, medication regimen, and compliance with medications. Laboratory examinations, chest radiographs (CXRs), electrocardiograms (ECGs), neuroimaging, and a complete psychiatric and neurologic evaluation along with a Mini Mental Status Exam usually are indicated. Careful attention must be paid to signs and symptoms of elder abuse or neglect (see Chapter 5.3.2).

Management in the ED, besides the diagnostic workup and evaluation, may hinge on the immediate treatment of certain symptoms, especially psychosis and agitation. A general rule is to remember that in the geriatric population, because of polypharmacy and increased sensitivity to medication effects and side effects, caution must be used with psychopharmacologic agents. **Remember: go slow and start low! Use the lowest effective dose.**

Typical and atypical neuroleptics are widely used as long as they are given in small doses. Although similar in response, atypicals have the added advantage of a more favorable side-effect profile, especially important in this population.

haloperidol (Haldol), 0.5 to 2 mg, PO/IM; monitor carefully for side effects
risperidone (Risperdal), 0.25 to 1 mg, PO (oral solution)
olanzapine (Zyprexa), 2.5 to 5 mg, PO.

Try to stay away from low-potency neuroleptics such as chlorpromazine (Thorazine) or thioridazine (Mellaril) because of the increased risk of side effects. Benzodiazepines should be used judiciously because the longer-acting benzodiazepines, like diazepam, can accumulate and cause more serious side effects, such as incoordination, confusion, rebound anxiety, or sedation. This is commonly called "sundowner syndrome."

Disposition planning in the ED typically involves making a decision to admit the patient (medical/surgical or psychiatric unit) to monitor and stabilize the immediate presentation. Psychiatric inpatient admission is reserved for those patients who have serious psychiatric symptoms, requiring increased provision of safety and management. Depression, suicidality, agitation, wandering and other unsafe and risky behaviors at home, anxiety, withdrawal and isolation, and decreased self-care are many of the reasons that would prompt a hospitalization. The determination of legal status might be a challenging situation. If the patient is cognitively intact and understands the need for hospitalization and his or her rights, a voluntary admission would suffice. Conversely, if the patient is cognitively impaired and does not have the capacity to make such a decision, an involuntary hospitalization is warranted. The more ambiguous cases pose the challenge: patients willing to be admitted and wanting to sign in voluntarily, but cognitively impaired, or the cognitively intact persons unwilling to be admitted despite apparent dangers to themselves. Family, caretakers, guardians, healthcare proxies, and powers of attorney should be checked into and involved in any of the decision making. Discharge plans from the ED should involve a carefully detailed plan for aftercare services and even the possibility of visiting medical service (if available), home attendants, determination of need for special equipment or home features (adjustable toilet seat, railings, hand-grips, etc.), or even a discussion with the family about possible placement options. Referral to senior citizen centers or other community-based support services can be quite important as well. Long-term placement seldom if ever occurs from the ED, but many patients arriving from an adult home, nursing home, or other forms of long-term care facilities, when discharged, will return to the home.

SUICIDE AND THE ELDERLY

Suicide rates increase with age and are highest in people aged 65 and older, especially elderly white men. In 1998, men accounted for 83% of the suicides among this group. The most common method of suicide, in both men and women, was with firearms. Suicide rates among the elderly are highest for those who are divorced or widowed. In 1992, the suicide rate for elderly divorced or widowed men was 2.7 times that for married men, 1.4 times that for never-married men, and more than 17 times that for married women. The rate for divorced or widowed women was 1.8 times that for married women and 1.4 times that for never-married women. Additionally, as seen in the general population, depression is manifested differently in women than in men; elderly women tend to have more appetite disturbances, whereas elderly men seem to have more associated agitation when depressed.

Risk factors for suicide among the elderly differ from those in other age groups. Elderly people have a higher prevalence of depression, have more physical illnesses, experience more social isolation, and have more cognitive impairments and sleep disruptions. The elderly make fewer attempts but use more lethal methods—more access to firearms—with higher rates of completed suicides.

BIBLIOGRAPHY

Centers for Disease Control and Prevention. Surveillance for injuries and violence among older adults. *MMWR* 1999;48(SS-8):27–34.

Conwell Y, Duberstein PR, Connor K, et al. Access to firearms and risk for suicide in middle-aged and older adults. *Am J Geriatr Psychiatry* 2002;10:407–416.

Kindermann SS, Dolder CXR, Bailey A, et al. Pharmacological treatment of psychosis and agitation in elderly patients with dementia: four decades of experience. *Drugs Ageing* 2002;19:257–276.

Kirchner V, Kelly CA, Harvey RJ. Thioridazine for dementia. *Cochrane Database Syst Rev* 2001;3:CD000464.

Kockler M, Hueun R. Gender differences of depressive symptoms in depressed and nondepressed elderly persons. *Int J Geriatr Psychiatry* 2002;17:65–72.

Laks J, Engelhardt E, Marinho V, et al. Efficacy and safety of risperidone oral solution in agitation associated with dementia in the elderly. *Arch Neuropsychiatry* 2001;59:859–864.

Lang AJ, Stein MB. Anxiety disorders: how to recognize and treat the medical symptoms of emotional illness. *Geriatrics* 2001;56:24–27, 31–34.

Lavretsky H, Kumar A. Clinically significant non-major depression: old concepts, new insights. *Am J Geriatr Psychiatry* 2002;10:239–255.

Madhusoodannan S, Sinha S, Brenner R, et al. Use of olanzapine for elderly patients with psychotic disorders: a review. *Ann Clin Psychiatry* 2001;13:201–213.

Neugroschl J. Agitation: how to manage behavior disturbances in the older patient with dementia. *Geriatrics* 2002;54:33–37.

Oxman TE, Sengupta A. Treatment of minor depression. *Am J Geriatr Psychiatry* 2002;10:256–264.

Parnetti L, Amici S, Lanari A, et al. Pharmacological treatment of non-cognitive disturbances in dementia disorders. *Mech Ageing Dev* 2001;122:2063–2069.

Turvey CL, Conwell Y, Jones MP, et al. Risk factors for late-life suicide: a prospective, community-based study. *Am J Geriatr Psychiatry* 2002;10:398–406.

Chpater 6-4 Mental Retardation and Developmental Disabilities

Patients with mental retardation (MR) or other developmental disabilities are often seen in the ED, usually accompanied by a parent, guardian, or other primary caretaker. Those with MR are a heterogeneous group of patients, arbitrarily defined by functional levels, with significant social stigma and popular misconceptions. Patients with MR must have below-average intellectual functioning, determined by standardized testing and with onset before age 18 years. Common differential diagnoses for MR are

- Learning disorders
- Communications disorders
- Pervasive developmental disorders
- Dementias.

Estimates range from 10% to 70% that patients with MR have an Axis I disorder. Patients with MR can exhibit the full range of psychiatric disorders and are at higher risk for certain disorders, such as posttraumatic stress disorder, oppositional defiant disorder, depression, anxiety, or Alzheimer disease—especially true for patients with Down syndrome. These patients often do not fall neatly into the DSM-IV criteria, making difficult the diagnosis of a comorbid psychiatric disturbance. Often abnormal behaviors are thought to be the by-product of the MR rather than a possible psychiatric condition meriting investigation and treatment; this is known as diagnostic overshadowing. Many times a psychiatrist will have to infer the symptoms based on the behaviors or changes in behaviors noted by family or caretakers. As with children and adolescents, the symptoms may not conform to the DSM standards, but they may be *equivalent* for a given disease state. Examples of these inferences or equivalents are loss of happy mood or humor, tearfulness, irritability, and somatic complaints for the more standard DSM depressed episode criteria. Comments such as "No one likes me," or "I can't do this right" may be considered equivalent to feelings of worthlessness. Classic neurovegetative symptoms may look like refusal to eat, to go to bed, or to get up in the morning. Deliberate dangerous acts or lack of response to an attack or other aggressive confrontation can be considered suicidality for that patient. Excess silliness and laughing, loudness in speech, hyperactivity, and difficulty being redirected may all be signs of mania or hypomania in patients with MR. Research has demonstrated that patients with MR, even severe to profound, can exhibit the full range of positive symptoms of schizophrenia, including hallucinations, delusions, and disorganization. Catatonia, sleep problems and nightmares, mutism, flat affect, social withdrawal, anxiety, somatic complaints, psychomotor agitation, echolalia, hypersexuality, aggressiveness, and self-injurious behaviors may all be symptom equivalents of schizophrenia. Unfortunately, many physicians, because of lack of experience and expertise in this area, faced with a nonverbal patient who has some degree of MR, find it hard to diagnose a primary psychiatric condition.

Most ED visits are secondary to exacerbation of underlying psychiatric or medical conditions, usually accompanied by the parent, guardian, or caretaker. Depending on the severity of the MR and ability to communicate (see Table 6-4.1 for levels of severity), agitation or excitement can be a manifestation of psychosis, depression, anxiety, or even a urinary tract infection (UTI) or medication side effect. Hardly ever will the diagnosis of MR be made primarily in an ED setting, but certainly the management of the behavioral or emotional acute manifestations will be commonplace. These behaviors must be understood from the perspective that through them, the patient may be receiving more attention, or avoiding a negative outcome, or either increasing or decreasing internal stimulation, or it may be a way of communicating needs. In the assessment process, collateral sources of data are fundamental. A detailed family and personal developmental history are needed, as well as a current understanding of the patient's functioning and *ANY* change in behavior, interests, mood, or activities. Inquire about the home or agency environment: have there been changes, stressor, or problems; fear from abuse can be manifested as agitation and other disruptive behaviors. Patients with MR are very sensitive to changes and may be reacting to

Table 6-4.1.   Mental retardation severity

Mild mental retardation	IQ level, 50–55 to 70
	Mental age (MA), 9–12 yr
Social and vocational skills for minimal self-support, although may require assistance when under stress	
Moderate mental retardation	IQ level, 35–40 to 50–55
	MA, 6–9 yr
Needs more structured and sheltered conditions and can achieve a 2nd-grade academic level	
Severe mental retardation	IQ level, 20–25 to 35–40
	MA, 3–6 yr
Poor motor/language development, requires full supervision and very little autonomous self-care.	
Profound mental retardation	IQ level, <20 or 25
	MA, less than 3 yr
Needs constant supervision, aid, and skilled nursing care	
Severity unspecified	
Strong presumption of mental retardation, but the person's intelligence is untestable by standard tests	

stressors, especially changes in caregivers from burnout. Modeling of behavior also is something to inquire about: have other peers been recently behaving similarly? When interviewing the patients, make sure they understand what you are asking; keep it simple; and avoid open-ended questions. Ask them what they mean if they are using idiosyncratic words or phrases, and do not steer the patient or "fish" for the answer you want to hear. Beware of "yesing." Patients will have more exaggerated affect and more posturing and child-like behaviors; under stress, stereotypes may become more pronounced or apparent. Patients' thoughts may be more concrete and literal; be cautious about diagnosing psychosis, because patients with MR may have more magical thinking, misreport sensory perceptions as hallucinations, and confusion under stress may appear to be a thought disorder. Complete workup should include medical and neurologic examinations as well as basic laboratories values and urine/serum toxicologic values, if clinically warranted. Many patients with MR have comorbid seizures and other motor and sensory disorders.

Treatment is focused on determining the cause of the disruptive behavior or symptom profile and treating accordingly. Psychotropic medication in patients with MR may have paradoxic and idiosyncratic effects. For aggression, most studies have shown that neuroleptics, such as thioridazine, risperidone, fluphenazine, or haloperidol, can be effective. Additionally, some studies have found that lithium·and propranolol are useful. Self-injurious behaviors require immediate control and protection; restraints may be used until psychopharmacologic agents become effective. Mittens, helmets, and other devices may be needed at times to ensure protection. These behaviors in the ED can respond well to typical or atypical antipsychotics, such as those mentioned earlier, and also clozapine or chlorpromazine. Other agents reported to be effective and to be used judiciously are benzodiazepines, naltrexone, clonidine, and anticonvulsants such as valproate, topiramate, and gabapentin.

Severity of symptomatic presentation and other related variables will decide the dispositions. Many times, agencies and parents/caretakers may seek hospitalization for the disruptive behavior and also for a respite for themselves. Caregiver burnout is a major problem and should be factored into the decision-making process. Inpatient psychiatric hospitalization is not without its difficulties; many times inpatient staff are not prepared or experienced in dealing with patients with MR. One-on-one observation is often required with these patients; many hospitals have arrangements with the patient's agencies to have their staff provide the needed one-on-one observation while the patient is hospitalized. These patients require significant staff time and energy and can be a drain on inpatient resources. Otherwise you must discharge the patient back to the home or the agency, with appropriate psychiatric follow-up as soon as possible. A note or a call to the treating psychiatrist can assist in the continuity of care. Other community-based treatment options include habilitation programs, day-treatment programs, employment or vocational services, residences, respite care for the caregiver (in-home, out-of-home, overnight), crisis teams, visiting nurse or medical services, home aides or attendants, etc.

BIBLIOGRAPHY

Borthwick-Duffy SA. Epidemiology and prevalence of psychopathology in people with mental retardation. *J Consult Clin Psychol* 1994;62:17–27.

Cherry KE, Penn D, Matson JL, et al. Characteristics of schizophrenia among persons with severe or profound mental retardation. *Psychiatr Serv* 2000;51:922–924.

Parmlee DX. Child and adolescent psychiatry. In: Parmlee DX, ed. *Mosby's neurology psychiatry access series.* St. Louis, MO: Mosby, 1996.

Reid AH. Schizophrenia in mental retardation: clinical features. *Res Dev Disabil* 1989;10:241–249.

Turner TH. Schizophrenia and mental handicap: an historical review, with implications for further research. *Psychol Med* 1989;19:301–314.

Wiener JM, ed. *Textbook of child and adolescent psychiatry.* 2nd ed. Washington, DC: American Academy of Child and Adolescent Psychiatry, 1997.

Legal/Forensic Issues

CONFIDENTIALITY

In general, confidentiality is a given when it comes to the patient–doctor relationship. Confidentially, as stipulated by Hippocrates onward, is a basic tenet of the relationship between a doctor and a patient. The American Medical Association (AMA), American Psychiatric Association (APA), and the American Academy of Psychiatry and the Law (AAPL) have specific codes of ethics regarding confidentiality. It is understood that a clinician will keep private all of the information shared in a clinical setting and will not divulge any of it unless permitted by the patient. This is an ethical obligation, with many far-reaching and complex legal ramifications. Additionally, it is a patient's privilege that bars a physician from testifying about the clinical information in a judicial or quasi-judicial setting, unless the patient relinquishes this privilege or the courts override it. The ultimate inclusion of this information as evidence is a decision made by a judge. Remember: the patient owns the privilege, not the physician.

In an acute care setting, issues about physician–patient privilege are commonplace and quite confusing. A general rule is that if the information is made within the patient–physician relationship, during the course of treatment, and the information gathered was necessary for treatment, the communication is confidential unless it falls into an exception category. The exceptions to these provisions include the mandatory reporting of child abuse (see Chapter 5-3.1), reporting of infectious diseases as part of public health policy, court-ordered examinations, and in cases in which a patient makes the psychiatric history an issue, called the patient litigant exception. Other exceptions to confidentiality include most forensic examinations—it is understood *a priori* that there is no doctor–patient relationship—and the presence of dual agencies, such as prisons, schools, military settings, or a company psychiatrist. Additionally, certain emergencies and the duty to warn and protect others against a potentially violent patient are other instances of exceptions to confidentiality.

Common exceptions to confidentiality:

- Child abuse
- Competency proceedings
- Court-ordered examination
- Danger to self/others
- Patient-litigant exception
- Intent to commit a crime or harmful act
- Civil commitment proceedings
- Communication with other treatment providers.

The duty to warn and protect third parties from violence or homicidal acts is a complex yet legal obligation of the clinician to take any reasonable measures to protect others from foreseeable harm. Starting with *Tarasoff v Regents of University of California* and the subsequent Tarasoff cases of the 1970s, a legal duty-to-protect standard was established.

What is now known as the Tarasoff principle states:

When a psychotherapist determines, or pursuant to the standards of his profession should determine, that his patient presents a serious danger of violence to another, he incurs an obligation to use reasonable care to protect the intended victim against such danger. The discharge of this duty may require the therapist to take one or more of various steps, depending upon the nature of the case. Thus, it may call for him to warn the intended victim or others likely to apprize the victim of the danger, to notify the police, or to take whatever steps are reasonably necessary under the circumstances.

The breach of patient confidentiality implicit in this principle places the public's safety above the patient's confidentiality. The key elements of Tarasoff are the "duty to protect" and the use of "reasonable standards of profession." The standard of care speaks to the assessment of dangerousness not the prediction of violence.

Further, to complicate matters, in 1991 in Florida, the District Court of Appeals ruled in *Boynton v Burglass* that a psychiatrist did not have the duty to protect, claiming it was "neither reasonable . . . and is potentially fatal to the effective patient-therapist relationship." Unfortunately, no single legal duty exists in all states, making it very important for all physicians to understand the ethical codes, practice standards, and moral underpinnings involved with protecting third parties while protecting a patient's confidentiality in the place where they practice. However, increasingly many states have adopted Tarasoff-like principles in either statutes or case law.

When confronted in the ED with a potentially homicidal patient (see Chapter 4-12), it is imperative that you assess their dangerousness carefully.

- Is the patient a real and serious danger to someone else?
- Have there been recent acts of violence or aggression?
- Has the patient made serious threats of harm?
- How likely is the patient to commit an act of harm?
- Is there a psychiatric disorder?

Remember that the potential for violence, like suicide or safety considerations, is fluid and can fluctuate and change quite rapidly. It requires a thorough understanding of the patient's current condition, historical risk factors, available social supports, and appropriate disposition options. One of the hardest assessments for an ED clinician to make regards the degree of a patient's dangerousness and the appropriateness of admitting to the hospital or discharging and notifying the identified victim and/or police. Often clinicians are uncomfortable with assessing violent patients, and most are unsure of the legal, ethical, and risk-management issues involved. Determination of specific ("I'm gonna kill my girlfriend") versus generalized ("I'm gonna kill the first person I see outside") risks is difficult. Determination of the "imminent" nature of the danger also is a complex concept about which many clinicians are unclear. How soon is imminent: very, very soon or "on the point of happening"? As set forth in the ethical codes of the APA, the American Psychological Association, the Canadian Psychiatric Association, and the Declaration of Madrid of the World Psychiatric Association, the danger does not need to be imminent to breach confidentiality. The standard dictates that there be a substantial risk of harm to another person if no intervention is made.

In most ED settings, hospitalization solves many of these dilemmas, affording protection and maintaining confidentiality. The issue that comes up at that juncture is whether to hospitalize the patient voluntarily or involuntarily. Another dilemma that can arise is the need to transfer if no locked psychiatric units are available. This must be done with utmost care and making sure that all the necessary precautions are taken to ensure the safe transportation of the patient. If the risk is not deemed to be imminent or the threat serious enough to warrant hospitalization, several outpatient interventions can be used before resorting to more restrictive measures. These include:

- Enforced medication compliance
- Increased frequency of outpatient visits
- Involvement of family or friends
- Medication adjustment or change
- Removal of weapons
- Addressed substance-use disorders.

If the need arises to disclose the patient's threats to the police or the victim, it is important that this be explained to the patient. In any of these complicated situations, it is crucial that the clinician be familiar with the local commitment laws, confidentiality statutes, protective disclosures statutes, reporting responsibilities, the Tarasoff principle and how it applies in the jurisdiction, and ethical position statements.

INFORMED CONSENT

Over the years, the notion of medical paternalism was modified significantly to respect the patient's autonomy—this was ultimately achieved through informed consent. The idea and the importance of informed consent dates to the late 1950s, and now it is established dogma, both legally and medically, that a patient must give informed consent to receive or refuse any medical treatment. If a patient does not give consent, even life-saving treatment must be withheld. The caveat is that for a patient to give informed consent, he or she must be:

- Competent or at least deemed to have decision-making capacity
- Have the needed information
- Be free from coercion.

Recent research has raised practical problems about obtaining informed consent. Many patients, because of emotional, cultural, cognitive, spiritual, or medical problems either have difficulty understanding clinical information or do not wish to participate in making decisions about their treatment. Another confounding factor in this clinical dilemma is the apparent lack of adequate communication skills among clinicians and culturally sensitive and linguistically adequate, effective educational materials for patients.

It is extremely important that a patient's decision-making capacity be determined with the greatest possible degree of sensitivity and specificity, although the clinical reality is quite different. Patients are deemed incompetent on a daily basis in courts of law, losing their autonomy, and the standards of competence, incompetence, and informed consent are blurry to even the most seasoned physician. To give informed consent, a patient must have adequate information, capacity to decide, and absence of coercion.

The standard for the amount of information required before being able to make an informed consent is now considered the information that a "reasonable person" would want to know before having to make a decision. The information should entail:

- Description of the patient's diagnosis
- The nature of the patient's illness and the proposed treatment
- The potential benefits of the proposed treatment
- The potential risks of the proposed treatment
- Alternative treatment options, including no treatment
- Prognosis with or without proposed treatment

In 1997 the American Psychiatric Association determined that under four circumstances, a physician could treat a patient without first obtaining his or her informed consent.

1. Incompetence of the patient, in which case, the physician has to seek consent from the patient's guardian or other decision maker.
2. An emergency situation in which serious risk to self or others is at stake, without consent, if the treatment given represents the standard of emergency care.
3. Competent patients who voluntarily determine that the physician should make the medical decision for them, known as therapeutic waivers. These must be carefully documented, and the patient must still be informed of the right to participate and make the decision.
4. Therapeutic privilege allows a physician to withhold information from a patient if that information would constitute a threat to the patient's health or would impair the ability to be effective decision makers. This privilege must be carefully thought out clinically and ethically, as well as clearly documented, and cannot be used to withhold information simply because it might make the patient less likely to accept a proposed treatment.

Exceptions to informed consent:

- Emergencies
- Incompetence determination
- Therapeutic privilege
- Therapeutic waiver

COMPETENCE

Competence is considered the capacity to understand and make decisions about particular issues, in our setting, particularly about medical issues. Everyone is deemed to have competence to make decisions for himself or herself unless proven otherwise by judicial determination.

Competence requires that the individual:

- Understand relevant information about the specific task or issue
- Communicate a choice regarding the situation in question
- Appreciate the relevance of the situation and its consequences
- Manipulate the information provided rationally
- Make a decision based on established higher-order values, which are consistent with life-long beliefs and desires.

Competence is task specific; a person may have the competence to make a decision regarding one task but lack competence for another.

The determination of lack of competence is usually called into question when a person is trying to make a "wrong" decision about a proposed treatment. It seldom is called into question that a person making a "right" decision might not be competent to be making that decision. Both legal and ethical considerations dictate that competence or capacity is just as relevant when a patient agrees with treatment recommendations as when he or she disagrees. Currently there is a sense that determination of competency has different thresholds and can change depending on the context, the treatment proposed, or the risks. The President's Commission for the Study of Ethical Problems in Medicine and Biomedical and Behavioral Research recommended that the level of competence to make medical decisions be linked to the risk involved in the proposed treatment.

The determination of incompetence is a judicial one, and a patient must have due process, right to a notice of a hearing, a hearing, and, preferably access to legal counsel. The legal counsel usually acts as the patient's guardian. Patients in the ED with obvious lack of competence will have decision made by either an appointed decision maker or a guardian. Family and friends should be called to determine if there is a guardian or if there are advanced directives. Advanced directives are made by a competent individual who directs and/or authorizes certain actions or treatments in the event that he or she becomes incapacitated or unable to make decision.

RIGHT TO TREATMENT AND THE RIGHT TO REFUSE TREATMENT

In the last 30 years or so, the age-old notion that mentally ill patients, especially those hospitalized—voluntarily or even involuntarily—lacked the capacity to make decision about the treatment, has changed dramatically due to litigation and changing social notions. As the concept that mentally ill patients have the right to treatment has taken hold, conversely, it has been argued that these patients also have the right to refuse treatment. Despite the lack of a national or constitutionally based right to treatment, several legally determined outcomes, via judicial imposition, malpractice suits, or legislative bills of right have helped define a patient's right to treatment. The right of patients to refuse treatment is an offshoot of the concept of the right to treatment. A patient has the right:

- To the least restrictive conditions
- To not be exposed to unnecessary and excessive medications
- To not be subjected to experimental research without informed consent.

A patient is thought to have the right to refuse treatment as accorded under the Constitution (Amendments I, V, VIII, and XIV), as well as under other models and legal concepts. The ongoing debate about a patient's right to refuse treatment is largely limited to nonemergency situations, voluntarily or involuntarily hospitalized patients, and treatment refusal. Treatment refusal is an unfortunate but common occurrence in clinical practice. Whatever the reason, it is a source of concern, affects treatment outcomes and prognosis, and can affect morbidity and mortality in some cases. Nonadherence is a major dilemma for practitioners, with some estimates at more than 50% nonadherence with psychopharmacologic agents. This is especially true and concerning for patients with chronic illnesses, psychiatric or otherwise, and in light of the increasing number of medications that are shown to be efficacious when taken as prescribed.

Nonadherence can be directly related to the patient–doctor relationship or can be owing to concerns about the treatment itself and adverse consequences. Nonadherence can be related to the stigma attached to certain illnesses or needing to take medications—this is especially true for psychiatric disorders and the medication used to treat these disorders; denial of illness is a major component in many of these cases. Occasionally treatment refusal or noncompliance occurs because of religious beliefs. Harder to determine is treatment refusal for secondary gain, as in patients seeking financial or legal gains from being ill.

In an ED setting, the outcomes of medication or treatment noncompliance can be quite visible. It is commonly understood and accepted that an exception occurs to requiring informed consent before instituting treatment. Many patients will have exacerbation of their underlying psychiatric disorder—manic, depressed, psychotic, anxious—because of medication noncompliance. In these types of presentations, noncompliance as an issue will be addressed in the ED. It has been deemed acceptable for physicians in EDs to provide standard treatment despite treatment refusal intervention to patients to prevent or minimize harm to the patient or others. The decision to treat a patient over his or her objection in an emergency setting is permissible, although the legal definition of an emergency is still rather unclear. It is a difficult task in an emergency setting to perform a thorough exploration to determine a patient's competence and possible reasons for treatment refusal. Despite the lack of clear and concise rules, it is important that the practitioner base the decision on strong clinical knowledge and a practical case-by-case understanding of the patient's situation.

Patients with mental disorders can pose specific consent difficulties, depending on whether the proposed treatment is directly related to the mental disorder. Problems also may arise from adult patients who refuse treatment because of undue influence from others. Obtaining consent for treatment of children depends on their age, maturity, and understanding. Specific difficulties may arise if the child's wishes conflict with those with parental consent, or when those with parental responsibility unreasonably refuse to give consent.

In settings such as the ED, making competence decisions can be quite difficult. The determination of a patient's decision-making capacity, an indirect and nonjudicial assessment of competence, is an essential component of securing voluntary informed consent for either treatment or refusal of care. Decision-making capacity should be determined on some level during each patient encounter and requires that a patient be able to

- Receive, process, and understand information
- Weigh the risks and benefits
- Make choices consistent with his or her values and life-long expressed wishes
- Communicate those preferences.

For patients and in situations in which this may be questionable, a thorough assessment of the decision-making capacity is expected as long as it does not delay needed urgent care or place the patient at risk. Always inquire about alternatives decision-making persons for the patient, such as a surrogate, a consultant, or another clinician—usually psychiatrists—who can assist in making a reasonable clinical decision.

A key consideration is the need to document carefully, especially

- The patient's condition
- Reasons provided for refusal
- Staff interventions at alternative and least-restrictive measures used
- Involvement of family or others
- Risks and benefits as well as alternatives to treatment discussed with patient.

Remember that you must document as much as possible, always with an eye on medicolegal implications of the decisions you make, explaining your decision-making process as you go along.

RELEASE-OF-INFORMATION STANDARDS

In August 1996, the Health Insurance Portability and Accountability Act (HIPAA) was signed into law, establishing national standards for healthcare transactions, as determined by the Department of Health and Human Services (DHHS). One of its major goals was to simplify and standardize common electronic transactions in the healthcare industry as well as protect the security and privacy of patient's health information. These standards apply to all healthcare providers and institutions, so it is important that you be familiar with your institution's internal HIPAA-compliant policies.

Confidential patient information normally includes all clinical and psychosocial information gathered during the diagnostic/therapeutic process, all financial information related to a patient's or employee's personal financial status, credit or insurance information, and any information, including the treatment, regarding a patient receiving psychiatric or substance abuse–related treatment.

Usually all medical records, radiology films, and pathology slides are considered confidential records and must be maintained in a secure environment, being kept for the benefit of the patient but the legal property of the hospital. These originals cannot be taken off-site, and authorization of the patient, surrogate, or legal guardian is required for release of copies off-site except to comply with a regulation; in response to a subpoena; or to allow continued patient care, for example, in the event of a direct transfer.

According to HIPAA, you may not disclose or use any protected health information (written, oral, or electronic) except when permitted or required uses and disclosures exist. These required disclosures include

- The individual who is the subject of the information. That person has a right to inspect and obtain copies of his or her records, which includes medical, billing, financial records, and other records used, on request. The patient is not entitled to psychotherapy notes, information compiled in anticipation of litigation, and certain protected laboratory information. The institution may deny a request if it may endanger the life or physical safety of the individual or others or cause substantial harm.
- The DHHS on request, if it is conducting an investigation or compliance review.

Certain permitted uses and disclosures of information for treatment, payment, or other health-related functions (quality assurance, physician reviews, planning and development, customer service, etc.) require a patient's consent. A consent must be in plain language and spell out what information will be used and allow restrictions, and be signed and dated, becoming part of the patient's medical records. Once again, the exception to this is emergency-treatment situations, provided that the physician has made all efforts to obtain consent as soon as reasonably possible after the delivery of treatment. Other exceptions include

- Treatments required by law
- Barriers to communication because of which a provider will have to make a professional decision and infer consent to treatment from the circumstance if no translator is available
- Indirect providers, such as a radiologist or pathologist who are providing service or reports directly to the ordering physician
- Public health reasons
- Health oversight by public agency
- Certain legal proceedings in which the medical information is an issue
- Law-enforcement or military purposes.

Whenever information about a patient is requested from another institution, a release of information should be obtained from the patient and faxed to the requesting institution. The general rule of thumb is that the information to be provided be the "minimum necessary" to accomplish the intended purpose of the use, disclosure, or request. The patient must sign the form after understanding what the procedure is for obtaining or releasing the personal requested information. Many institutions have separate release-of-information forms for general medical information, psychiatric and substance abuse–related information, and authorization of release of HIV-related material. The electronic transmission of confidential patient information, whether internally or externally, will be governed by tight security standards, as determined by HIPAA. Each institution will have a distinct policy and procedure for electronic transmission, with which you should be familiar.

LEGAL STATUS

Once a disposition has been reached that a patient seen in the ED requires an inpatient psychiatric hospitalization, determination of the admission legal status is the next order of business. Because most psychiatric inpatient facilities are locked units and are governed by the local or state mental hygiene laws and regulations, the patient's legal status of admission is important. It is imperative that every clinician be familiar with the local or state mental hygiene laws regarding admission of psychiatric patients. The types of admissions are either involuntary or voluntary admissions.

Voluntary Psychiatric Hospitalizations

Some units have an informal process of admission, in which a patient will voluntarily sign into the hospital and leave without any notice, commonly seen in certain general hospital psychiatric units and detoxification units.

Other facilities require a more formal voluntary admission. To be eligible for a voluntary psychiatric admission, a patient must have a mental illness for which care and treatment in a mental hospital is appropriate. The person must be suitable for admission on a voluntary basis and have the capacity to understand his or her status and rights as a voluntary patient. If the patient is unable to demonstrate a working understanding of the rights as a voluntary patient, he or she should not be signed in under this status. These rights, for example, may include that the patient must notify the staff in writing of a request to leave the hospital.

In 1990, *Zinermon v Burch,* the court found that voluntary hospitalization requires "express and informed consent" and stated that either following through was necessary with existing state procedures, or each state must develop appropriate safeguards in the admission process to determine if the patient's consent was provided in the admission process. A general consensus exists that all patients, even those who meet criteria for involuntary hospitalization, should be offered the possibility of a voluntary admission to demonstrate a more active participation in the treatment process. The American Psychiatric Association has made recommendations about patients who are not competent to sign themselves into a psychiatric hospital but do not meet criteria for involuntary hospitalization; these patients or "assenters" are considered impaired and warranting a hospitalization but requiring heightened review and monitoring during their hospitalization.

Certain jurisdictions have additional voluntary admission statuses, such as temporary or emergency holds, which have different criteria and procedural aspects for admission.

Involuntary Psychiatric Hospitalization

Involuntary commitment of psychiatric patients is an extremely controversial and legally fraught concept with many social misconceptions and debates. A clinician's ability in an ED to predict dangerousness or potential for violence in patients is notoriously low and inaccurate. Notwithstanding this, courts have upheld the use of commitment by psychiatrists as a way of dealing with this issue.

The involuntary commitment of a psychiatric patient currently rests on two legal principles: *parens patriae,* or the state's responsibility to care for the individuals who cannot care for themselves; and *police powers,* the state's responsibility to protect its people and society at large from dangerous (psychiatric) patients.

A general rule of thumb is always to attempt the least restrictive treatment alternative and afterward to be conservative when it comes to involuntary hospitalization. In cases in which it is hard to determine whether involuntary commitment is required, the admission usually provides a safe environment and allows a more thorough clinical assessment. Additionally, because these types of admissions are through an ED or emergency setting, many emergency situations require a decisive and safe action, so involuntary commitment becomes a viable choice.

The APA model commitment law set some clinical standards about involuntary commitment. Most jurisdictions since then have incorporated parts of it into their mental hygiene law. Often these local laws, as in the case of New York State Mental Hygiene Laws, require that one or more physicians determine that:

- The patient has a severe mental illness
- It is the least restrictive treatment alternative, and appropriate care and treatment will reasonably improve the patient's condition
- Because of the mental condition, the patient poses a substantial threat to self or others
- The patient has impaired judgment or lacks capacity to understand the need for such care and treatment
- The patient is unable to survive safely in the community
- The hospitalization will reasonably improve the patient's condition or at least prevent deterioration

Substantial threat of harm or the likelihood of serious harm, depending on the wording of the law, can include:

- Substantial risk of physical harm to the person, as manifested by threats of or attempts at suicide or serious bodily harm
- Substantial risk of physical harm to other persons, as manifested by homicidal or other violent behavior by which others are placed in reasonable fear of serious physical harm
- A person's refusal or inability to meet the essential need for food, shelter, clothing, or health care, provided that such refusal or inability is likely to result in serious harm if the person is not hospitalized immediately
- A person's history of dangerous conduct associated with noncompliance with mental health treatment programs

The physicians normally will have to document that they have considered less restrictive and alternative forms of care and treatment that are deemed inadequate to provide for the needs of the patient. All patients being admitted to a hospital for the mentally ill as involuntary patients are entitled to certain rights, provided in a written notice, usually including the right to appeal the decision for involuntary care and treatment and the ability to request a court hearing and representation by a lawyer.

A recent Supreme Court case, *Addington v Texas,* set the standard of proof for the determination of a patient's dangerousness as clear and convincing evidence (in other words, about 75% certainty), compared with preponderance of the evidence (51%) and beyond a reasonable doubt (95%).

BIBLIOGRAPHY

Addington v Texas, 99 SCt 1804 (1979).

American Psychiatric Association. Resource document on principles of informed consent in psychiatry. *J Am Acad Psychiatry Law* 1997;25: 121–125.

American Psychiatric Association. *Task Force Report 34: consent to voluntary hospitalization.* Washington, DC: American Psychiatric Association, 1992.

American Psychiatric Association. *Diagnostic and statistical manual of mental disorders.* 4th ed, revised. Washington, DC: American Psychiatric Association, 1999.

Appelbaum P, Gutheil T. *Clinical handbook of psychiatry and the law.* 2nd ed. Baltimore: Williams & Wilkins, 1991.

Bernat JL. Informed consent. *Muscle Nerve* 2001;24:614–621.

Black's Law Dictionary. 4th ed, rev. St. Paul, MN: West Publishing, 1968.

Burglass BV. 590 502d 446 (Fla App 3 Dist (1991)).

Cramer J, Rosenheck R. Compliance with medication regimens for mental and physical disorder. *Psychiatr Serv* 1998;49:196–201.

Doyal L. Informed consent: moral necessity or illusion? *Qual Health Care* 2001;10(suppl 1):29–33.

Ethical principles of psychologists and code of conduct (Section 5.05 Disclosures). *Am Psychol* 1992;47:1597–1611.

Felthous AR. The clinician's duty to protect third parties. *Psych Clin North Am* 1999;22:49–59.

Gutheil TG, Appelbaum PS. *Clinical handbook of psychiatry and law.* 3rd ed. Baltimore: Lippincott Williams & Wilkins, 2000.

Kaplan HI, Sadock BJ, eds. *Comprehensive textbook of psychiatry.* 8th ed. Baltimore: Williams & Wilkins, 1999.

Larkin GL, Marco CA, Abbott JT. Emergency determination of decision-making capacity: balancing autonomy and beneficence in the emergency department. *Acad Emerg Med* 2001;8:282–284.

Leung WC. Consent to treatment in the A&E department. *Accid Emerg Nurs* 2002;10:17–25.

Markson LJ, Kern DC, Annas GJ, et al. Physician assessment of patient competence. *J Am Geriatr Soc* 1994;42:1074–1080.

Naess AC, Foerde R, Steen PA. Patient autonomy in emergency medicine. *Med Health Care Philos* 2001;4:71–77.

NYS Mental Hygiene Law. MHL Article 9—Hospitalization of Mentally Ill. McKinney's Consolidated Laws of New York Annotated, West Publishing Co.

President's Commission for the Study of Ethical Problems in Medicine and Biomedical and Behavioral Research. *Making healthcare decisions: the ethical and legal implications of informed consent in the patient-practitioner relationship.* Vol. 1. Washington, DC: Superintendent of Documents, 1982.

Roth LH, Meisel A, Lidz CW. Test of competency to consent to treatment. *Am J Psych* 1977;134:279–284.

Rundell JR, Wise MG, eds. *Textbook of consultation-liaison psychiatry.* Washington, DC: American Psychiatric Press, 1996.

Schwartz HI. Informed consent and competency. In: Rosner R, ed. *Principles and practice of forensic psychiatry.* New York: Chapman & Hall, 1994.

Simon RI. *Concise guide to psychiatry and law for clinicians.* Washington, DC: American Psychiatric Press, 1992.

Tarasoff v Regents of University of California, 17 Cal3d 425 (1976).

The Canadian Medical Association Code of Ethics annotated for psychiatrists: the position of the Canadian Psychiatric Association (1978). *Can J Psychiatry* 1980;25:432–438.

The Declaration of Madrid (approved by the World Psychiatric Association General Assembly in Madrid, Spain, 25 August, 1996). http://www.wpanet.org/generalinfo/ethic1.html.

Opinions of the Ethics Committee on the principles of medical ethics: with annotations especially applicable to psychiatry. Washington, DC: American Psychiatric Association, 2001.

Vermeire E, Hearnshaw H, Van Royen P, et al. Patient adherence to treatment: three decades of research: a comprehensive review. *J Clin Pharm Ther* 2001;26:331–342.

Weiner B, Wettstein R. *Legal issues in mental health care.* New York: Plenum, 1993.

Welie JV, Welie SP. Patient decision making competence: outlines of a conceptual analysis. *Med Health Care Philos* 2001;4:127–138.

Wettstein RM. The right to refuse psychiatric treatment. *Psych Clin North Am* 1999;22:173–182.

Wyatt v Stickney, 344 F Supp 373 (1972).

Zinermon v Burch, 494 US 113 (1990).

Appendix A

General Assessment Guidelines

Patients can present with or manifest acute psychiatric symptomatology with a wide variety of signs and symptoms; I have taken the most common types of acute psychiatric symptoms and divided them into four presentation categories for easier classification and understanding: psychotic, behavioral, emotional, and cognitive.

See Table A.1.

- **Psychotic presentations** are all those patients with complaints of illusions, hallucinations (auditory, gustatory, olfactory, tactile, visual), and delusions (erotomanic, grandiose, jealous, persecutory, somatic, mixed).
- **Behavioral presentations** are all those patients with suicidal or homicidal ideation, acute agitation, threatening violence or other forms of aggressive manifestations.
- **Emotional presentations** are all those patients with symptoms of agoraphobia, anxiety, depression, depersonalization, derealization, hypomania or mania, panic.
- **Cognitive presentations** are all those patients with confusion, disorientation, and/or other forms of memory impairments.

Figure A-1 has a list of the symptom categories and the possible psychiatric and medical causes. As evidenced by the number of psychiatric and/or medical causes for each type of acute presentation it is fundamental that an adequate assessment be made in order to diagnose and initiate treatment appropriately. Unfortunately, patients will rarely present with symptoms as easily categorized as above and in reality frequently present with a more complex combination of "classic" psychiatric as well as medical symptoms. Patients presenting acutely with any of the above mentioned symptoms could have either a primary medical illness and associated psychiatric symptoms or a primary psychiatric disorder with associated medical findings.

The diagnostic interface of medical, substance-related, and primary psychiatric illness is complex and confusing at times. The areas of intersection and probability of causal effects are numerous. The diagram below illustrates the multiple interfaces and the possible diagnostic causes of certain psychiatric presentations.

Table A.1. Presentations of psychiatric and medical conditions

Presentation	Psychiatric Disorders (DSM-IV)	Medical Conditions
Psychotic (hallucinations, delusions)	Atypical psychosis, brief psychotic disorder, conversion disorder with sensory symptoms or deficits, delusional disorder, dementia, delirium, factitious disorder, malingering, mood disorders, personality change due to a general medical condition (paranoid type), personality disorders, shared psychotic disorder, schizoaffective disorder, schizophrenia, schizophreniform disorder, substance-related disorders	Hyper/hypothyroidism, AIDS, SLE, Cushing syndrome, brain neoplasms, postpartum psychosis, Addison disease, seizure disorders, hyperparathyroidism, acute intermittent porphyria, hepatic encephalopathy, Wilson disease, vitamin deficiencies, infections, tertiary syphilis, tumors (i.e., occipital lobe), hyperparathyroidism
Behavioral (agitation, violence)	Adjustment disorder, conduct and oppositional defiant disorder, dementia, delirium, intermittent explosive disorder, mental retardation, personality change due to a general medical condition (aggressive type), personality disorders, posttraumatic stress disorder, premenstrual dysphoric disorder, schizophrenia, and other psychotic disorders (especially with paranoia), substance-related disorders	Hyper/hypothyroidism, hypo/hyperglycemia, brain neoplasms and other intracranial processes (trauma, infection, anatomic defects, vascular malformations, cerebrovascular accidents), seizure or seizure-like syndromes (ictal, postictal, and interictal periods), AIDS, acute intermittent porphyria, Cushing disease, hepatic encephalopathy, vitamin deficiencies, tertiary syphilis
Emotional (anxiety, panic, agoraphobia, depersonalization, derealization, affective states)	Acute stress disorder, adjustment disorder, depersonalization disorder, generalized anxiety disorder, mood disorders,	Hyper/hypothyroidism, hypo/hyperglycemia, brain neoplasms, AIDS, pancreatic carcinoma, Cush-

Table A.1. *Continued*

Presentation	Psychiatric Disorders (DSM-IV)	Medical Conditions
	panic disorder, obsessive–compulsive disorder, personality disorders, posttraumatic stress disorder, substance-related disorders	ing syndrome, Addison disease, seizure disorders, hypo/hyperparathyroidism, SLE, multiple sclerosis, acute intermittent porphyria, hepatic encephalopathy, pheochromocytoma, Wilson disease, Huntington disease, tertiary syphilis
Cognitive (confusion, disorientation, memory impairment)	Amnestic disorders, dissociative amnesia, dementia, delirium, substance-induced persisting dementia	Hypo/hyperglycemia, head trauma, AIDS, hyponatremia, Cushing syndrome, seizure disorders, hypo/hyperparathyroidism, vitamin deficiencies, tertiary syphilis

AIDS, acquired immunodeficiency syndrome; SLE, systemic lupus erythematosus.

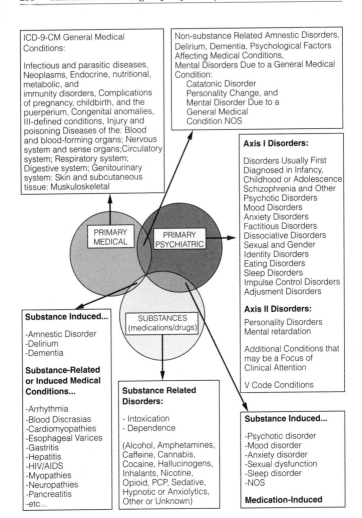

ICD-9-CM General Medical Conditions:

Infectious and parasitic diseases, Neoplasms, Endocrine, nutritional, metabolic, and immunity disorders, Complications of pregnancy, childbirth, and the puerperium, Congenital anomalies, Ill-defined conditions, Injury and poisoning Diseases of the: Blood and blood-forming organs; Nervous system and sense organs;Circulatory system; Respiratory system; Digestive system; Genitourinary system: Skin and subcutaneous tissue: Muskuloskeletal

Non-substance Related Amnestic Disorders, Delirium, Dementia, Psychological Factors Affecting Medical Conditions, Mental Disorders Due to a General Medical Condition:
    Catatonic Disorder
    Personality Change, and
    Mental Disorder Due to a
    General Medical
    Condition NOS

Axis I Disorders:

Disorders Usually First Diagnosed in Infancy, Childhood or Adolescence Schizophrenia and Other Psychotic Disorders Mood Disorders Anxiety Disorders Factitious Disorders Dissociative Disorders Sexual and Gender Identity Disorders Eating Disorders Sleep Disorders Impulse Control Disorders Adjusment Disorders

Axis II Disorders:

Personality Disorders Mental retardation

Additional Conditions that may be a Focus of Clinical Attention

V Code Conditions

PRIMARY MEDICAL

PRIMARY PSYCHIATRIC

SUBSTANCES (medications/drugs)

Substance Induced...

-Amnestic Disorder
-Delirium
-Dementia

Substance-Related or Induced Medical Conditions...

-Arrhythmia
-Blood Discrasias
-Cardiomyopathies
-Esophageal Varices
-Gastritis
-Hepatitis
-HIV/AIDS
-Myopathies
-Neuropathies
-Pancreatitis
-etc...

Substance Related Disorders:

- Intoxication
- Dependence

(Alcohol, Amphetamines, Caffeine, Cannabis, Cocaine, Hallucinogens, Inhalants, Nicotine, Opioid, PCP, Sedative, Hypnotic or Anxiolytics, Other or Unknown)

Substance Induced...

-Psychotic disorder
-Mood disorder
-Anxiety disorder
-Sexual dysfunction
-Sleep disorder
-NOS

Medication-Induced

Figure A-1. Symptom Categories and the Possible Psychiatric and Medical Causes

Appendix B

Partial List of Controlled Substances by Schedule

UNITED STATES CODE SECTION 801, TITLE II OF THE
COMPREHENSIVE DRUG ABUSE PREVENTION AND
CONTROL ACT OF 1970

Schedule I: The drug or other substance has a high potential for abuse. The drug or other substance has no currently accepted medical use in treatment in the United States. There is a lack of accepted safety for use of the drug or other substance under medical supervision.

Substance	Other Names
1-Methyl-4-phenyl-4-propionoxypiperidine	MPPP, synthetic heroin
3,4-Methylenedioxyamphetamine	MDA, Love Drug
3,4-Methylenedioxymethamphetamine	MDMA, Ecstasy, XTC
4-Bromo-2,5-dimethoxyphenethylamine	Nexus, 2-CB, sold as Ecstasy, i.e. MDMA
Aminorex	Sold as methamphetamine
Codeine methylbromide/ Codeine-N-oxide	Codeine
Gama Hydroxybutyric Acid (GHB)	GHB, gamma hydroxy-butyrate
Heroin	Diacetylmorphine, diamorphine
Lysergic acid diethylamide	LSD, lysergide
Marihuana	Cannabis, marijuana
Mescaline	Constituent of "Peyote" cacti
Methaqualone	Quaalude, Parest, Somnafac, Opitimil, Mandrax
Morphine	Morphine
Nicomorphine	Vilan
Peyote	Cactus which contains mescaline
Psilocyn	Psilocin, constituent of "Magic mushrooms"

Schedule II: The drug or other substance has a high potential for abuse. The drug or other substance has a currently accepted medical use in treatment in the United States or a currently accepted medical use with severe restrictions. Abuse of the drug or other substances may lead to severe psychological or physical dependence.

Substance	Other Names
1-Phenylcyclohexylamine	Precusor of PCP
1-Piperidinocyclohexanecarbonitrile	Precusor of PCP
Amobarbital	Amytal, Tuinal
Amphetamine	Dexedrine, Biphetamine
Benzoylecgonine	Cocaine metabolite
Cocaine	Crack
Codeine	Methyl morphine
Dihydrocodeine	Didrate, Parzone
Ecgonine	Cocaine precursor in coca leaves
Fentanyl	Innovar, Sublimaze, Duragesic
Glutethimide	Doriden, Dorimide
Hydrocodone	dihydrocodeinone
Hydromorphone	Dilaudid, dihydromorphinone
Levo-alphacetylmethadol	LAAM, long acting methadone
Meperidine	Demerol, Mepergan, pethidine
Methadone	Dolophine, Methadose, Amidone
Methamphetamine	ICE, Crank, Speed
Methylphenidate	Ritalin
Morphine	MS Contin, Roxanol, Duramorph
Opium derivatives	Papaver somniferum, Laudanum, raw opium, gum opium, powdered opium, granulated opium
Oxycodone	OxyContin, Percocet, Tylox, Roxicodone, Roxicet,
Oxymorphone	Numorphan
Pentobarbital	Nembutal
Phenazocine	Narphen, Prinadol
Phencyclidine	PCP, Sernylan
Secobarbital	Seconal, Tuinal
Thebaine	Precursor of many narcotics

Schedule III: The drug or other substance has a potential for abuse less than the drugs or other substances in schedules I and II. The drug or other substance has a currently accepted medical use in treatment in the United States. Abuse of the drug or other substance may lead to moderate or low physical dependence or high psychological dependence.

Substance	Other Names
Amobarbital	Amobarbital/ephedrine capsules
Anabolic steroids	"Body Building" drugs
Aprobarbital	Alurate
Butabarbital	Butisol, Butibel
Butalbital	Fiorinal, Butalbital with aspirin

Substance	Other Names
Codeine combination product	Empirin, Fiorinal, Tylenol, ASA or APAP w/codeine
Dihydrocodeine combination product	Synalgos-DC, Compal
Drostanolone	Drolban, Masterid, Permastril
Fluoxymesterone	Anadroid-F, Halotestin, Ora-Testryl
Hydrocodone combination product	Tussionex, Tussend, Lortab, Vicodin, Hycodan, Anexsia
Ketamine	Ketaset, Ketalar, Special K, K
Lysergic acid/Lysergic acid amide	LSD precursor
Mesterolone	Proviron
Methyltestosterone	Android, Oreton, Testred, Virilon
Opium combination product	Paregoric
Oxandrolone	Anavar, Lonavar, Provitar Oxymesterone
Other barbiturates	Pentobarbital, Secobarbital
Stanolone	Anabolex, Andractim, Pesomax, dihydrotestosterone
Talbutal	Lotusate
Testosterone	Android-T, Androlan, Depotest
Thiopental	Pentothal

Schedule IV: The drug or other substance has a low potential for abuse relative to the drugs or other substances in schedule III. The drug or other substance has a currently accepted medical use in treatment in the United States. Abuse of the drug or other substance may lead to limited physical dependence or psychological dependence relative to the drugs or other substances in schedule III.

Substance	Other Names
Alprazolam	Xanax
Barbital	Veronal, Plexonal, barbitone
Bromazepam	Lexotan, Lexatin, Lexotanil
Chloral hydrate	Noctec
Chlordiazepoxide	Librium, Libritabs, Limbitrol
Clobazam	Urbadan, Urbanyl
Clonazepam	Klonopin, Clonopin
Clorazepate	Tranxene
Dexfenfluramine	Redux
Dextropropoxyphene dosage forms	Darvon, propoxyphene, Darvocet, Dolene, Propacet
Diazepam	Valium, Valrelease
Estazolam	ProSom, Domnamid, Eurodin
Ethchlorvynol	Placidyl
Ethinamate	Valmid, Valamin
Fencamfamin	Reactivan
Fenfluramine	Pondimin, Ponderal
Fenproporex	Gacilin, Solvolip

Substance	Other Names
Flunitrazepam	Rohypnol, Narcozep, Darkene, Roipnol
Flurazepam	Dalmane
Lorazepam	Ativan
Lormetazepam	Noctamid
Mazindol	Sanorex, Mazanor
Mefenorex	Anorexic, Amexate, Doracil, Pondinil
Meprobamate	Miltown, Equanil, Deprol, Equagesic, Meprospan
Methohexital	Brevital
Methylphenobarbital (mephobarbital)	Mebaral, mephobarbital
Midazolam	Versed
Modafinil	Provigil
Nimetazepam	Erimin
Nitrazepam	Mogadon
Nordiazepam	Nordazepam, Demadar, Madar
Oxazepam	Serax, Serenid-D
Oxazolam	Serenal, Convertal
Paraldehyde	Paral
Pemoline	Cylert
Pentazocine	Talwin, Talwin NX, Talacen,
Petrichloral	Pentaerythritol chloral, Periclor
Phenobarbital	Luminal, Donnatal, Bellergal-S
Phentermine	Ionamin, Fastin, Adipex-P, Obe-Nix, Zantryl
Pinazepam	Domar
Prazepam	Centrax
Quazepam	Doral, Dormalin
Temazepam	Restoril
Triazolam	Halcion
Zaleplon	Sonata
Zolpidem	Ambien, Stilnoct, Ivadal

Schedule V: The drug or other substance has a low potential for abuse relative to the drugs or other substances in schedule IV. The drug or other substance has a currently accepted medical use in treatment in the United States. Abuse of the drug or other substance may lead to limited physical dependence or psychological dependence relative to the drugs or other substances in schedule IV.

Substance	Other Names
Buprenorphine	Buprenex, Temgesic
Codeine preparations	Cosanyl, Robitussin A-C, Cheracol, Cerose, Pediacof
Difenoxin preparations	Motofen
Dihydrocodeine preparations	Cophene-S, various others
Diphenoxylate preparations	Lomotil, Logen
Opium preparations	Parepectolin, Kapectolin PG, Kaolin Pectin P.G.

Appendix C

Commonly Used Psychiatric Medications

Commonly Used Psychiatric Medications

Brand®	Generic	Approximate Daily Dosage (mg/day)	How Supplied
ANTIDEPRESSANT AGENTS			
Monoamine Oxidase Inhibitors (MAOI)			
Nardil	phenelzine	15–90	15mg tablets
Parnate	tranylcypromine	30–60	10mg tablets
Tricyclic Agents (TCA)			
Ascendin	amoxapine	50–600	25, 50, 100, 150mg tablets
Anafranil	clomipramine	25–250	25, 50, 75mg tablets
Desyrel	trazodone	150–600	50, 100, 150, 300mg tablets
Elavil	amitriptyline	50–300	10, 25, 50, 75, 100, 150mg tablets
Norpramin	desipramine	25–300	10, 25, 50, 75, 100, 150mg tablets
Pamelor	nortriptyline	75–150	10, 25, 50, 75mg capsules
Sinequan	doxepin	25–300	10, 25, 50, 75, 100mg capsules, 10mg/ml concentrate
Surmontil	trimipramine	50–300	25, 50, 100mg capsules
Tofranil	imipramine	50–300	75, 100, 125, 150,mg capsules, 10, 25, 50mg tablets
Serotonin/Norepinephrine Selective Reuptake Inhibitors (SSRI)			
Celexa	citalopram	20–40	10, 20, 40mg tablets, 10mg/5 ml solution
Effexor/(XR)	venlafaxine	75–375/(37.5–225)	25, 37.5, 50, 75, 100mg tablets
Lexapro	escitalopram	10–20	10, 20mg tablets
Luvox	fluvoxamine	50–300	25, 50, 100mg tablets
Paxil	paroxetine	10–60	10, 20, 30, 40mg tablets

Prozac	fluoxetine	20–80	10, 20, 40mg capsules, 20mg/5 ml solution, 10mg tablets
Remron	mitrazapine	15–45	15, 30, 45mg tablets
Serzone	nefazadone	200–600	50, 100, 150, 200, 250mg tablets
Wellbutrin/(SR)	bupropion	200–450/(150–400)	75, 100mg tablets, (100, 150, 200mg tablets)
Zoloft	sertraline	50–200	25, 50, 100mg tablets, 20mg/ml concentrate
Zyban	bupropion SR	150–300	150mg tablets
MOOD STABILIZERS			
Eskalith/ Eskalith-CR, Lithonate, Lithobid, Lithotabs	lithium	600–1800	300mg capsules/450mg tablets, 300mg capsules, 300mg tablets
Depakote/ Depakote ER, capsules Depakene, Depakote Sprinkles	valproic acid	750–4200	125, 250, 500mg tablets/500mg tablets, 250mg capsules, 250mg/5 ml syrup, 125mg
Tegretol/ Tegretol XR	carbamazepine	400–1600	200mg tablets, 100mg chewable tablets, 100mg/5 ml suspension/100, 200, 400mg tablets
Lamictal	lamotrigine	50–500	25, 100, 150, 200mg tablets, 5, 25mg chewable tablets
Neurontin	gabapentin	300–3600	100, 300, 400mg capsules, 600, 800mg tablets
Topamax	toprimate	200–400	15, 25mg capsules, 25, 100, 200mg tablets

continued

Commonly Used Psychiatric Medications (*Continued*)

Brand®	Generic	Approximate Daily Dosage (mg/day)	How Supplied
ANXIOLYTICS			
Benzodiazepine			
Ativan	lorazepam	1–10	0.5, 1, 2mg tablets
Klonopin	clonazepam	1.5–2.0	0.5, 1, 2mg tablets
Librium	chlordiazepoxide	15–100	5, 10, 25mg capsules, 100mg powder (IM)
Tranxene	clorazepate	15–60	3.75, 7.5, 7.5, 15, 22.5mg tablets
Valium	diazepam	4–40	2, 5, 10mg tablets, 5mg/ml solutions
Xanax	alprazolam	0.75–10	0.25, 0.5, 1, 2mg tablets
Serax	oxazepam	30–120	10, 15, 30mg capsules, 15mg tablets
Non-benzodiazepine			
Buspar	buspirone	15–60	5, 10, 15, 30mg tablets (dividoses)
Vistaril/Atarax	hydroxyzine	50–300	25, 50, 100mg capsules, 50mg/ml solution, 25/5 ml suspension
HYPNOTICS			
Benzodiazepines			
Dalmane	flurazepam	15–30	15, 30mg capsules
Doral	quazepam	7.5–15	
Halcion	triazolam	0.125–0.5	0.125, 0.25mg tablets
Prosom	estazolam	1–2	1, 2mg tablets
Restoril	temazepam	7.5–30	7.5, 15, 30mg capsules

Non-benzodiazepines

Ambien	zolpidem	5–10	5, 10mg tablets
Noctec	chloral hydrate	500–2000	500mg capsules, 500mg suppositories, 250mg/5 ml, 500mg/5 ml syrup
Sonata	zaleplom	5–10	5, 10mg capsules

ANTIPSYCHOTICS
Typical Antipsychotics

Haldol/decanoate(IM)	haloperidol	1–100/20 × oral dose IM	0.5, 1, 2, 5, 10, 20mg tablets, 5mg/ml 50mg/ml, 100mg/ml solution
Loxitane	loxapine	20–250	5, 10mg capsules
Mellaril	thioridazine	20–800	10, 15, 25, 50, 100, 150, 200mg tablets, 30mg/ml concentrate
Moban	molindone	15–225	5, 10, 25, 50, 100mg tablets, 20mg/ml concentrate
Navane	thiothixene	6–60	1, 2, 5, 10, 20mg capsules
Prolixin/ decanoate(IM)	fluphenazine	1–40/1.2 × oral dose IM	1, 2.5, 5, 10mg tablets, 5mg/ml concentrate, 2.5mg/5 ml elixir, 2.5mh/ml, 25mg/ml solution
Serentil	mesoridazine	30–400	10, 25, 50, 100mg tablets, 25mg/ml concentrate & solution
Stelazine	trifluoperazine	2–40	1, 2, 5, 10mg tablets, 10mg/ml concentrate, 2mg/ml solution
Trilafon	perphenazine	12–64	2, 4, 8, 16mg tablets, 16mg/5 ml concentrate, 5mg/ml solution
Thorazine	chlorpromazine	30–800	10, 25, 50, 100, 200mg tablets, 30mg/ml 100mg/ml concentrate, 25mg/ml solution, 25, 100mg suppositories, 10mg/5 ml syrup

continued

Commonly Used Psychiatric Medications (*Continued*)

Brand®	Generic	Approximate Daily Dosage (mg/day)	How Supplied
Atypical Antipsychotics			
Abilify	Aripiprazole	10–30	10, 15, 20, 30mg tablets
Clozaril	clozapine	12.5–900	25, 100 tablets
Risperidal	risperidone	2–16	0.25, 0.5, 1, 2, 3, 4mg tablets, 1mg/ml solution
Seroquel	quetiapine	50–750	25, 100, 200, 300mg tablets
Zyprexa	olanzapine	5–10	2.5, 5, 7.5, 10, 15, 20mg tablets
Geodon	ziprasidone	40–160	20, 40, 60, 80mg capsules
ANTIPARKINSONIAN AGENTS			
Akineton	biperiden	2–8	2mg tablets
Artane	trihexyphenidyl	2–15	2, 5mg tablets, 0.4mg/ml elixir
Benadryl	diphenhydramine	50–400	25mg capsules, 6.25mg/5 ml, 12.5mg/5 ml liquid, 50mg/ml solution, 25mg tablets, 12.5mg chewable tablets
Cogentin	benztropine	1–8	0.5, 2mg tablets, 1mg/ml solution
Symmetrel	amantadine	100–400	100mg tablets, 50mg/5 ml syrup
PSYCHOSTIMULANTS			
Dexedreine	dextroamphetamine	5–40/5–60	5, 10, 15mg capsules, 5mg tablets
Adderall/ Adderall XR	dextroamphetamine + amphetamine	5–40/5–60	1.875, 3.125, 3.27mg tablets
Ritalin/Ritalin XR	methylphenidate	10–40/10–60	5, 10, 20mg tablets, 20mg tablets (XR)
Provigil	modafinil	200–400	100, 200mg tablets
Cylert	pemoline	37.5–112.5	18.75, 37.5, 75mg tablets, 37.5mg chewable tablets

Abnormal Involuntary Movement Scale (AIMS) Examination Procedure

ABNORMAL INVOLUNTARY MOVEMENT SCALE (AIMS) EXAMINATION PROCEDURE

	0	1	2	3	4
Have the patient sit in chair with their hands on their knees, legs slightly apart, and feet flat on floor. Look at the entire body for movements while in this position.					
Ask the patient to sit with their hands hanging unsupported. If male, between their legs, or if female and wearing a dress, hanging over knees. Observe their hands and other body areas.					
Ask patient to open their mouth. Observe tongue at rest within mouth. Do this twice.					
Ask patient to stick out their tongue. Observe any abnormalities of tongue movement. Do this twice.					
Ask the patient to tap their thumb with each finger, as rapidly as possible for 10 to 15 seconds; first with the right hand and then with the left hand. Observe facial and leg movements.					
Flex and extend patient's left and right arms. (One at a time.)					
Ask the patient to stand up. Observe in profile. Observe all body areas again, hips included.					
Ask patient to extend both arms out in front of them with palms down. Observe trunk, legs and mouth.					
Have patient walk a few paces; turn and walk back to the chair. Observe hands and gait. Do this twice.					

Score: _____

BRIEF PSYCHIATRIC RATING SCALE

Rate patient's current condition as:

1 = not present
2 = very mild
3 = mild
4 = moderate
5 = moderately severe
6 = severe
7 = extremely severe

Items	Description	Score
Somatic Concern	Degree of concern over present bodily health. Rate the degree to which physical health is perceived as a problem for the patient, whether complaints have a realistic basis of not.	
Anxiety	Worry, fear, or over-concern for present or future, Rate solely on the basis of verbal report of patient's own subjective experiences. Do not infer anxiety from physical signs or from neurotic defense mechanisms.	
Emotional Withdrawal	Deficiency in relating to the interviewer and to the interview or situation. Rate only the degree to which the patient gives the impression of failing to be in emotional contact with other people in the interview situation.	
Conceptual Disorganization	Degree to which the thought processes are confused, disconnected, or disorganized. Rate on the basis of integration of the verbal products of the patient; do not rate on the basis of patient's subjective impression of his own level of functioning.	
Guilt Feelings	Over-concern or remorse for past behavior. Rate on the basis of the patient's subjective experiences of guilt as evidenced by verbal report with appropriate affect; do not infer guilt from feelings from depression, anxiety, or neurotic defenses.	
Tension	Physical and motor manifestations of tension, 'nervousness', and heightened activation level. Tension should be rated solely on the basis of physical signs and motor behavior and not on the basis of subjective experiences of tension reported by the patient.	
Mannerisms	Unusual and unnatural motor behavior, the type of motor behavior that causes certain mental patients to stand out	

Items	Description	Score
	and Posturing in a crowd of normal people. Rate only abnormality of movements; do not rate heightened motor activity here.	
Grandiosity	Exaggerated self-opinion, connection of unusual ability or powers. Rate only on the basis of patient's statements about himself not on the basis of his demeanor in the interview situation.	
Depressive Mood	Despondency in mood, sadness. Rate only degree of despondency; do not rate on the basis of inferences concerning depression based on general retardation and somatic complaints.	
Hostility	Animosity, contempt, belligerence, disdain for other people outside the interview situation. Rate solely on the basis of the verbal report of feelings and actions of the patient toward others; do not infer hostility from neurotic defenses, anxiety, nor somatic complaints. (Rate attitude toward interviewer under 'uncooperativeness.')	
Suspiciousness	Belief (delusional or otherwise) that others have now, or have had in the past, malicious or discriminatory intent toward the patient. On the basis of verbal report, rate only those suspicions that are currently held whether they concern past or present circumstances.	
Hallucinatory Behavior	Perceptions without normal external stimulus correspondence. Rate only those experiences that are reported to have occurred within the last week and that are described as distinctly different from the thought and imagery processes of normal people.	

continued

Items	Description	Score
Motor Retardation	Reduction in energy level evidenced in slowed movements. Rate on the basis of observed behavior of the patient only; do not rate on the basis of the patient's subjective impression of own energy level.	
Uncooperativeness	Evidence of resistance, unfriendliness, resentment, and lack of readiness to cooperate with the interviewer. Rate only on the basis of the patient's attitude and responses to the interviewer and the interview situation; do not rate on basis of reported resentment or uncooperativeness outside the interview situation.	
Unusual Thought Content	Unusual, odd, strange, or bizarre thought content. State here the degree of unusualness, not the degree of disorganization of thought processes.	
Blunted Affect	Reduced emotional tone, apparent lack of normal feeling or involvement.	
Excitement	Heightened emotional tone, agitation, increased reactivity.	
Disorientation	Confusion or lack of proper association for person, place, or time.	

Score: _____

HAMILTON DEPRESSION RATING SCALE

Depressed Mood	0 ☐	Absent.
	1 ☐	Indicated only on questioning.
	2 ☐	Reported spontaneously.
	3 ☐	Communicated non-verbally—weeping, facial expressions, posture, voice, etc.
	4 ☐	Reports only these feelings in spontaneous and non-verbal communication.
Feelings of Guilt	0 ☐	Absent.
	1 ☐	Self-reproach, feels he/she has let people down.
	2 ☐	Ideas of guilt of rumination over past errors or sins.

	3	☐	Present illness is punishment. Delusions of guilt.
	4	☐	Has accusatory or denunciatory voices and/or threatening visual hallucinations.
Suicide	0	☐	Absent.
	1	☐	Feels life is not worth living.
	2	☐	Wishes he/she were dead or thoughts of possible death to self.
	3	☐	Suicide ideas or gestures.
	4	☐	Serious attempts at suicide.
Insomnia—early	0	☐	No difficulty.
	1	☐	Complains of occasional difficulty falling asleep (more than 1/2 hour).
	2	☐	Complains of nightly falling asleep.
Insomnia—middle	0	☐	No difficulty.
	1	☐	Complains of being restless and disturbed during the night.
	2	☐	Waking or getting out of bed during the night (except for voiding).
Insomnia—late	0	☐	No difficulty.
	1	☐	Waking in early hours of the morning but can go back to sleep.
	2	☐	Unable to fall asleep again if gets out of bed.
Work and Activities	0	☐	No difficulty.
	1	☐	Thought and feelings of incapacity, fatigue or weakness related to activities.
	2	☐	Loss of interest in activities, hobbies or work (reported directly or indirectly).
	3	☐	Decreased time spent in activities or decreased productivity.
	4	☐	Stopped working because of present illness.
Retardation	0	☐	Normal speech and thought.
	1	☐	Slight retardation at interview.
	2	☐	Obvious retardation at interview.
	3	☐	Interview difficult.
	4	☐	Complete stupor.
Agitation	0	☐	None
	1	☐	"Playing with" hands, hair, handkerchief, etc.
	2	☐	Hand-wringing, nail-biting, hair-pulling, biting of lips, etc.
Anxiety (psychic)	0	☐	No difficulty.
	1	☐	Subjective tension and irritability.
	2	☐	Worrying about minor matters.
	3	☐	Apprehensive attitude apparent in face or speech.
	4	☐	Fears expressed without questioning.
Anxiety (Somatic)	0	☐	Absent
	1	☐	Mild

	2	☐	Moderate
	3	☐	Severe
	4	☐	Incapacitating
Somatic	0	☐	None
Symptoms	1	☐	Loss of appetite but eating.
(Gastro-	2	☐	Difficulty eating without encouragement.
intestinal)			
Somatic	0	☐	None
Symptoms	1	☐	Heaviness in limbs, back or head. Loss
(General)			of energy or fatigue.
	2	☐	Any clear-cut symptoms rate a 2.
Symptoms	0	☐	Absent
(Genital)	1	☐	Mild
	2	☐	Severe
Hypochondriasis	0	☐	Not present
	1	☐	Self-absorption (bodily)
	2	☐	Preoccupation with health.
	3	☐	Frequent complaints, requests
			for help, etc.
	4	☐	Hypochondriacal delusions

Loss of Weight (only A or B)

A. When rating by history:

	0	☐	No weight loss
	1	☐	Probable weight loss associated with present illness.
	2	☐	Definite (according to patient) weight loss.

B. On weekly ratings by ward staff, when actual weight change present:

	0	☐	Less than 1lb weight loss in week.
	1	☐	Greater than 1 lb weight loss in week.
	2	☐	Greater than 2 lb weight loss in week.

Insight	0	☐	Acknowledges being depressed and ill.
	1	☐	Acknowledges illness but attributes cause to bad food, climate, overwork, need for rest, etc.
	2	☐	Denies being ill at all.

Diurnal Variation Note whether symptoms are worse in morning or evening.

		☐	No variation
		☐	Worse in AM
		☐	Worse in PM

When present rate the variation:

	1	☐	Mild
	2	☐	Severe

Depersonalization	0	☐	Absent
and	1	☐	Mild
Derealization	2	☐	Moderate
	3	☐	Severe
	4	☐	Incapacitating
Paranoid	0	☐	None
symptoms	1	☐	Suspicious
	2	☐	Ideas of reference

	3	☐	Delusions of reference and persecution.
Obsessional and	0	☐	Absent
Compulsive	1	☐	Mild
Symptoms	2	☐	Severe

Score: _____

HAMILTON ANXIETY RATING SCALE

0-Not Present
1-Mild (occurs irregularly and for short periods of time)
2-Moderate (occurs more constantly and of longer duration, requiring considerable effort on part of patient to cope)
3-Severe (continuous, dominates patient's life)
4-Very Severe (incapacitating)

Symptom	0	1	2	3	4
ANXIOUS MOOD: Worries, anticipation of the worst, fearful anticipation, irritability.					
TENSION: Feelings of tension, fatigability, startle response, moved to tears easily, trembling, and feelings of restlessness, inability to relax.					
FEARS: Of dark, of strangers, of being left alone, of animals, of traffic, of crowds.					
INSOMNIA: Difficulty in falling asleep, broken sleep, unsatisfying sleep and fatigue on waking, dreams, nightmares, night terrors.					
INTELLECTUAL (cognitive): Difficulty in concentration, poor memory.					
DEPRESSED MOOD: Loss of interest, lack of pleasure in hobbies, depression, early waking, diurnal swing.					
SOMATIC (muscular): Pains and aches, twitching, stiffness, myoclonic jerks, grinding of teeth, unsteady voice, increased muscular tone. (sensory): Tinnitus, blurring of vision, hot and cold flashes, feelings of weakness, prickling sensation.					
CARDIOVASCULAR SYMPTOMS: Tachycardia, palpitations, pain in chest, throbbing of vessels, fainting feelings, missing beat.					
RESPIRATORY SYMPTOMS: Pressure or constriction in chest, choking feelings, sighing, dyspnea.					
GASTROINTESTINAL SYMPTOMS: Difficulty in swallowing, wind, abdominal pain, burning sensations, abdominal fullness, nausea, vomiting, looseness of bowels, loss of weight, constipation.					

Symptom	0	1	2	3	4
GENITOURINARY SYMPTOMS: Frequency of micturition, amenorrhea, menorrhagia, development of frigidity, premature ejaculation, loss of libido, impotence.					
AUTONOMIC SYMPTOMS: Dry mouth, flushing, pallor, tendency to sweat, giddiness, tension headache, raising of hair.					
BEHAVIOR AT INTERVIEW: Fidgeting, restlessness or pacing, tremor of hands, furrowed brow, strained face, sighing or rapid respiration, facial pallor, swallowing, belching, brisk tendon jerks, dilated pupils, exophthalmos.					

OVERT AGGRESSION SCALE (OAS)

Check all that apply: Each type of aggressive behavior and intervention is given a weighted score, from 1 to 6.

☐ No aggressive incidents (verbal or physical) against self, others, or objects during the shift.

Verbal Aggression
☐ Makes loud noises, shouts angrily 1
☐ Yells mild personal insults (e.g., "You're stupid!") 2
☐ Curses viciously; uses foul language in anger, makes moderate threats to others or self 3
☐ Makes clear threats of violence toward others or self (e.g., "I'm going to kill you") or requests help to control self 4

Physical aggression against objects
☐ Slams door, scatters clothing, makes a mess 2
☐ Throws objects down, kicks furniture without breaking it, marks the wall 3
☐ Breaks objects, smashes windows 4
☐ Sets fires, throws objects dangerously 5

Physical aggression against self
☐ Picks or scratches skin, hits sell, pulls hair (with no or minor injury only) 3
☐ Hangs head, hits fist into objects, throws self onto floor or into objects (hurts self without serious injury) 4
☐ Small cuts or bruises, minor burns 5
☐ Mutilates self, makes deep cuts, bites that bleed, internal injury, fracture, loss of consciousness, loss of teeth 6

Physical aggression against other people
☐ Makes threatening gesture, swings at people, grabs at clothes 3
☐ Attacks others causing mild-moderate physical injury (bruises, sprains, welts) 4

☐ Attacks others causing severe physical injury
    (broken bones, deep lacerations, internal injury)   5
☐ Strikes, kicks, pushes, pulls hair (without injury
    to them)   6

INTERVENTION
☐ None
☐ Talking to patient   1
☐ Closer observation   2
☐ Holding patient   3
☐ Isolation without seclusion (time-out)   3
☐ Immediate medication given by mouth   4
☐ Immediate medication given by injection   4
☐ Seclusion   5
☐ Use of restraints   5
☐ Injury requires immediate medical treatment
    for patient
☐ Injury requires immediate treatment for other
    person

Reproduced with permission from the American Psychiatric Association.

YALE-BROWN OBSESSIVE COMPULSIVE SCALE
Time occupied by obsessive thoughts
0 = None
1 = Mild (less than 1 hr/day), or occasional intrusion (occur no more than 8 times a)
2 = Moderate (1 to 3 hrs/day), or frequent intrusion (occur more than 8 times a day, but most hours of the day are free of obsessions).
3 = Severe (greater than 3 and up to 8 hrs/day), or very frequent intrusion (occur more than 8 times a day and occur during most hours of the day).
4 = Extreme (greater than 8 hrs/day), or near constant intrusion (too numerous to count and an hour rarely passes without several obsessions occurring)

Interference due to obsessive thoughts
0 = None
1 = Mild, slight interference with social or occupational activities, but overall performance not impaired.
2 = Moderate, definite interference with social or occupational performance, but still manageable.
3 = Severe, causes substantial impairment in social or occupational performance.
4 = Extreme, incapacitating.

Distress associated with obsessive thoughts
0 = None
1 = Mild, infrequent, and not too disturbing.
2 = Moderate, frequent, and disturbing, but still manageable.
3 = Severe, very frequent, and very disturbing.
4 = Extreme, near constant, and disabling distress.

Resistance against obsessive thoughts
0 = Makes an effort to always resist, or symptoms so minimal doesn't need to actively resist.
1 = Tries to resist most of the time.
2 = Makes some effort to resist.
3 = Yields to all obsessions without attempting to control them, but does so with some reluctance.
4 = Completely and willingly yields to all obsessions.

Control over obsessive thoughts
0 = Complete control.
1 = Much control, usually able to stop or divert obsessions with some effort and concentration.
2 = Moderate control, sometimes able to stop or divert obsessions.
3 = Little control, rarely successful in stopping obsessions, can only divert attention with difficulty.
4 = No control, experienced as completely involuntary, rarely able to even momentarily divert thinking.

Time spent performing compulsions
0 = None
1 = Mild (less than 1 hr/day performing compulsions), or (occasional performance of compulsive behaviors no more than 8 times a day).
2 = Moderate (1 to 3 hrs/day performing compulsions), or frequent performance of compulsive behaviors (more than 8 times a day, but most hours are free of compulsive behaviors).
3 = Severe (spends more than 3 and up to 8 hrs/day performing compulsions), or very frequent performance of compulsive behaviors (occur more than 8 times a day and compulsions performed during most hours of the day).
4 = Extreme (more than 8 hrs/day performing compulsions), or near constant compulsive behaviors (too numerous to count and an hour rarely passes without several compulsions being performed).

Interference due to compulsive behaviors
0 = None
1 = Mild, slight interference with social or occupational activities, but overall performance not impaired.
2 = Moderate, definite interference with social or occupational performance, but still manageable.
3 = Severe, causes substantial impairment in social or occupational performance.
4 = Extreme, incapacitating.

Distress associated with compulsive behaviors
0 = None
1 = Mild, only slightly anxious if compulsions prevented, or only slight anxiety during performance of compulsions.
2 = Moderate, reports that anxiety would mount but remain manageable if compulsions prevented, or that anxiety increases but remains manageable during performance of compulsions.

3 = Severe, prominent, and very disturbing anxiety if compulsions interrupted, or prominent and very disturbing anxiety when performing compulsions.
4 = Extreme, incapacitating anxiety from any intervention aimed at modifying activity, or incapacitating anxiety develops during performance of compulsions.

Resistance against compulsions
0 = Makes an effort to always resist, or symptoms so minimal doesn't need to actively resist.
1 = Tries to resist most of the time.
2 = Makes some effort to resist.
3 = Yields to all compulsions without attempting to control them, but does so with some reluctance.
4 = Completely and willingly yields to all compulsions.

Degree of control over compulsive behaviors
0 = Complete control.
1 = Much control, experiences pressure to perform the behavior, but usually able to voluntarily control it.
2 = Moderate control, strong pressure to perform behavior, must be carried to completion, can only delay with difficulty.
3 = Little control, very strong drive to perform behavior, can only delay with difficulty.
4 = No control, drive to perform behavior experienced as completely involuntary and overpowering, rarely able to even momentarily delay activity.

Total Score:

  0–7   Subclinical
  8–15 Mild
16–23 Moderate
24–31 Severe
32–40 Extreme

Y-BOCS SYMPTOM CHECKLIST
Contamination Obsessions
Concerns or disgust with bodily waste or secretions
Concerned with dirt or germs
Excessive concern with environmental contaminants
Excessive concern with household items (cleaners)
Bothered by sticky substances or residues
Concerned will get ill (e.g., AIDS)
Concerned will get others ill by spreading germs
Somatic obsessions
Other
Sexual Obsessions
Personally unacceptable sexual thoughts
Hoarding/Saving Obsessions
Collects useless items, e.g., old newspapers (distinguish from hobbies; concern with objects of monetary or sentimental value)

Concerned with losing or throwing out items by mistake
Other

Obsession With Need for Symmetry or Exactness
Bothered by things not being lined up or being in order
Other

Aggressive Obsessions
Violent or horrific images
Fear will act on unwanted impulses leg, to stab friend
Fear will harm others because not careful enough leg, hit and run
    motor vehicle accident, putting poison in food
Fear will be responsible for something else terrible happening leg,
    fire, burglary
Other

Religious Obsessions (Scrupulosity)
Concerned with sacrilege and blasphemy
Excess concern with right and wrong, morality

Pathological Doubt
After completing routine activities, doubts whether performed or
    not leg, whether signed check to pay bill
Other

Other Obsessions
Superstitious fears (e.g., lucky or unlucky numbers or colors)
Other

Cleaning/Washing Compulsions
Excessive or ritualized hand washing
Excessive or ritualized showering, bathing, tooth brushing,
    grooming
Cleaning of household items or other inanimate objects
Other measures to prevent or remove contact with contaminants
Other

Repeating Rituals
Rereading or rewriting Repeats same questions
Need to repeat routine activities leg, in and out door
Other

Ordering/Arranging Compulsions
Lines up clothes, canned goods, shoes in fixed order
Need for symmetry (e.g., shoelaces must be at same tension, socks
    at same height)
Can't complete activity until "Just right"

Other Compulsions
Mental rituals (e.g., silently reciting prayers to neutralize a bad
    thought)
Counting compulsions (e.g., count ceiling tiles)
Excessive list making Pathological slowness (pervades most rou-
    tine activities)
Need to tell, ask, confess Need to touch, tap, or rub[a]

Checking Compulsions
Checking locks, stove, appliances, water faucets, emergency brake
Checking that did not harm others
Checking that did not make mistake (e.g., balancing checkbooks
    over and over)

Checking tied to somatic obsessions (e.g., checking self for signs of cancer)
Other

Hoarding/Collecting Compulsions
Inspecting household trash and accumulating useless objects
Superstitious behaviors (e.g., stepping on sidewalk cracks, bed-time rituals)
Asking for reassurance over and over
Self-damaging behaviors[a]
Rituals involving blinking or staring[a]
Other

[a] May or may not be OCD phenomena.

Appendix E

Additional Information on Suicide

STATISTICS
- eighth leading cause of death for all Americans
- third leading cause of death for people aged 15 to 24
- more people die from suicide than homicide in the U.S.
- 86 people commit suicide and 1,500 attempt suicide every day
- there were 30,575 suicide deaths in 1998
- annual rate of 11.3 per 100,000 population - rate has remained constant over the years.
- it is believed that the number of suicide attempts is 8 to 10 times the number of actual completed suicides
- The Surgeon General's Call to Action to Prevent Suicide has estimated that there are 4.5 million suicide-attempt survivors nationwide. (When compiling such data, one must factor in possible misclassifications of certain causes of death, such as accidents of undetermined cause, and "chronic suicides," such as deaths through alcohol and substance dependence, or deliberate poor adherence to medical regimens for diabetes, obesity, and hypertension.)
- U.S. suicide rates, when compared to other industrialized nations, fall in the middle:
  - highest rates (>25/100,000) are Scandinavian countries, Switzerland, Germany, Austria, Eastern European countries ("suicide belt"), and Japan,
  - lowest rates (<10/100,000) are Spain, Italy, Ireland, Egypt, and Holland
- suicide rates are generally higher in the western states, when compared to the national average, and lower in the eastern and midwestern states.
- New Jersey has the reported lowest suicide rate for both sexes in the country
- Golden Gate Bridge in San Francisco is considered the number one suicide spot in the world.
- statistics indicate that males were four times more likely to die from suicides than females, and account for $\frac{3}{4}$ of all completed suicides—because men use more lethal means when attempting suicide.
- over $\frac{1}{2}$ of suicides (in both men and women) are committed with a firearm.
- females are more likely to attempt suicide than males
- 90% of all completed suicides are committed by Caucasian males and females
- suicide risk increases with age:
  - in men, rates peak after age 45, and in women, after age 55
  - elderly people account for 25% of all suicides.
- it is estimated that 90%–95% of all suicides have a DSM-IV Axis-I psychiatric diagnosis:
  - 60% have a depressive disorder,
  - 10% to 15% have schizophrenia,
  - 15% to 25% have a alcohol or substance-related disorder.

- more than 50% of all suicides have alcohol in their blood.
- patients with psychiatric diagnoses have lifetime risks of suicide as follows:
  - affective disorders 15%,
  - schizophrenia 10%,
  - panic disorder 7%–15%,
  - alcohol and substance-related disorders 2%–3%.
- patients with Axis-I psychiatric disorders are 3 to 12 times more at risk for suicide than the general population.

BIOLOGY

Research into the biology of suicide shows some evidence in alterations in the serotonin and norepinephrine neurotransmitter systems. Depressed patients who attempted suicide have deficiencies in their serotonin systems, which might be related to impulse control and impulsivity. There have been some studies into the genetics of suicide providing evidence that suicide can run in families and possibly might be related to genetic factors involved in the transmission of other mental disorders.

RISK FACTORS/PREDICTORS

Suicide cuts across the spectrum of psychiatric disorders. Over 90% of completed suicides have a psychiatric diagnosis of alcoholism, depression, schizophrenia, or some combination of these. Suicide is not predictable, and the goal of the physician in the acute setting is to adequately assess the potential of future suicidality. There are some known associated findings, factors, and predictors, which can assist in the assessment of suicidality.

Psychiatric Disorders

- Patients diagnosed with **mood disorders** have a 15% lifetime risk of suicide. There are several concurrent symptoms, which are known to increase the likelihood of suicide in this population: panic attacks and anxiety, anhedonia, and concomitant alcohol abuse. Long-term suicide risk is known to be aggravated in patients with mood disorders when there is recurrent suicidal ideation, increased hopelessness, and a prior history of suicide attempts. Hopelessness has been found to be one of the most accurate indicators of long-term suicide risk.
- **Panic disorder** patients have a 7%–15% lifetime risk of suicide. Risk is related to the severity of illness and/or comorbid conditions. Patients with anxiety or agitation have increased risk, as they are vulnerable to acting impulsively. It should be noted that suicide among such patients does not usually occur during an actual panic episode.
- There is a 10% lifetime risk for suicide in patients with **schizophrenia:** 60%–80% experience suicidal ideation, with 30–55% actually attempting suicide. Suicide is less common during psychotic episodes, although the relationship between command auditory hallucinations and suicide has not been confirmed. Nonetheless, psychosis is a risk factor, and in an acute setting command auditory hallucinations should be viewed as high-risk and an indication of severity. There are certain risk factors for individuals with schizophrenia that include: early phase of illness, persistence of illness, numerous ex-

acerbations, severe functional impairments, awareness of the deteriorative effects of the illness, excessive treatment dependence, perception of an unsuccessful future, loss of faith in treatment services, or high achievement prior to illness onset. Schizophrenic males under the age of 30 with concurrent symptoms of depression and chronic relapsing are at higher risk, and are less likely to report suicidal ideation.

- **Substance users** have a 3% lifetime risk of suicide and this group comprises about 15%–25% of all completed suicides. The correlation between alcoholism and increased suicide risk are: active abuse, adolescence, second or third decade of illness, comorbid psychiatric illness, recent or anticipated interpersonal loss. It is thought that substance abuse might be a form of self-medication to reduce the anxiety or affective dysregulation associated with an underlying and often untreated psychiatric disorder.
- Patients with **borderline personality disorder** have a 7% lifetime risk of suicide. There is higher risk with the presence of other comorbid psychiatric conditions, especially mood disorders and substance abuse or dependence. Key characteristics that increase risk are: impulsivity, maladaptive coping mechanisms, feelings of emptiness and despair, poor interpersonal connections, and self-mutilatory behaviors.

Additional factors that have been shown to increase suicide risk are as follows:

- first week after discharge from the hospital,
- non-adherence with medications,
- under-diagnosed or under-treated bipolar disorder—especially mixed states—and severe depression.

GENDER

Gender plays a significant role in suicide risk. Prior suicide attempts are more of an acute predictor in women, although it does not predict suicide within one year, prior suicide attempts are predictive within 2 to 10 years. Suicide risk is greater among people in higher socioeconomic categories. Notably, when there is a downward economic change for such people, risk is increased. Professionals, especially physicians, (psychiatrists, ophthalmologists, and anesthesiologists) are at greater risk for suicide, as well as psychiatric disorders, such as substance abuse and depression. Other at-risk professions include musicians, dentists, law enforcement agents, lawyers, and insurance agents. Other conditions that increase risk are: family history of psychiatric illness (especially suicide), dysfunctional family interactions, life stressors (e.g., divorce, bereavement), the presence of firearms in the home, history of a near-fatal suicide attempts, acute suicidal ideation, severe hopelessness, attraction to death, and acute overuse of alcohol.

GENERAL PHYSICAL HEALTH

Physical health status is considered a risk factor for suicide. More than 30% of people who committed suicide have had medical attention within six months of their death and 25% to 75% have had a medical illness. Physical illnesses, especially those with chronic pain, increase risk. In several studies, the findings indicate that these patients had visited a physician prior to their attempt and had voiced their intent to a physician, but no intervention or prevention was done. Additionally, there are medications that can be depressogenic and increase suicide risk. These include: reserpine, corticosteroids, antihypertensives, etc.

SUICIDE ATTEMPTS AND COMPLETED SUICIDES

- 7%–10% greater risk for future attempts when compared to the general population.
- Although 90% will never complete the act, it is estimated that 1% will kill themselves yearly.
- It is estimated that 18%–38% of those who had completed suicide, had made at least one prior attempt.
- Prior suicidal ideation or attempts are an important predictive factor when assessing suicidality.

Subject Index

Page numbers followed by f indicate a figure; t following a page number indicates tabular material